Occupational Therapy: Advanced Techniques

Occupational Therapy: Advanced Techniques

Editor: Oscar Alvarez

AMERICAN
MEDICAL PUBLISHERS
www.americanmedicalpublishers.com

AMERICAN
MEDICAL PUBLISHERS
www.americanmedicalpublishers.com

Cataloging-in-Publication Data

Occupational therapy : advanced techniques / edited by Oscar Alvarez.
p. cm.
Includes bibliographical references and index.
ISBN 978-1-63927-175-7
1. Occupational therapy. 2. Physical therapy. 3. Therapeutics, Physiological. 4. Psychotherapy.
5. Medical care. I. Alvarez, Oscar.
RM735 .O23 2022
615.851 5--dc23

American Medical Publishers,
41 Flatbush Avenue,
1st Floor, New York,
NY 11217, USA

ISBN 978-1-63927-175-7 (Hardback)

Contents

Preface

This book was inspired by the evolution of our times; to answer the curiosity of inquisitive minds. Many developments have occurred across the globe in the recent past which has transformed the progress in the field.

Occupational therapy is an allied health care profession that makes the use of assessment and intervention to maintain, develop or recover the meaningful activities of individuals, groups, or communities. Occupational therapy focuses on treating people with mental health problems, injuries, impairments or disabilities. Occupational therapy also aims to help children with disabilities to participate in school and social activities or situations, to provide support for older adults who experience physical and cognitive changes and injury rehabilitation. Physical therapy, nursing, psychiatry, orthopedics and social work are some disciplines from where occupational therapy borrowed its principles and techniques. This book unravels the recent studies in the field of occupational therapy and its utmost significance in modern times. It is compiled in such a manner, that it will provide an in-depth knowledge about the theory and practice of occupational therapy. Researchers and students actively engaged in this field will find this book full of crucial and unexplored concepts.

This book was developed from a mere concept to drafts to chapters and finally compiled together as a complete text to benefit the readers across all nations. To ensure the quality of the content we instilled two significant steps in our procedure. The first was to appoint an editorial team that would verify the data and statistics provided in the book and also select the most appropriate and valuable contributions from the plentiful contributions we received from authors worldwide. The next step was to appoint an expert of the topic as the Editor-in-Chief, who would head the project and finally make the necessary amendments and modifications to make the text reader-friendly. I was then commissioned to examine all the material to present the topics in the most comprehensible and productive format.

I would like to take this opportunity to thank all the contributing authors who were supportive enough to contribute their time and knowledge to this project. I also wish to convey my regards to my family who have been extremely supportive during the entire project.

Editor

Spanish Transcultural Adaptation and Validity of the Behavioral Inattention Test

Ángel Sánchez-Cabeza,[1,2] Elisabet Huertas-Hoyas,[2] Nuria Máximo-Bocanegra,[2] Rosa María Martínez-Piédrola,[2] Marta Pérez-de-Heredia-Torres,[2] and Jorge Alegre-Ayala[2]

[1] *Hospital Universitario Fundación Alcorcón, Madrid, Spain*
[2] *Department of Physiotherapy, Occupational Therapy, Rehabilitation and Physical Medicine, Universidad Rey Juan Carlos, Madrid, Spain*

Correspondence should be addressed to Jorge Alegre-Ayala; jorge.alegre@urjc.es

Academic Editor: Lynette A. MacKenzie

Objective. To adapt, validate, and translate the Behavioral Inattention Test as an assessment tool for Spanish individuals with unilateral spatial neglect. *Design.* A cross-sectional descriptive study. *Setting.* University laboratories. *Participants.* A sample of 75 Spanish stroke patients and 18 healthy control subjects. *Interventions.* Not applicable. *Main Outcome Measures.* The Behavioral Inattention Test. *Results.* The Spanish version of the Behavioral Inattention Test shows a high degree of reliability both in the complete test ($\alpha = .90$) and in the conventional ($\alpha = .93$) and behavioral subtests ($\alpha = .75$). The concurrent validity between the total conventional and behavioral scores was high ($r = -.80$; $p < 0.001$). Significant differences were found between patients with and without unilateral spatial neglect ($p < 0.001$). In the comparison between right and left damaged sides, differences were found in all items, except for article reading ($p = 0.156$) and card sorting ($p = 0.117$). *Conclusions.* This measure is a useful tool for evaluating unilateral spatial neglect as it provides information on everyday problems. The BIT discriminates between stroke patients with and without unilateral spatial neglect. This measure constitutes a reliable tool for the diagnosis, planning, performance, and design of specific treatment programs intended to improve the functionality and quality of life of people with unilateral spatial neglect.

1. Introduction

Unilateral spatial neglect (USN) is a cognitive spatial disorder that can affect perception and the mental representation of spatial information, as well as the ability to plan and perform motor actions. This is, in addition to, the inability to respond, orientate, or react to stimulation received on the opposite side of the damaged hemisphere [1]. This disorder is experienced by 23–43% of stroke survivors and is most common in right hemisphere strokes (43% right hemisphere; 20% left hemisphere) [2, 3]. Interestingly, although some patients with neglect recover completely within the acute poststroke period, in other cases, neglect persists [4, 5]. This impairment is one of the most disruptive factors affecting the recovery of functional independence in stroke patients [1, 6].

Functional Implications of Unilateral Spatial Neglect. Patients with neglect suffer from problems which affect their daily activities, including difficulties with personal hygiene, dressing, eating, swallowing, movement and mobility, understanding, and reading [7]. The behavioral signs most commonly associated with neglect include, amongst others, an inability to communicate with people on the neglected side, attending to only one side of the body as far as hygiene and personal cleanliness are concerned (such as only shaving one side of the face or only washing one side of the body), and bumping into people and objects on the affected side. Patients frequently get lost and are unable to find their way. Also, they ignore food on one side of their plate and cannot copy or draw an object without omitting or distorting a part of it. Furthermore, many patients fail to read letters or words on one side of the page.

Evaluation of Unilateral Spatial Neglect. The neuropsychological evaluation of neglect is complex, as patients often have other associated cognitive disorders that hamper examination and diagnosis [8]. Several types of tests have been used to assess neglect, mainly based on visual scanning activities [9, 10], as well as line bisection tests [11], cancellation tests [12], drawing tests [13], reading tests [14], and bilateral simultaneous stimulation [15]. None of these tests evaluate aspects relating to everyday life.

The Behavioral Inattention Test. The original Behavioral Inattention Test (BIT) was designed by Wilson, Cockhurn, and Halligan in 1987, based on proven graphic visual scanning tests, complemented by a series of tests based on everyday tasks, in order to provide a more natural and ecological testing environment. The BIT is divided into two sections, the first of which is conventional and comprises six tests: line bisection, star cancellation, copying figures and shapes, line cancellation, representational drawing, and letter cancellation. The second behavioral section comprises nine tests selected by psychologists and occupational therapists and based on specific difficulties faced by patients with visual neglect in everyday life situations, such as picture scanning, phone dialing, menu reading, article reading, telling and setting the time, coin sorting, address and sentence copying, map navigation, and card sorting. The BIT therefore combines a series of parameters capable of providing accurate data to reflect the functional incapacity of a person suffering from neglect [16].

The information provided by the BIT is important for the recovery of stroke patients, whose difficulties extend hospital stays and impact the recovery of motor skills [17]. It is also fundamental for proper planning of occupational therapy treatment, as it deals with the functional consequences caused by cognitive deficits [18].

When this instrument is used to evaluate non-English speaking patients (the language in which the BIT was designed), transcultural adaptation is required to ensure semantic, linguistic, and cultural equivalence, particularly regarding items that have a clear and specific cultural background (coins, cards, food, etc.). This article describes the process of academic translation and transcultural adaptation of the BIT to Spanish and analyzes the validity and reliability of the BIT in Spanish stroke patients with, and without, USN. Our work hypothesis is that this adaptation of the scale will enable clinicians to detect neglect in Spanish stroke patients. Also, we hypothesize that the scores in conventional and behavioral test in patients with USN will be significantly worse than stroke patients without neglect.

2. Material and Methods

2.1. Study Design. This is a cross-sectional descriptive study designed to adapt, translate, and validate a Spanish version of the BIT.

2.2. Sample. The study was carried out in the Autonomous Community of Madrid, Spain, and included a sample of 93 subjects, of whom 75 were patients and 18 were healthy controls. Patients were recruited from various multidisciplinary neurological rehabilitation centers: POLIBEA, Centro Estatal de Atención al Daño Cerebral, and the Amma Home for the Elderly (Alcorcón). The inclusion criteria for the study group consisted of a diagnosed stroke with minimal evolution of 6 months and proven unilateral damage and being over the age of 18 years. The doctors and neuropsychologists at the centers were in charge of selecting the sample. The exclusion criteria were the presence of other central nervous system disorders (tumors, anoxia, etc.), cardiorespiratory or neurodegenerative conditions, severe brain damage, and severe awareness deficits. Healthy subjects were recruited from the researcher's social environment and the relatives of the stroke patients. The inclusion criteria included subjects over the age of 18 years and exempt from any condition that may limit their functional capacity. Participants with USN were distinguished by a neuropsychologist and an occupational therapist who participated in the intervention according to daily performance after stroke.

2.3. Adaptation Process. Permission was firstly obtained from the authors of the test for the translation and validation of the same to the Spanish population. We then obtained authorization from the Rey Juan Carlos University Ethics Committee.

The translation process was carried out according to the study published by Beaton et al. [19] as follows:

(i) Translation into Spanish: the test was translated by two native-speaking Spanish translators, resulting in translations T_1 and T_2.

(ii) Analysis: both translations were analyzed to reach a consensus on a single translation (T_{12}).

(iii) Back translation to English: native-speaking English translators, who were unaware of the process carried out, then translated T_{12} into two new English versions (RT_1 and RT_2).

(iv) Revision by an expert committee: the committee was comprised of four occupational therapists, two translators, and two researchers familiar with the tool. After analyzing all the versions (T_1, T_2, T_{12}, RT_1, and RT_2), a prefinal Spanish version was chosen.

(v) Pilot testing of the prefinal version: in this phase, the prefinal version was used on a sample of patients (30–40), who were subsequently interviewed regarding any difficulties they had in understanding the meaning of the questions and the responses. We also analyzed incidents of noncompleted and repeated replies (i.e., when all patients provide the same response to a specific question).

(vi) Use of the tool: the present pilot test was designed and the tool was administered to 93 people, including 75 patients and 18 healthy control subjects.

(vii) Conclusions: we checked for errors and typing mistakes which derived in the final version of the test. This version was then sent to the authors of the original test.

With regard to the changes made to the test for the Spanish population, firstly, all the tests requiring words in Spanish

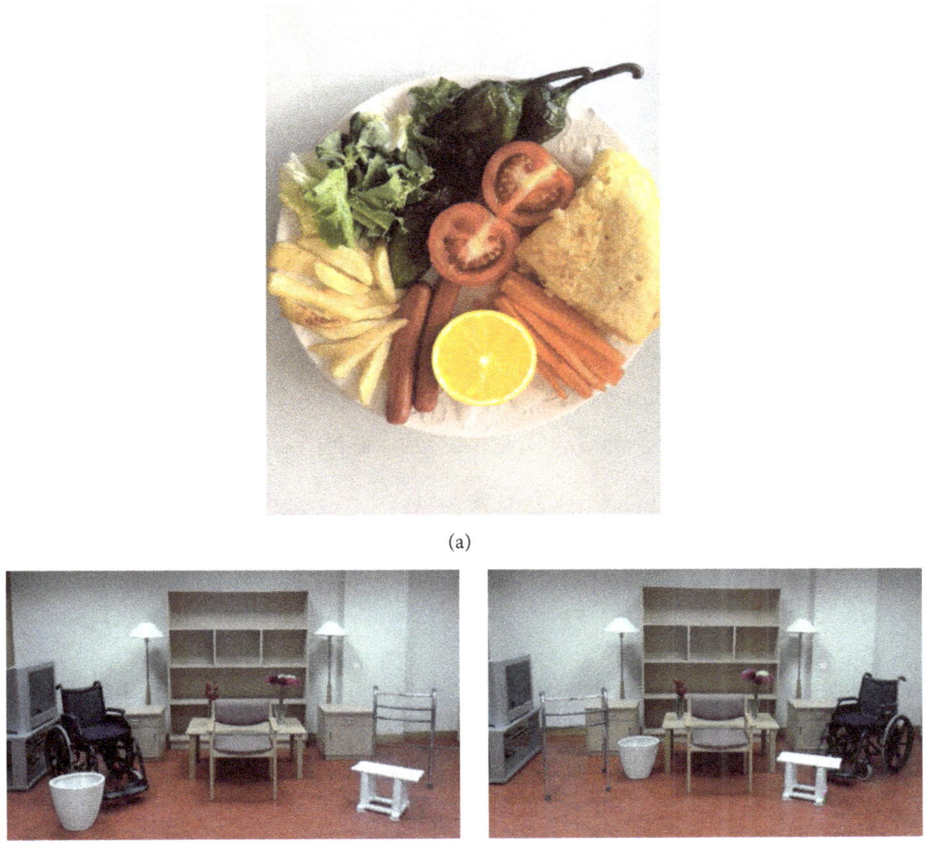

(a) (b) (c)

FIGURE 1: Picture scanning test. Adaptation to the Spanish population (authorized by Pearson Assessment).

were translated, as follows: for the conventional subtests: star cancellation (*cancelación de estrellas*); for the behavioral subtests: menu reading (*lectura de un menú*), article reading (*lectura de un artículo*), coin sorting (*clasificación de monedas*), and address and sentence copying (*copia de una dirección y una frase*). Adaptations to the behavioral picture scanning test were made for the Spanish population: specifically, we adapted picture scanning test. In Figure 1(a), the most common Spanish foods were added, such as green peppers, Spanish omelette, French fries, and lemon (Figure 1). In Figures 1(b) and 1(c), an attempt was made to use the same original furniture, although other simple elements are added (Figure 1). Changes were made in the coin sorting (*clasificación de monedas*) test and the euro was featured, which is the currency used in Spain. Finally, the card sorting (*clasificación de cartas*) test was changed and a Spanish deck of cards was used instead of a poker deck.

2.4. Statistical Analysis. Given that the size of the compared groups did not comply with consistency criteria, the Mann–Whitney nonparametric test was used to study the differences between independent samples.

Firstly, we obtained descriptive data, which shows the frequency of the categorical variable, the median, and the interquartile range (q1–q3) of the other continuous variables, as well as the estimated reliability of the assessment tool using the Cronbach α test, which indicated adequate reliability (Table 4). Secondly, we analyzed the dependent variables to determine the differences between groups in a cross-sectional manner for all the subjects included in the study. Results with p values < 0.05 were considered statistically significant.

All computations were conducted using IBM SPSS Statistics 19 for Windows (IBM Corporation, Armonk, NY, US).

3. Results

Table 1 shows the sociodemographic data of the entire sample, divided into the following subgroups: right stroke, left stroke, and healthy control subjects. Table 2 presents the sociodemographic data of participating patients with and without unilateral spatial neglect.

Table 3 displays the means and standard deviations of the data obtained from the healthy control subjects, as well as the cut-off point. The scores obtained by the control group were used to establish the limits of the normal distribution and determine the score that would serve as a cut-off point for the individual test components.

With regard to the reliability of the scale, the complete test was found to be highly reliable (α = .90) as were the conventional (α = .93) and behavioral subtests (α = .75)

TABLE 1: Sociodemographic data. Complete sample.

	Left stroke	Right stroke	Total	Healthy controls	p value
n	17	58	75	18	
Age	53.29 ± 10.31	58.52 ± 12.58	55.77 ± 13.40	47.28 ± 15.25	**0.011***
Age range	39–79	32–91	23–91	26–74	
Sex					0.193
Male	5 (29.4%)	38 (65.5%)	43 (57.3%)	7 (38.9%)	
Female	12 (70.6%)	20 (34.5%)	32 (42.7%)	11 (61.1%)	
Education level					0.842
Basic	1 (5.9%)	8 (13.8%)	9 (12%)	2 (11.1%)	
Primary	8 (47.1%)	22 (37.9%)	30 (40%)	6 (33.3)	
Secondary	8 (47.1%)	28 (48.3%)	36 (48%)	10 (55.6%)	
With unilateral spatial neglect	4 (23.5%)	37 (63.8%)	41 (54.7%)	—	
Without unilateral spatial neglect	13 (76.5%)	21 (36.2%)	34 (45.3%)	—	

Note. Values are expressed as mean ± SD and frequency is expressed as a percentage (%). *Significant with $p < 0.05$. Differences between stroke patients and healthy controls.

TABLE 2: Data on stroke patients with and without unilateral spatial neglect.

	With USN	Without USN	p value
n	41	34	
Age	60.61 ± 11.76	53.38 ± 11.79	**0.004***
Age range	33–91	32–81	
Sex			0.035
Male	28 (68.3%)	15 (44.1%)	
Female	13 (31.7%)	19 (55.9%)	
Diagnosis of stroke	41 (93.2%)	34 (87.2%)	
Damaged side			**0.003***
Right	37 (90.2%)	21 (61.8%)	
Left	4 (9.8%)	13 (38.2%)	
Stroke onset (years)	3.20 ± 3.77	4.32 ± 4.70	0.124
Range of evolution time	1–14	0–19	

Note. Values are expressed as mean ± SD and frequency is expressed as a percentage (%). *Significant with $p < 0.05$. Differences between patients with Unilateral spatial neglect and without Unilateral spatial neglect.

(Table 4). The concurrent validity of the test as a measure of spatial neglect was determined by the relationship between the conventional and behavioral total scores obtained by the 75 stroke patients, with a correlation of −0.80 ($p < 0.001$).

Finally, we found statistically significant differences between patients with and without unilateral spatial neglect in all the items on the BIT ($p < 0.001$) (Table 5). In the comparison between right and left brain injury, we found differences in all the items except article reading ($p = 0.156$) and card sorting ($p = 0.117$) (Table 6).

4. Discussion

The objective of this study was to create a Spanish adaptation and translation of the BIT (BIT-E) for use by patients with USN and to analyze the validity and reliability of the same in Spanish stroke patients with and without USN. Moreover, we hypothesized that the conventional and behavioral scores of USN patients would be worse than the remaining stroke participants.

This study enabled us to follow a scientific and valid process at both a theoretical and methodological level for adapting a diagnostic tool. Our findings revealed high reliability for the complete BIT (α = .90), as well as for the conventional (α = .93) and behavioral subtests (α = .75). Also, internal consistency was considered good to excellent. These findings contrast with those reported for the Turkish adaptation of the BIT [20], for which the conventional test was less valid (α = .77); however, the validity of the behavioral section was greater (α = .91), compared to our findings.

In addition, in our study, concurrent validity was observed between conventional and behavioral sections (r = −.80). The concurrent validity was less than that of the original BIT [21].

In the comparison between stroke patients with, and without, USN, our study showed significant differences between both groups in all the items on the BIT. According to the results obtained, there are statistically significant differences between subgroups in all the BIT-E variables, therefore enabling the conclusion that the BIT-E detects problems of neglect and attention problems between patients with and without unilateral spatial neglect. An Israeli version has also been adapted, reporting similar results in the behavioral test except for article reading and telling and setting the time, where no differences were found [22].

The translation procedure employed in this study is commonly used. The translation, cultural adaptation, and validation processes were based on the recommendations by Beaton et al. [19]. During the adaptation process, the translation of the tests that required words in Spanish did not give rise to discussion, given that the concepts were

TABLE 3: Results obtained by healthy control participants in conventional and behavioral tests ($n = 18$).

Subtest	Maximum score	Cut-off point (acceptable range)	Median (q1–q3)	Min–max	Cut-off score
Conventional subtest					
Line cancellation	36	34 (35-36)	36 (36-36)	23–36	34
Letter cancellation	40	32 (33–40)	40 (40-40)	36–40	32
Star cancellation	54	51 (52–54)	54 (54-54)	4–54	51
Copying figures and shapes	4	3 (4)	4 (4-4)	4–8	3
Line bisection	9	7 (8-9)	9 (8-9)	3–9	7
Drawing	3	2 (3)	3 (3-3)	3–9	2
Total Conventional subtest	146	129	146 (144.75–146)	132–146	129
Behavioral subtest					
Picture scanning	9	5 (6–9)	9 (8-9)	7–9	5
Phone dialing	9	7 (8-9)	9 (9-9)	9-9	7
Menu reading	9	8 (9)	9 (9-9)	9-9	8
Article reading	9	8 (9)	9 (9-9)	9-9	8
Telling and setting the time	9	8 (9)	9 (9-9)	9-9	8
Coin sorting	9	8 (9)	9 (9-9)	9-9	8
Address and sentence copying	9	7 (8-9)	9 (9-9)	9-9	8
Map navigation	9	8 (9)	9 (9-9)	9-9	7
Card sorting	9	8 (9)	9 (9-9)	9-9	8
Total behavioral subtest	81	67	81 (80-81)	79–81	67

Note. Values expressed as median (q1–q3).

TABLE 4: Descriptive data on scales and reliability ($n = 75$).

Scale	Median (q1–q3)	Min–max	α
Conventional Test	136 (115–142)	61–146	0.93
Behavioral Test	70 (50–76)	3–81	0.75

Note. Values expressed as median (q1–q3).

TABLE 5: Comparison of groups of patients with and without USN ($n = 75$).

	With USN Median (q1–q3)	Without USN Median (q1–q3)	p value
Conventional test	115 (93.5–132)	141 (138–144)	**<0.001***
Line cancellation	33 (24–36)	36 (36-36)	**<0.001***
Letter cancellation	30 (25–37.5)	38 (36 75–40)	**<0.001***
Star cancellation	44 (34–51)	53.5 (52–54)	**<0.001***
Copying figures and shapes	3 (0.5–4)	4 (3-4)	**<0.001***
Line bisection	5 (4–7.5)	8 (7–9)	**<0.001***
Drawing	2 (0–3)	3 (3-3)	**<0.001***
Behavioral test	50 (25.5–65.5)	75.5 (72.75–79)	**<0.001***
Picture scanning	3 (0–6)	7 (6–8)	**<0.001***
Phone dialing	8 (5.5–9)	9 (9-9)	**<0.001***
Menu reading	7 (1–9)	9 (9-9)	**<0.001***
Article reading	5 (0–9)	9 (9-9)	**<0.001***
Telling and setting the time	8 (6–9)	9 (8-9)	**<0.001***
Coin sorting	3 (1–7)	7 (7–9)	**<0.001***
Address and sentence copying	6 (0–9)	9 (9-9)	**<0.001***
Map navigation	7.5 (4–9)	9 (9-9)	**<0.001***
Card sorting	3 (1–6)	9 (9-9)	**<0.001***

Note. Values expressed as median (q1–q3). *Significant with $p < 0.05$. Differences between patients with unilateral spatial neglect and without unilateral spatial neglect.

simple and easy to translate. The majority of the discussion focused on certain photographs and tests including Spanish food (Figure 1(a)), coins (*coin sorting* test), and objects (*card sorting* test). Certain simple nominated elements were added to Figures 1(b) and 1(c). In the prefinal version of the questionnaire used with a sample of stroke patients, the pilot study showed an optimal degree of understanding.

The BIT has also been translated and validated for other populations. The adaptation of the tool to the population of Turkey was carried out by applying the Rasch model. The reported findings showed a lack of reliability and validity of the internal construct, given that although, in certain aspects, the results were considered adequate, there were problems relating to certain tests that clearly failed to achieve the expectations of the model [20]. In contrast, the results of the Israeli adaptation of the test [22] support the predictive and construct validity in the majority of behavioral and functional BITs for measuring unilateral neglect. The number of participants in this study was smaller than those participating in the Turkish BIT adaptation ($n = 118$), although higher than the Israeli version ($n = 40$). The time since stroke onset varied considerably in our study compared to the Israeli study (mean: 11 months) and the Turkish study (median: 38 days). Our sample presents a greater chronicity in comparison with the remaining BIT adaptation studies and possibly the severity of the participants' neglect in the present study was greater.

TABLE 6: Comparison of groups according right or left damaged side ($n = 75$).

	Right stroke Median (q1–q3)	Left stroke Median (q1–q3)	p value
Conventional test	130.50 (102.25–140)	140 (136–144.5)	**0.007***
Line cancellation	36 (31–36)	36 (36-36)	**0.028***
Letter cancellation	35.50 (26–38)	38 (36–39)	**0.033***
Star cancellation	50 (38.75–53)	54 (52.5–54)	**0.002***
Copying figures and shapes	3 (2–4)	4 (3-4)	**0.001***
Line bisection	6.5 (4–8)	9 (7.5–9)	**0.009***
Drawing	2 (1–3)	3 (3-3)	**0.002***
Behavioral test	66.5 (42.75–74.25)	75 (67.5–78.5)	**0.010***
Picture scanning	5 (1–7)	8 (6.5–8.5)	**<0.001***
Phone dialing	9 (7–9)	9 (9-9)	**0.009***
Menu reading	8 (3–9)	9 (9-9)	**0.006***
Article reading	9 (3–9)	9 (7–9)	0.156
Telling and setting the time	8 (7–9)	9 (9-9)	**0.005***
Coin sorting	6 (3–7)	7 (7–9)	**0.012***
Address and sentence copying	9 (2–9)	9 (9-9)	**0.018***
Map navigation	9 (6.75–9)	9 (9-9)	**0.009***
Card sorting	6 (3–9)	9 (4.5–9)	0.117

Note. Values expressed as median (ql–q3). *Significant with $p < 0.05$. Differences between right and left stroke patients.

4.1. Study Limitations. This study presents important limitations. Firstly, the sample comes from the same Spanish region (Community of Madrid). Furthermore, the number of women was higher than men, and the level of education of women was also higher; therefore, there could be a selection bias. Also, the psychometric properties of the scale were not analyzed in depth; thus data for test-retest reliability, construct validity, and interrater reliability is not presented at this time.

5. Conclusions

The BIT is a tool used to evaluate unilateral spatial neglect which provides information on everyday problems faced by patients who have suffered from a stroke. We translated the BIT into Spanish, elaborating a Spanish version conceptually equivalent to the English version which was understood by our patients with unilateral spatial neglect, thanks to the academic translation methods employed. The availability of an adapted and validated Spanish version of the tool (BIT-E) provides professionals with a reliable instrument that contributes to the effective diagnosis, planning, and design of individualized treatment interventions that will no doubt improve the functionality and quality of life of patients with unilateral spatial neglect.

Consent

All participants provided written informed consent.

Competing Interests

The authors have declared no competing interests.

Acknowledgments

Thanks are due to Polibea Rehabilitación, Centro Estatal de Atención al Daño Cerebral, and AMMA Home for the Elderly (Alcorcón).

References

[1] P. Chen, K. Hreha, Y. Kong, and A. M. Barrett, "Impact of spatial neglect on stroke rehabilitation: evidence from the setting of an inpatient rehabilitation facility," *Archives of Physical Medicine and Rehabilitation*, vol. 96, no. 8, pp. 1458–1466, 2015.

[2] T. Ogourtsova, P. Archambault, and A. Lamontagne, "Impact of post-stroke unilateral spatial neglect on goal-directed arm movements: systematic literature review," *Topics in Stroke Rehabilitation*, vol. 22, no. 6, pp. 397–428, 2015.

[3] D. S. J. Ting, A. Pollock, G. N. Dutton et al., "Visual neglect following stroke: current concepts and future focus," *Survey of Ophthalmology*, vol. 56, no. 2, pp. 114–134, 2011.

[4] R. M. Umarova, K. Nitschke, C. P. Kaller et al., "Predictors and signatures of recovery from neglect in acute stroke," *Annals of Neurology*, vol. 79, no. 4, pp. 673–686, 2016.

[5] M. Bonato, "Unveiling residual, spontaneous recovery from subtle hemispatial neglect three years after stroke," *Frontiers in Human Neuroscience*, vol. 9, article 413, 2015.

[6] N. Katz, A. Hartman-Maeir, H. Ring, and N. Soroker, "Functional disability and rehabilitation outcome in right hemisphere damaged patients with and without unilateral spatial neglect," *Archives of Physical Medicine and Rehabilitation*, vol. 80, no. 4, pp. 379–384, 1999.

[7] E. W. M. Herman, "Spatial neglect: new issues and their implications for occupational therapy practice," *American Journal of Occupational Therapy*, vol. 46, pp. 207–216, 1992.

[8] A. B. Lindell, M. J. Jalas, O. Tenovuo, T. Brunila, M. J. M. Voeten, and H. Hämäläinen, "Clinical assessment of hemispatial neglect: evaluation of different measures and dimensions," *Clinical Neuropsychologist*, vol. 21, no. 3, pp. 479–497, 2007.

[9] D. T. Wade, V. A. Wood, and R. Langton-Hewer, "Recovery of cognitive function soon after stroke: a study of visual neglect, attention span and verbal recall," *Journal of Neurology Neurosurgery and Psychiatry*, vol. 51, no. 1, pp. 10–13, 1988.

[10] S. Egelko, D. Simon, E. Rilev, W. Gordon, M. Ruckdeschel-Hibbard, and L. Diller, "First year after stroke: tracking cognitive and affective deficits," *Archives of Physical Medicine and Rehabilitation*, vol. 70, pp. 297–392, 1989.

[11] T. Schenkenberg, D. C. Bradford, and E. T. Ajax, "Line bisection and unilateral visual neglect in patients with neurologic impairment," *Neurology*, vol. 30, no. 5, pp. 509–517, 1980.

[12] M. L. Albert, "A simple test of visual neglect," *Neurology*, vol. 23, no. 6, pp. 658–664, 1973.

[13] J. C. Marshall and P. W. Halligan, "Visuo-spatial neglect: a new copying test to assess perceptual parsing," *Journal of Neurology*, vol. 240, no. 1, pp. 37–40, 1993.

[14] M. Kinsbourne and E. K. Warrington, "A variety of reading disability associated with right hemisphere lesions," *Journal of Neurology, Neurosurgery, and Psychiatry*, vol. 25, pp. 339–344, 1962.

[15] M. B. Bender and C. T. Furlow, "Phenomenon of visual extinction in homonymous fields and psychologic principles involved," *Archives of Neurology And Psychiatry*, vol. 53, no. 1, pp. 29–33, 1945.

[16] V. S. Mercer, J. K. Freburger, Z. Yin, and J. S. Preisser, "Recovery of paretic lower extremity loading ability and physical function in the first six months after stroke," *Archives of Physical Medicine and Rehabilitation*, vol. 95, no. 8, pp. 1547–1555.e4, 2014.

[17] J. A. Semrau, J. C. Wang, T. M. Herter, S. H. Scott, and S. P. Dukelow, "Relationship between visuospatial neglect and kinesthetic deficits after stroke," *Neurorehabilitation and Neural Repair*, vol. 29, no. 4, pp. 318–328, 2015.

[18] J. Poole, W. Dunn, B. Schell, K. Tiernan, and J. M. Barnhart, "Statement: occupational therapy services management of persons with cognitive impairments," *The American Journal of Occupational Therapy*, vol. 45, no. 12, pp. 1067–1068, 1991.

[19] D. E. Beaton, C. Bombardier, F. Guillemin, and M. B. Ferraz, "Guidelines for the process of cross-cultural adaptation of self-report measures," *Spine*, vol. 25, no. 24, pp. 3186–3191, 2000.

[20] S. Kutlay, A. A. Küçükdeveci, A. H. Elhan, and A. Tennant, "Validation of the Behavioural Inattention Test (BIT) in patients with acquired brain injury in Turkey," *Neuropsychological Rehabilitation*, vol. 19, no. 3, pp. 461–475, 2009.

[21] B. A. Wilson, J. Cockburn, and P. W. Halligan, "Development of a behavioral test of visuospatial neglect," *Archives of Physical Medicine and Rehabilitation*, vol. 68, no. 2, pp. 98–102, 1987.

[22] A. Hartman-Maeir and N. Katz, "Validity of the behavioral inattention test (BIT): relationships with functional tasks," *The American Journal of Occupational Therapy*, vol. 49, no. 6, pp. 507–516, 1995.

2

Principal Approaches to Understanding Occupation and Occupational Science Found in the Chilean Journal of Occupational Therapy (2001–2012)

Rodolfo Morrison,[1,2] Silvia Gómez,[1,2] Enrique Henny,[2,3] María Jesús Tapia,[1,2] and Laura Rueda[1,2]

[1]*Department of Occupational Therapy and Occupational Science, Faculty of Medicine, University of Chile, Santiago, Chile*
[2]*Chilean Society of Occupational Science, Santiago, Chile*
[3]*Tedes Center, Santiago, Chile*

Correspondence should be addressed to Rodolfo Morrison; morrison.rodolfo@gmail.com

Academic Editor: Claudia Hilton

Background. The progression of occupational science in Chile is documented in the main scientific publication of the field, the Chilean Journal of Occupational Therapy (RChTO). *Objective.* Identify approaches to understanding and applying occupation and occupational science as elucidated in the RChTO. *Methodology.* A systematic qualitative review of the journal (2001–2012) identified articles elucidating an approach to understanding and application operationally defined as references to specific authors, theories, models/paradigms, definitions, and other fields that support approaches to O/OS. *Results.* The study identified two main approaches. The first considers occupation/occupational science from a practical perspective or as a means to explain human behavior; the second considers occupation/occupational science as an object of study. Each approach is further divided into categories. *Conclusion.* This study provides a novel perspective on regional use of occupational science concepts. These findings contribute to our understanding of this science in context and to recognition of the cultural relevance of these scientific concepts.

1. Introduction

Rapid technological advances and the emergence of the information society have changed the landscape for the scientific community. It is more important than ever to elucidate the international perspectives and bodies of knowledge that form the foundation of any discipline. Given the abundance of information available, it is essential to provide clear guidelines for discourse and academic research.

Occupational therapy in Chile has been influenced by occupational science concepts that were developed in other regions but are applicable to the Chilean context. However, undergraduate occupational therapy programs tend to teach a limited number of theoretical frameworks [1]. Moreover, within our country there has been little discussion of the various ways that occupational science and occupation can be understood and the local implications of these alternative perspectives [2–4].

The challenge for Chilean occupational therapists is to stimulate local discussion of these ideas and develop a theoretical framework that will support undergraduate and postgraduate occupational science/occupational therapy education. This content would provide students with a sound theoretical foundation, strengthen professional identity, and create effective connections between theory and practice [5–11].

Meeting this challenge requires recognizing the place of occupational science in professional education. Studies have shown that occupational therapists rarely use occupational therapy-specific theories to justify their practices, depending instead on concepts borrowed from other disciplines. This situation can be improved if occupational science concepts, foundations, and theories are taught explicitly [12] in occupational therapy education programs, along with their therapeutic applications to occupational behaviors.

As members of the Occupational Science Education Committee, we propose that it is essential to analyze the Chilean understanding of occupational science. Chilean perspectives are reflected in the Chilean Journal of Occupational Therapy (RChTO), which is our highest-impact scientific journal in the discipline [13]. This study explores the question: What approaches to understanding and applying occupational science/occupation are referenced in RChTO articles?

Theoretical Framework. As the objective of this study is to identify approaches to understanding and applying occupational science, we will define some relevant concepts.

Occupational science is the academic study of occupation [14]. It provides a theoretical and scientific foundation for occupational therapy practice, approaching occupation as an inherent human phenomenon. Because of its focus on human behavior, occupational science is considered a social science, like anthropology, psychology, or sociology [15].

One of the first approaches used in occupational science was to study the form, function, and meaning of occupation [14]. Form references to directly observable aspects of occupation. For example, occupational scientists may compare how different cultures or social groups perform a given occupation. Function refers to the contributions of an occupation to human development, health, or quality of life. Meaning refers to the subjective experience of participating in an occupation, which is constructed symbolically within a culture.

Understanding the evolution of occupational science/occupational therapy requires epistemological reflection. Contemporary analysis also involves social, economic, and political dimensions, as the discipline has broadened from an individual-centered perspective to consider the contribution of the community and context [16].

Occupational science/occupation is addressed in many ways in the literature. One way to sift through these perspectives is to investigate how concepts are applied, understood, and studied within the field, seeking to identify different approaches to understanding and application.

Several authors [17–19], reflecting on currents of thought, define approaches to understanding and application as ideologies, viewpoints, or theoretical concepts which explain phenomena that are shared, followed, and reproduced [18] within a discipline [19] through conferences, scientific journals, or other means. Authors sharing an approach may develop their own branches of the fundamental theory but use a common explanatory model [17]. Therefore, an approach is distinctive within a discipline [20], and there is general agreement on the basic conceptual elements and theoretical foundations [18].

Occupational therapy paradigms represent unified concepts set forth by authors seeking to define the nature and purpose of the discipline. These concepts are based on the principles articulated in publications such as those listed in the bibliography. Paradigms provide conceptualizations that organize theories and explain their applications [20].

Approaches to understanding and application represent a distinctive vision of the world. Different approaches may share instruments or theoretical categories. The procedures used in different approaches are based on their underlying world view [18]. Authors sometimes explicitly identify an approach as separate from another approach to understanding and application, alluding to the controversies over different approaches [19].

2. Methods

A systematic qualitative review [21] of the RChTO was performed. This method is based on grounded theory [22], which identifies the core concepts within systematically collected data on a topic. Such an approach does not require an a priori hypothesis but rather seeks to identify a new theory, in this case, approaches to the study of occupation. Other reviews have found this method effective for discovering patterns in the occupational science literature [23].

Inclusion criteria for articles were as follows: (a) keyword(s) and/or title referring to OS/O concepts; (b) published articles between 2001 and 2012; and (c) being available in full-text format.

Articles were analyzed using the operational definition of approach to understanding and application:

(i) *Authors refer explicitly* to a viewpoint on occupational science/occupation.

(ii) *Theories are explicitly identified*, such as epistemological assumptions in the context of a given paradigm; general theories on society or history; theories or assumptions on measurement, observation, data collection, or empirical evidence; theoretically based inferences; or construction of theoretical concepts [24].

(iii) *Conceptual models and paradigms are used.* For instance, theoretical or conceptual elements extracted from a general theory are cited; a model is used to understand an issue; or an explicit theoretical position from a specific approach is applied.

(iv) *Definitions of occupational science/occupation are provided.* A definition is an attempt to explain an idea or term by providing a precise and exhaustive reflection. Therefore, a definition is a cohesive description of the complex state of an object, circumstance, or idea that can be validated through examination.

(v) *Conceptualizations of occupational science/occupation are developed.* A conceptualization is an abstract, simplified perspective on our understanding of some aspect of the world. These abstract ideas stem from the experience and conscious understanding of the world [24, 25]. Conceptualizations may include new propositions and concepts or syntheses of existing ideas on occupational science/occupation.

The research team held several meetings to agree on our understanding and synthesis of the content and capture the issues highlighted by the authors. Finally, the articles were categorized according to similarities and differences.

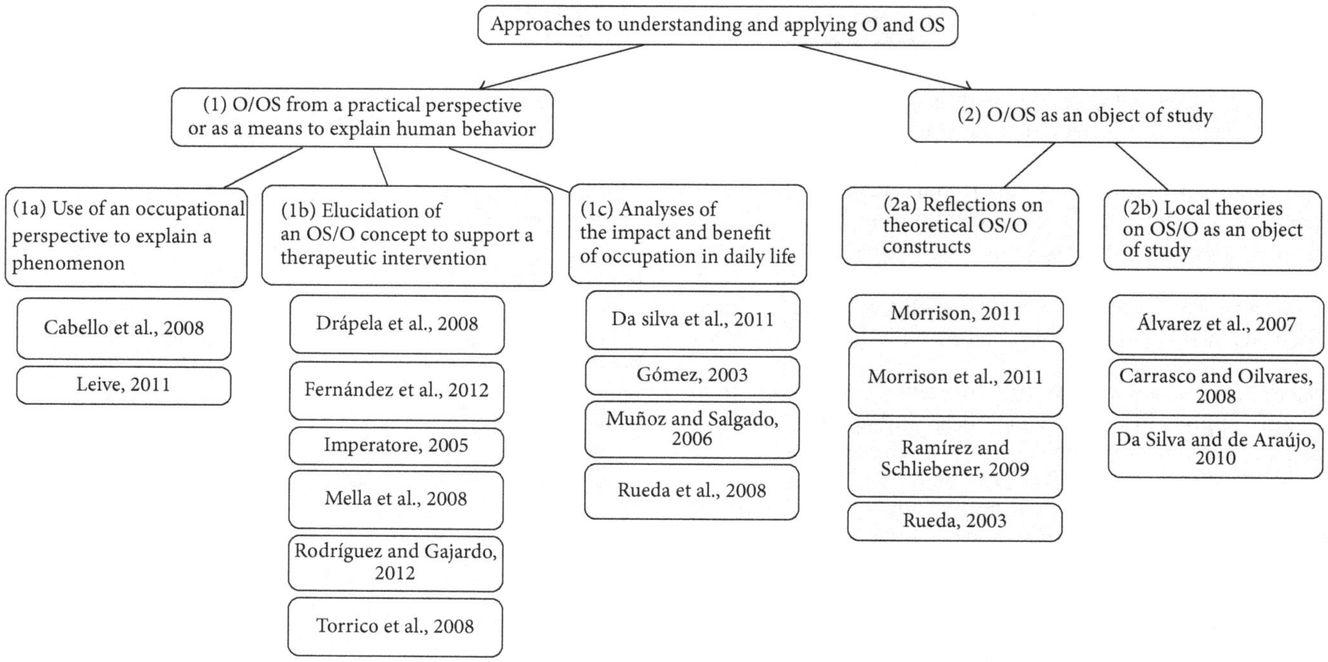

FIGURE 1: Approaches used by various authors, highlighting the two main approaches and the categories.

The research team systematically carried out specific tasks, including cross-reviewing notes, working in parallel and in dyads, outlining meeting minutes, summarizing findings, and critically reviewing these summaries.

The process can be summarized as follows:

(i) Article selection.
(ii) Identification and labeling of references to occupational science/occupation, including authors referenced, in each full-text article.
(iii) Summaries of findings regarding the approaches cited, including the key ideas and citations to support each point.
(iv) Triangulation of information gathered by the research team.
(v) Analysis and synthesis of articles in weekly meetings.
(vi) Categorization of articles.
(vii) Naming the approach to understanding and application for each group.

3. Analysis and Results

Of the 95 articles published in the journal between 2001 and 2012, 19 met the inclusion criteria. The analysis identified two main approaches. The first considers occupation/occupational science from a practical perspective or as a means to explain human behavior (12 articles); the second considers occupation/occupational science as an object of study (7 articles). Both approaches were then divided into categories, as shown in Figure 1 and described below.

(1) Occupation or Occupational Science Considered from a Practical Perspective or as a Means to Explain Human Behavior. These approaches represent first-order analyses, that is, studies performed by authors who instead of asking "what is occupation?" attempt to assign attributes to the concept and provide bibliographic references to support their analysis. These authors approach occupational science/occupation from a practical standpoint and as a way to explain human behavior.

This approach is divided into categories: (a) use of an occupational perspective to explain a phenomenon; (b) elucidation of an occupational science/occupation concept to support a therapeutic intervention; and (c) analyses of the impact and benefit of occupation in daily life.

(1a) Use of an Occupational Perspective to Explain a Particular Phenomenon. This category is based on a concrete situation, a specific conception of occupation, or a local reality. Occupation is used to explain a social behavior from the perspective of a previously defined theoretical construct. Authors that use this approach include Leive [26] and Cabello et al. [27].

In terms of conceptualizations and definitions of occupational science/occupation, Leive [26] focuses on the occupations of families. Occupations are evolving, flexible, orchestrated in parallel with other occupations, and purposeful. Therefore, behaviors that are involuntary, such as sleeping, are not occupations. However, going to sleep and waking up are occupations, as these acts possess a temporal-spatial structure, organization, and biological dimension.

To support this idea, Leive cites the following: Pierce's [28] concept of cooccupation, an occupation that requires synchrony within the occupational patterns of a cohabitating group; Zemke and Clark [14], emphasizing the crucial role of the environment in the construction of occupation, especially the family environment for children; Esdaile and Olson [29], noting that if occupational problems occur, the family dynamic is affected, including the orchestration of caregiver-child cooccupations and other familial roles; and Evans and Rodger [30], noting that the degree of synchronization between the caregiver and child impacts the construction of everyday occupations.

Occupations are performed as part of a routine that depends partly on others. An occupation has a name provided by society that reflects its meaning, is flexible in the face of daily requirements, is performed at a given time, and can be executed with mastery.

Occupations are made up of various tasks. Performing these tasks impacts growth and development. The conditions for existence underlying an occupation include the presence of cooccupations, such as a child going to sleep, which require a certain profile of person, such as a caregiver, to assist in performing them.

Leive asserts that it is necessary to develop certain behaviors before performing some occupations (e.g., going to sleep independently) and that synchrony between the caregiver and child constructs the child's occupation. Moreover, a suitable environment is required (such as the environment surrounding a child and caregiver). Finally, a routine is necessary to configure an occupation, which occurs through a progressive process.

For Cabello et al. [27], occupations are understood as part of everyday life and are performed habitually. Occupations are influenced by the occupations of others and modeled over time. As such, parents influence their children's occupations. The structure of an occupation impacts the family and children, driving behaviors. Occupational modeling consists of imitation (acting; doing) and imagination (preparing for action; thinking) and is influenced by interpersonal relationships. When there is disequilibrium, such as when a family member has a disability, occupations can become risk factors.

The authors cite concepts from Christiansen [31] to suggest that occupations impact social development and the emergence of habits and personal identity. Problems with participation in occupations are risk factors that affect the health of family members, especially children. The authors draw upon Nelson and Jepson-Thomas [32], noting that learning is an adaptive process that occurs through the performance of occupations.

Occupations and occupational knowledge impact a person's health. Occupations influence one's ability to adapt to society, develop habits, and identity and maintain relationships. Occupational modeling arises through interactions between people.

This perspective differs from those that follow because it does not (explicitly) take occupation as a therapeutic tool, but it allows accounting for different phenomena, a function that is also taken by authors in the following categories.

(1b) Elucidation of an Occupational or Occupational Science Concept to Support a Specific Therapeutic Intervention. This group of authors proposes that a theoretical construct of occupation can be used to explain a behavior and perform a therapeutic intervention in a particular population. Authors using this approach include Drápela et al. [33]; Fernández et al. [34]; Imperatore [35]; Mella et al. [36]; Rodríguez and Gajardo [37]; and Torrico et al. [38].

In terms of definitions and conceptualizations of occupational science/occupation, Drápela et al. [33], in their investigation of persons deprived of their liberty, where they identified the meanings associated with criminal activity, indicate that occupation is human performance in response to the vital needs of an individual that allows one to meet social demands, express oneself, and develop an identity. Occupations provide a path towards meaning in life and the development of personal, cultural, and social identity. Occupations consist of meaningful activities; their effects include a sense of efficacy, and they are essential for achieving personal objectives and forging a strong self-concept. These elements are therefore developed through occupation in an occupational therapy intervention. In this way, in occupational therapy intervention, through the occupation, the previous elements are identified.

Fernández et al. [34] suggest that, in order for an occupation to be meaningful, it should support identity construction, provide a sense of belonging, and promote empowerment. This research is focused on productive enterprises of people suffering from mental health problems and shows how therapeutic intervention favors these enterprises and contributes to social rehabilitation.

Imperatore [35] reflects on occupation as the object of occupational science study in the context of sensory integration disorders, especially the impact of such disorders on occupation selection. The author notes that occupation consists of form, function, and meaning, based on concepts [14]. The author presents factors that influence occupation selection, with an emphasis on the "occupational metamorphosis" concept [39], which explains relationships among biological factors such as sensory-seeking behaviors. Thus, occupation functions as a therapeutic tool that affects a person's biology as well as their occupational performance. For this reason, therapeutic intervention by means of the occupation is a central axis in the treatment of sensory integration disorders.

The author cites Zemke [40], reflecting on the organization of occupation in space and time and its relationship with sensory processing. Time is described as the perception of change, including perception of simultaneity, subjective present, sequencing, and duration.

Mella et al. [36], in their investigation of persons deprived of liberty, focus on other considerations regarding occupation. For these authors, occupation (a) is a right and a fundamental element of society in everyday life; (b) has individual meaning and value provided by one's culture and context; (c) includes everyday tasks (self-care, leisure, and contributions to social and economic development of one's community); and (d) represents an intervention space for occupational therapy, as it serves as a potential rehabilitation tool consisting of an organized set of specific tasks and activities.

In the process of therapeutic intervention, the occupation guarantees the right to social integration, allows for emergence of a social order, and supports individual and social wellbeing (including for persons deprived of liberty). Its conditions for existence include everyday activities, which change according to the context and are structured as a function of a person's external conditions.

The authors assert that occupational science conceptualizations are relevant to occupational therapy practice. Theoretical occupational science foundations can be applied to interventions, including in the population of persons deprived of liberty. The authors suggest that these conceptualizations can be used to establish foundations for interventions. Outlining the stages of the intervention based on occupational science concepts ensures that the process will reflect a focus on occupational elements.

Rodríguez and Gajardo [37], in their research into the perceptions of elderly people about their use of public transport, note that occupation provides structure to life, drives habit development, and regulates affective relationships both with others and with the context. Occupation also offers a means to address psychological and behavioral symptoms. Therefore, its conditions for existence are the demands of the environment and the conditions of the person. The relevance of therapeutic intervention in this context is crucial to increase the quality of life of elderly people.

Torrico et al. [38] in their study on the occupational performance of a group of women note that occupations are affected by the rhythms of daily life and are expressed in both work and family contexts. The authors reflect on whether occupation arises from an individual or is determined by historical or cultural context. Occupation consists of form, function, and meaning.

In the intervention process, the occupation increases productivity; affects a person's life satisfaction; satisfies basic survival needs (self-care, shelter, safety, and sustenance); supports social structures (defense against predators and the environment); develops personal abilities; and affects health. Occupations may also generate or be influenced by risk factors including hardship, marginalization, alienation, and inequality [41], as well as gender prejudices that limit the occupations of women.

The principal condition for existence of occupation is the person, that is, the human as an occupational being in a sociocultural context. Occupational choices are determined by economic, political, social, and cultural conditions and are associated with social justice and equality.

To summarize, authors in this category consider occupation and occupational science in terms of therapeutic interventions with specific groups of users or patients. Like category (1a), this category uses occupational terminology to account for a problem, but it differs by proposing a specific therapeutic intervention. Thus, occupational science constructs are present in the intervention processes.

(1c) Analysis of the Impact and Benefit of Occupation in Daily Life. This category is used by a group of authors who address the benefits of occupation in general rather than for a particular population. These authors include Gómez [42]; Da Silva et al. [43]; Muñoz and Salgado [44]; and Rueda et al. [45].

In terms of the definition and conceptualization of occupation, Gómez [42] argues that occupation is a powerful agent capable of driving significant life changes. Occupations organize life, create a day-to-day identity, and provide existence with meaning.

Occupation has both a purpose and meaning. Purpose initiates the activity of occupation, and meaning is a complex, unconscious process mediated by affective and social elements.

Gómez notes that the study of occupation reveals the practical dimension of individuality that emerges through performing an occupation. That is, the concept of individuality is fundamental to the theoretical foundation of occupational science. The author emphasizes that the practice of individual occupations overlaps and intersects with other occupations, making it impossible to understand an occupation as an isolated entity. The intersections between occupations are evident in family, social, and work environments.

Da Silva et al. [43] understand occupation as a therapeutic strategy and central element in the development of occupational therapy. They note that the meaning of occupation changes according to the cultural context. For example, roles that are significant in occidental societies may have no meaning in nonoccidental societies. The authors point out that participating in occupations positively impacts a person's health.

In terms of the conceptualization and definition of occupational science/occupation, Muñoz and Salgado [44] propose that occupation includes a person's everyday tasks and may include activities performed during one's free time, such as relaxation, recreation, or leisure. Occupation has form, function, and meaning. In this approach to understanding occupation, the physical context is crucial and an object of occupational science investigation.

For Rueda et al. [45], occupation differentiates persons from other living beings and is constitutive of humanity. Participation in occupations can (a) generate an occupational equilibrium or disequilibrium; (b) emerge as the product of the time and place in which a person performs his or her activities; (c) provide an individual and collective sense to human groups; and (d) promote social belonging and strengthen the bonds among persons. In conclusion, occupations help to make sense of the project of life.

Authors in this category evaluate occupational context from various perspectives. They address the benefits of occupation in general. Thus, this category provides universal characteristics of the occupation applicable to every person. It does not focus on a specific population, as in category (1b), nor does it only explain a phenomenon such as in category (1a).

This approach, which views occupation and occupational science from a practical perspective or as a means to explain human behavior, differs from the next approach, which employs epistemological and theoretical elements to explain and analyze occupation and occupational science.

(2) Occupation and Occupational Science as an Object of Study. This approach is characterized by (1) reflection on occupational science/occupation concepts; (2) discussion of the approaches used to analyze these constructs; and (3) analysis of theoretical positions that impact practical occupational therapy knowledge and theory. These reflections are second-order analyses, associated with philosophy or epistemology.

This approach can be divided into the following categories: (a) reflections on theoretical occupational science/occupation constructs and (b) local theories on occupational science/occupation as an object of study.

(2a) Reflections on Theoretical Constructs of Occupation or Occupational Science. Authors in this category offer ways to understand occupational science/occupation from a reflective and epistemological perspective.

Morrison [46] offers a conceptual foundation based on philosophical methods which challenges occupational science to engage in a speculative and metareflective process. This philosophy of human occupation (Spanish acronym FOH, for *filosofía de la ocupación humana*) links rhetoric with science to analyze the development, structure, and dissemination of occupational science/occupational therapy knowledge, from an interpretive and critical position.

For Morrison, occupation is a phenomenon amenable to philosophical analysis, a component of clinical occupational therapy practice, a subject of occupational science investigation, and a political element. Morrison cites authors such as Wilcock [41], emphasizing her theory of the occupational nature of human beings, developed through reflections on policies, ecosystems, and relationships between the person and the environment; Kronenberg et al. [47], emphasizing their political-social perspective; and Carrasco and Olivares [2], noting that the construct of occupation implies interdependence between the subject and the constructed reality.

Morrison et al. [48] also conceptualize FOH as a discipline that studies the structure of occupational therapy/occupational science knowledge, developing metatheories that allude first to scientific knowledge and then to scientific practice. The authors support their propositions by citing Díez and Moulines [49], Echeverría [50], Longino [51], and Marcos [52].

FOH addresses knowledge, learning, and internalization of information. The process allows for a critical approach towards the acquisition of occupational therapy knowledge and its translation into actions within the context of professional practice.

Paradigms, therefore, operate within both theory and practice. Paradigms facilitate articulation of key occupational therapy/occupational science concepts and illustrate the evolution of scientific knowledge within the social context of the professionals who generate the findings.

The article also applies Morín's complexity paradigm [53] to the study of occupational therapy/occupation. The advantage of this approach is its divergence from linear, mechanistic paradigms [54]. The notion of complexity liberates the authors from the health-sickness dichotomy and accommodates the totality of factors affecting quality of life. Conceptualizations derived from the complexity paradigm can be applied to occupational science, including multidimensionality and the impulse towards multidimensionality and critical thinking that leads to the problematization of previously taken-for-granted concepts.

Finally, the authors propose a social paradigm of occupation, based on Kuhn [19]. This paradigm considers the evolution of scientific knowledge within the social context of the professionals who generate the findings. The paradigm remains in constant development, positioning occupation as a complex, systematic concept with economic, political, health-related, cultural, and social dimensions that affect the equity and wellbeing of communities.

Ramírez and Schliebener [55] propose the use of dialectics to generate occupational science research and analysis methods. These authors examine occupation in relation to existing narratives, including the occupational reflections of characters found in classical Chilean literature.

The authors consider occupation to be a complex phenomenon that undergoes constant transformation, as its medium (the environment and the person) also experiences continual change. Occupations are understood in the local context and performed by people in the here and now, but each occupation also has a history, essence, and distinctive character that differentiate it from other occupations. The concept, therefore, possesses both an objective dimension, based on reality, and a subjective dimension, based on individual learning. The occupational action executed by a person represents the synthesis of both factors. This action consists of individual elements, which have distinctive features, and common elements, which remain constant in different places and times.

Ramírez and Schliebener posit that occupations create and transform society, changing recursively in the face of emerging requirements. Occupations also influence personal identity, thereby changing the way that a person performs other occupations. Occupations are based on material and historical conditions but are also influenced by the ideas of the performer. That is, occupations are performed in given a space and time in a way that involves both objective (social) and subjective (individual) elements. Certain conditions are required for each occupation, which are determined by other, previously performed occupations, implying a historical development of occupation.

The authors also argue for the utility of historical materialism to justify interventions in a specific population (historical materialism is an epistemological explanation that accounts for how human history has developed. Based on the ideas of Karl Marx and Friedrich Engels, historical materialism positions material conditions of existence as a basis for understanding juridical relationships and forms of state and of all civil society [56]. Thus, to think of human occupation from this perspective implies understanding the material historicity of occupations and how this explains, for example, occupational performance). These authors use dialectics as a foundation to study occupation, noting that its complexity makes it useful for elucidating this multifaceted concept. The authors view dialectics as the science of the general laws governing nature, avoiding the partialities associated with the subject performing the occupation. The authors consider a materialist perspective to be essential for comprehending occupation and its inherently subjective elements from an objective standpoint [57].

Rueda [58] redefines the concept of occupation based on hermeneutic and phenomenological rules [59]. Hermeneutics is used to generate a new reading of occupation by examining previous texts from various authors. Phenomenology is used to understand occupation as a pivotal point of human experience as well as explore the significance of this experience.

The author interprets occupation as a concept that involves a speculative knowledge or an attempt to comprehend the world, including the facet of the world called occupation.

Based on historical texts, the author notes that occupational therapy brought together biomedical and humanist knowledge from different perspectives. These views included content from studies conducted outside of Chile, but applicable to the Chilean context through hermeneutics.

Rueda also considers occupation from a bioethical. The author underscores concepts essential to occupation as understood in occupational therapy: knowing, doing, formal education, professional practice, models, techniques, and praxis. These concepts are based on Lolas [60], who notes that some characteristics of professional practice are defined by society. Professional practice includes the translation of knowledge into action; moreover, the author distinguishes between those who create and those who apply knowledge. The latter group ultimately fulfills the goals of professional practice. Specific professional actions are expressed through models, which facilitate deeds well done that articulate the knowledge, techniques, and interests of a profession.

Rueda notes that, in generating a body of knowledge and validating scientific findings, it is important to remain conscious of the discipline's theoretical framework. Therefore, if occupational science is incorporated into occupational therapy, the development and evolution of the two fields go hand-in-hand.

Authors in this category use different theoretical and philosophical approaches to reflect on occupation and occupational science but do not propose a redefinition of concepts.

(2b) Local Theories on Occupation or Occupational Science as an Object of Study. This second category applies the study of occupational science/occupation to local realities and, unlike the previous category, proposes a redefinition of concepts. The authors that use this approach are Álvarez et al. [61], Carrasco and Olivares [2], and Da Silva and de Araújo [62].

Álvarez et al. (2010) propose a theoretical construction of occupation, with conceptual bases including (a) Latin American perspectives on knowledge and (b) the epistemology of historical consciousness, citing Zemelman in both instances [63, 64]. The first element suggests that Latin American concepts have developed out of investigations into the social world, incorporating components such as subjects, collective subjectivities, and social movements, and an awareness of history and politics. The second element focuses on the ethics and politics of generating knowledge, opening new, coherent horizons that contrast historically fragmented perspectives on knowledge.

The authors note that the reconceptualization of the term occupation provides opportunities for discussion and growth within the discipline. Recognizing that national conceptualizations are based largely on international works, they applied the international literature to the Latin American process, emphasizing the need to define occupational science in the national context. The authors propose a local definition that is the product of long-term reflection: occupation is a meaningful everyday activity, performed by a person and named by the culture.

Carrasco and Olivares [2] cite Kuhn's paradigm [19] to support the assertion that occupational science/occupational therapy professionals hold the concept of occupation central to their disciplines despite different nuances in interpretation. The authors propose that general systems theory (GST) [65, 66] supports a deep understanding of occupation, as it conceptualizes human beings as high-complexity systems and therefore drives articulation of social and natural scientific findings through multidisciplinary studies. They further suggest that dynamic systems theory (DST) [65, 67, 68] may facilitate a more comprehensive understanding of occupation. DST goes beyond the hierarchical relationships established by GTS to encompass heterarchical associations. Furthermore, DST captures the dynamic nature of complex systems. By citing the theoretical constructs used in the field, Carrasco and Olivares apply a constructivist approach [69], emphasizing the role of occupational therapists in developing the theoretical foundation of their discipline.

The authors approach occupation as an element that can be understood through human and social dimensions and as the object of occupational therapy investigations. Occupation is a phenomenon that can be studied and explained, as it is performed and observed in a given environment.

Carrasco and Olivares refer to authors who approach occupation as an object of occupational science investigations that consists of observable elements, such as form, as well as interpretable elements, such as meaning and purpose. The study of occupation promotes development of the academic discipline and clinical occupational therapy practice.

The authors also note that occupation is not synonymous with activity [28] as perceived by individuals or society in general. Occupation is a discrete act and experience perceived as distinct by the person who performs it. This experience is individual and singular. Occupations are different each time they are performed due to the interaction among the various components, evolving across the lifespan.

The authors reference Kielhofner [70] to illustrate that occupational therapy has a unique perspective shared across the discipline, despite nuances that surface in applications to different contexts. The authors also cite other sources that define occupation: (a) Nelson [71], who proposes that the significance of occupation lies in its symbolic meaning, which emerges in a given space and time, and is therefore singular, and (b) Iwama [72], who emphasizes the individual meanings of occupation that materialize in different cultural and social contexts.

Carrasco and Olivares conceptualize occupation as a result of dynamic interactions between activity, purpose, occupational form, and meaning.

In sum, the authors propose a concept of occupation based on three types of constructions: (a) the habitual and historic occupational therapy factors—that is, person, environment, and activity—which are not subject to direct observation or analysis, as it is impossible to separate the person from their environment or activity; (b) factors that can be perceived and analyzed by an observer, that is, the occupation's form, function, and meaning; and (c) factors only interpretable by the person performing the occupation.

Occupation also has certain conditions for existence, such as association with the human and social spheres. These factors are evident when occupation is approached from a subjective perspective. This means that there are many ways to understand occupation that depend on the observer's viewpoint and context and therefore many ways to explain reality. Categories, which emerge through interactions among people (intersubjectivity) in a given situation (context), can facilitate such understanding. These concepts explain "reality" but they are not reality.

The study by Da Silva and de Araújo [62] reflects on local contextualization of occupational science/occupation elements in the practice of occupational therapists working in the Amazon rainforest of Pará, Brazil. These authors cite Clark and Lawlor [73], noting that occupational science is an emerging discipline that understands human beings as occupational beings. The authors emphasize the associations between commitment in the context of occupation and the context of human life, especially the influence of this relationship on health, wellbeing, and social participation, citing Rudman et al. [74] to demonstrate the role of occupation in supporting health and participation.

These authors, therefore, view occupation as participation in everyday activities: self-care, leisure, work, and so forth. The definition of occupation is ambiguous within the discipline, and the term activity is sometimes used interchangeably with occupation. Occupation encompasses a diversity of actions carried out by people in a given context. It is a type of activity that occupies a person within a social context and integrates human expression.

Moreover, occupation includes the activities carried out by a person (who may vary according to age, race, sex, etc.) in the context of work, leisure, and social activities during one's everyday life (which in turn encompasses many contexts influenced by one's culture). Occupations are essential for a person's life, health, and wellbeing; they allow a person to organize his or her world; they are dynamic; and they evolve throughout the lifespan.

Occupation also has therapeutic value that transcends the everyday. Occupation in this sense can generate change, as it touches the social, cultural, economic, biological, and philosophical spheres. The authors approach occupation as a broad subject, noting that a clear description of occupation supports effective occupational therapy interventions.

Occupations consist of actions and meanings that evolve over a person's lifetime, generating change and transformation. Therefore, occupations have a meaning in a given context, provide structure, and endow a person with humanity; their social context is the condition for their existence.

Authors in this category, although employing a series of theoretical constructs that come from different fields of knowledge (especially in the United States), manage to reconstruct or contextualize the occupation for relevant perspectives with the local reality, which enriches regional theoretical and reflexive development.

4. Discussion and Conclusion

This study identified the main approaches to understanding and applying concepts of occupation and occupational science in the literature of the discipline as published in the RChTO between 2001 and 2012. These findings document the diversity of the discipline and contribute to the education of new occupational therapists.

This analysis made it clear that many positions can be used to study occupation. Approaches to understanding occupational science are informed by concepts of occupation, based on literature relevant to authors in occupational science and related fields. The analysis clearly revealed two different approaches. The first considers occupational science/occupation from a practical perspective and as a means to explain human behavior; the second considers occupational science/occupation as an object of study. These approaches were developed on a regional level and have been used as a foundation for local professional practice.

The first main approach is characterized by the application of occupational science/occupation constructions. This approach includes three categories: the use of an occupational perspective to explain particular phenomena; application of occupational science/occupation constructions to therapeutic interventions; and the study of the impact and benefits of occupational science/occupation in daily life.

The second main approach focused on occupational science/occupation as an object of study and can be divided into two branches. One is based on the global analysis of theoretical constructs while the other offers local perspectives on occupational science and occupation.

The latter refers rather to a reconstruction, contextualization, or adaptation of different international theoretical perspectives, and not to the creation of other theories to explain occupation. Thus, the value of this category is that it finds ways to apply international theories at a local level, making them culturally relevant.

A noteworthy finding of this study is that there were only two Latin American theoretical proposals offered in RChTO publications (2001–2012) [2, 55]. Likewise, only one original Latin American definition appeared [61].

In light of the above, we asked about the characteristics of the diffusion of knowledge of occupational therapy in Chile. In Chile and in neighboring countries, the theoretical contributions are generated by groups of academics from the main state universities. In the earlier publications, between the years 1960 and 1980 approximately, a reductionist biomedical paradigm is perceived, which has marked the pattern of practice of the profession in the region. However, the concern to include social participation spaces is not neglected. Later publications are concerned with the empowerment of individuals and groups in their own processes of health maintenance and recovery. In these later publications, the focus is not on the disease but on the person in his or her own context, and on the opportunities that context offers for activities that can be understood as healthy in terms of their meaning for the individual, linked to his or her history, beliefs, and life within a cultural environment.

These results lead to the following questions: What barriers to developing local knowledge do Latin American occupational therapists face? Do Latin American occupational therapists have the motivation, time, and training necessary to carry out research and publish manuscripts? Is the habit of reflecting on interventions an established part of professional practice? Does the discipline, on a Latin American level, place importance on the systematization of professional practices and development of evidence? On an institutional level, are there incentives and support to develop research competency and dissemination of knowledge?

Addressing these questions is crucial to supporting and promoting occupational science/occupational therapy research, a strong professional identity, evidence-based practice, continuing education, scientific societies, and application of research to professional practice. Academic staff responsible for developing occupational therapy curricula should review the competencies needed to improve the discipline and integrate research as a dimension of professional practice.

This study illustrates the recent directions of the discipline at the regional level, examining the written expressions in a particular Spanish-language occupational therapy journal. Therefore, the findings are applicable only to this specific geographic and cultural sphere. It would be interesting to ask the following question: What other fields and media develop and publish reflections and studies of occupational science/occupation?

It seems appropriate to investigate whether studies such as the present have been conducted in other Latin American countries since there are cultural similarities between them, due to their common history. In this way, it would contribute to a broader and deeper knowledge, possibly applicable to the reality of this region, in the areas of theory and practical knowledge. It is also clear, in our view, that the development of knowledge should consider the exercise of distinguishing local knowledge from universal disciplinary knowledge.

Thus, this study provides a new perspective on the way that authors in the field apply occupational science/occupation concepts. It is possible that other sources of literature would yield different approaches for understanding occupational science/occupation concepts.

This study focused on the historical context and temporal elements of the descriptions of occupation in each article. Research to address occupation from cross-sectional (social-historical-cultural) and longitudinal perspectives (current views, issues relevant to the "here and now," capturing unique and unrepeatable moments in time) would also be useful.

This article contributes to the systematization of data relevant to professional practice and provides insights on fundamental concepts such as occupation. The article illustrates current trends in the discipline in terms of research, practice, and education of occupational therapists.

New conceptualizations offered by Latin American authors enrich international development of occupational science and, therefore, the occupational therapy profession.

Conflicts of Interest

The authors declare that there are no conflicts of interest regarding the publication of this paper.

Acknowledgments

The present study is part of the research project "Updates in Occupational Science: A Contribution to Research-Based Teaching" and was funded by the "Fund for Applied Research in Occupational Therapy and Occupational Science of the Department of Occupational Therapy and Occupational Science of the University of Chile (2013)."

References

[1] M. Apablaza, "The challenge of training: a reflection from practice as trainer occupational therapists," *Chilean Journal of Occupational Therapy*, vol. 15, no. 2, 2015.

[2] J. Carrasco M and D. Olivares A, "Making way to go: construction and understanding of Occupation for research and practice in Occupational Therapy," *Chilean Journal of Occupational Therapy*, vol. 8, pp. 5–16, 2008.

[3] E. I. Blanche and E. Henny-Kohler, "Philosophy, science and ideology: a proposed relationship for occupational science and occupational therapy," *Occupational Therapy International*, vol. 7, no. 2, pp. 99–110, 2000.

[4] R. Morrison, "Pragmatist epistemology and Jane Addams: fundamental concepts for the social paradigm of occupational therapy," *Occupational Therapy International*, vol. 23, no. 4, pp. 295–304, 2016.

[5] P. Crist, M. Scaffa, and B. Hooper, "Occupational therapy education and the centennial vision: preface," *Occupational Therapy in Health Care*, vol. 24, no. 1, pp. 1–6, 2010.

[6] B. Hooper, "The occupation of teaching: elements of meaning portrayed through educators' teaching diagrams," *Journal of Occupational Science*, vol. 18, no. 2, pp. 167–181, 2011.

[7] B. Hooper, "On arriving at the destination of the centennial vision: navigational landmarks to guide occupational therapy education," *Occupational Therapy in Health Care*, vol. 24, no. 1, pp. 97–106, 2010.

[8] B. Hooper, "Shortening the distance between the 'i' and the 'it': a transformative approach to improving teaching," *Occupational Therapy in Health Care*, vol. 21, no. 1-2, pp. 199–215, 2007.

[9] B. Hooper and W. Wood, "Pragmatism and structuralism in occupational therapy: the long conversation," *American Journal of Occupational Therapy*, vol. 56, no. 1, pp. 40–50, 2002.

[10] C. Mattingly and M. H. Fleming, *Clinical Reasoning: Forms of Inquiry in A Therapeutic Practice*, Davis, F. A., Philadelphia, Pa, USA, 1994.

[11] E. J. Yerxa, "Infinite distance between the/and the it," *American Journal of Occupational Therapy*, vol. 63, no. 4, pp. 490–497, 2009.

[12] M. N. Ikiugu and H. M. Rosso, "Facilitating professional identity in occupational therapy students," *Occupational Therapy International*, vol. 10, no. 3, pp. 206–225, 2003.

[13] R. Bustos, "Chilean Journal of Occupational Therapy is the most consulted of Faculty of Medicine' jurnals in Internet," Faculty of Medicine, Universidad de Chile, http://noticias.med.uchile.cl/actividades-decanato/9588-revista-chilena-de-terapia-ocupacion-al-es-la-mas-consultada-en-internet-de-la-facultad-de-medicina.html.

[14] R. Zemke and F. Clark, *Occupational Science: The Evolving Discipline*, F. A. Davis Company, Philadelphia, Pa, USA, 1996.

[15] E. J. Yerxa, "Occupational science: a renaissance of service to humankind through knowledge," *Occupational Therapy International*, vol. 7, no. 2, pp. 87–98, 1998.

[16] G. Whiteford and C. Hocking, *Occupational Science: Society, Inclusion, Participation*, John Wiley & Sons, Milton, Australia, 2012.

[17] N. A. Casullo, R. Forster, and A. Kaufman, *Itineraries Modernity. Currents of thought and intellectual traditions from the Enlightenment to Postmodernism*, Eudeba, Buenos Aires, Argentina, 1999.

[18] J. García-Arias, "Could the theory of thought modes explain some of the differences between mainstream and keynesian/post-keynesian economics?" *Social Science Journal*, vol. 15, no. 4, pp. 573–585, 2010, http://www.redalyc.org/articulo.oa?id=28012285002.

[19] T. Kuhn, *The Structure of Scientific Revolutions*, University of Chicago Press, Chicago, Ill, USA, 2nd edition, 1970.

[20] G. Kielhofner, *Conceptual Foundations of Occupational Therapy Practice*, F. A. Davis, Philadelphia, Fla, USA, 4th edition, 2009.

[21] S. L. M. Letelier, M. J. J. Manríquez, and G. G. Rada, "Systematic reviews and metaanalysis: are they the best evidence?" *Medical Journal of Chile*, vol. 133, no. 2, pp. 246–249, 2005.

[22] A. L. Strauss and J. M. Corbin, *Bases of Qualitative Research: Techniques and Procedures for Developing Grounded Theory*, Univ. of Antioquia Press, Medellín, Colombia, 2002.

[23] D. Pierce, K. Atler, J. Baltisberger et al., "Occupational science: a data-based american perspective," *Journal of Occupational Science*, vol. 17, no. 4, pp. 204–215, 2010.

[24] R. Sautu, *Everything Is Theory: Research Objectives And Methods*, Lumiere, Buenos Aires, Argentina, 2005.

[25] Knowledge Master Corporation, "Conceptualization," http://conceptmaps.it/KM-Conceptualization-esp.htm.

[26] L. Leive, "Bedtime routine in the first years of life: first theoretical approach from an occupational Science perspective," *Chilean Journal of Occupational Therapy*, vol. 11, no. 2, pp. 70–83, 2011.

[27] P. A. Cabello, E. Henny, M. C. Hidalgo, and L. Vásquez, "The occupations of the children of parents with disabilities," *Chilean Journal of Occupational Therapy*, vol. 8, pp. 79–83, 2008.

[28] D. Pierce, "Untangling occupation and activity," *American Journal of Occupational Therapy*, vol. 55, no. 2, pp. 138–146, 2001.

[29] A. Esdaile and A. Olson, *Mothering Occupations. Challenge, Agency and Participation*, F.A. Davis, Philadelphia, 2004.

[30] J. Evans and S. Rodger, "Mealtimes and bedtimes: windows to family routines and rituals," *Journal of Occupational Science*, vol. 15, no. 2, Article ID 9686615, pp. 98–104, 2008.

[31] C. H. Christiansen, "Defining lives: occupation as identity: an essay on competence, coherence, and the creation of meaning [The Eleanor Clarke Slagle lecture]," *American Journal of Occupational Therapy*, vol. 53, no. 6, pp. 547–558, 1999.

[32] D. Nelson and J. Jepson-Thomas, "Occupational form, occupational performance, and a conceptual framework for therapeutic occupational," in *Perspectives in Human Occupation-Participation in Life*, P. Kramer, J. Hinojosa, and C. B. Royeen, Eds., pp. 87–155, Lippincott Williams and Wilkins, Baltimore, Md, USA, 2003.

[33] B. J. Drápela, G. M. d. Huidobro, S. J. Núñez, and T. M. Palacios, ""Meanings associated to criminal activities" in men who are deprived of their liberty in Centro de Detención Preventiva Santiago Sur," *Chilean Journal of Occupational Therapy*, vol. 8, pp. 47–58, 2008.

[34] M. M. E. Fernández, G. A. Gaviglio, and S. G. Adur, "An analysis on participation in productive enterprises in mental health area, in the context of social economy in Buenos Aires city-Argentina," *Chilean Journal of Occupational Therapy*, vol. 12, no. 2, 2012.

[35] E. Imperatore Blanche, "Deficit Sensory Integration: Long-term effects on occupation and play," *Chilean Journal of Occupational Therapy*, vol. 5, pp. 1–6, 2005.

[36] S. Mella, V. Villarroel, R. Sepúlveda, and G. Guzmán, "Occupation: a proposal for intervention with persons deprived of liberty based on occupation," *Chilean Journal of Occupational Therapy*, vol. 8, pp. 37–46, 2008.

[37] J. Rodríguez and J. Gajardo, "About the contribution of occupational therapy to non-pharmacologic approaches for the treatment of psychological and behavioral symptoms associated with dementia," *Chilean Journal of Occupational Therapy*, vol. 12, no. 2, 2012.

[38] P. Torrico, D. Urrutia, and M. Schliebener, "How meaningful is for the women themselves the activities they carry out?" *Chilean Journal of Occupational Therapy*, vol. 8, pp. 17–25, 2008.

[39] S.-P. C. Fanchiang, "The other side of the coin: growing up with a learning disability," *American Journal of Occupational Therapy*, vol. 50, no. 4, pp. 277–285, 1996.

[40] R. Zemke, *Time, Space and the Kaleidoscopes of Occupation*, The Eleanor Clarke Slagle Lecture, 2004 AOTA Conference, Minneapolis, MN, USA, 2004.

[41] A. Wilcock, *An Occupational Perspective of Health*, Slack Inc., Thorofare, NJ, USA, 2nd edition, 2006.

[42] L. S. Gómez, "The occupation and its significance as a factor of personal identity," *Chilean Journal of Occupational Therapy*, vol. 3, pp. 43–47, 2003.

[43] L. Da Silva Araújo, N. Fierro Jordán, P. Guitérrez Monclus, and O. Rodriguez, "Occupational science and occupational therapy: its relations and applications to clinical practice," *Chilean Journal of Occupational Therapy*, vol. 11, no. 1, pp. 79–87, 2011.

[44] E. I. Muñoz and G. P. Salgado, "Leisure occupations: approach from a perspective of development, life cycles and human needs," *Chilean Journal of Occupational Therapy*, vol. 6, pp. 39–45, 2006.

[45] L. Rueda, M. A. Montenegro, D. Poblete, and F. Traipe, "Post Traumatic Stress: interference and occupational adjustment," *Chilean Journal of Occupational Therapy*, vol. 8, pp. 27–35, 2008.

[46] R. Morrison J, "Rhetoric of science. Descriptions and critical reflection about creation of knowledge. Contributions to Occupational Therapy," *Chilean Journal of Occupational Therapy*, vol. 11, no. 1, pp. 89–101, 2011.

[47] F. Kronenberg, S. Simó Algado, and N. Pollard, *Occupational Therapy Without Borders: learning From The Spirit of Survivors*, Médica Panamericana, Buenos Aires, Argentina, 2006.

[48] R. Morrison, D. Olivares, and D. Vidal, "The Philosophy of Human Occupation and The Social Paradigm of the Occupation. Some reflections and suggestions on current epistemologies in Occupational Therapy and Occupational Science," *Chilean Journal of Occupational Therapy*, vol. 11, no. 2, pp. 102–119, 2011.

[49] J. Díez and C. Moulines, *Fundamentals of Philosophy of Science*, Ariel, Barcelona, Spain, 1997.

[50] J. Echeverría, *Philosophy of Science*, Akal, Madrid, Spain, 2nd edition, 1998.

[51] H. Longino, *The Fate of Knowledge*, Princeton University Press, NJ, USA, 2002.

[52] A. Marcos, *Science and Action. A Practical Philosophy of Science*, Fondo de Cultura Económica, Mexico City, Mexico, 2010.

[53] E. Morin, *Introduction to Complex Thought*, Gedisa, Barcelona, Spain, 1998.

[54] J. Solana, *With Edgar Morin, for a complex thought. Interdisciplinary implications*, Akal, Madrid, Spain, 2005.

[55] R. Ramírez P and M. Schliebener T, "Occupation and dialectics, an analysis from materialistic dialectic," *Chilean Journal of Occupational Therapy*, vol. 9, pp. 167–178, 2009.

[56] A. Giddens, *A Contemporary Critique of Historical Materialism*, vol. 1, Stanford University Press, Broadway, Calif, USA, 1995.

[57] A. Spirkin and O. Yajot, *Fundamentals of dialectical and historical materialism*, Austral, Santiago, Chile, 1972.

[58] L. Rueda Castro, "Occupation: science and technique of occupational therapy," *Chilean Journal of Occupational Therapy*, vol. 3, pp. 1–5, 2003.

[59] J. Acevedo, *Heidegger and the Technical Era*, Universitaria, Santiago, Chile, 2nd edition, 1999.

[60] F. Lolas, *Bioethics and Medical Anthropology*, Mediterráneo, Santiago, Chile, 2000.

[61] E. Álvarez, S. Gómez, I. Muñoz et al., "Concept of occupation: definition and development. Essay about an experience of theoretical construction from a local identity," *Chilean Journal of Occupational Therapy*, vol. 7, pp. 76–82, 2007.

[62] L. Da Silva and O. de Araújo, "Human occupation and occupational therapist practice's in Pará Amazon: a phenomenological perspective," *Chilean Journal of Occupational Therapy*, vol. 10, pp. 99–110, 2010.

[63] H. Zemelman, *The Horizons of Reason*, Anthropos, Madrid, Spain, 1992.

[64] H. Zemelman, *Subject: Existence and Power*, Anthropos/UNAM, Barcelona, Spain, 1998.

[65] M. Arnold and F. Osorio, *Introduction to Basic Concepts of General Systems Theory*, Möbius strip, 1998, http://www.redalyc.org/articulo.oa?id=10100306.

[66] L. Bertalanfly, *The General Systems Theory*, Fondo de Cultura Económica, Mexico City, Mexico, 1976.

[67] F. Capra, *The Web of Life*, Harper Collins, London, UK, 1997.

[68] J. A. S. Kelso and B. Tuller, "A dynamical basis for action systems," in *Handbook of Cognitive Neuroscience*, M. S. Gazzaniga, Ed., Plenum, New York, NY, USA, 1984.

[69] T. Ibáñez, *Social Psychology Constructionist*, Univ. de Guadalajara Press, Jalisco, México, 1994.

[70] G. Kielhofner, *Model of Human Occupation*, Médica Panamericana, Buenos Aires, Argentina, 3rd edition, 2004.

[71] D. L. Nelson, "Occupation: form and performance," *American Journal of Occupational Therapy*, vol. 42, no. 10, pp. 633–641, 1988.

[72] M. Iwama, *The Kawa Model, Culturally Relevant Occupational Therapy*, Churchill LivingstoneElsevier, New York, NY, USA, 2006.

[73] F. Clark and M. Lawlor, "The Making and mattering of occupational science," in *Willard and Spackman. Occupational Therapy*, E. Crepeau, E. Cohn, and B. Schell, Eds., pp. 14-11e, Wolters Klover Lippincott Williams and Wilkins, Philadelphia, Pa, USA, 2009.

[74] D. L. Rudman, J. V. Cook, and H. Polatajko, "Understanding the potential of occupation: a qualitative exploration of seniors' perspectives on activity," *American Journal of Occupational Therapy*, vol. 51, no. 8, pp. 640–650, 1997.

A Feasibility RCT Evaluating a Play-Informed, Caregiver-Implemented, Home-Based Intervention to Improve the Play of Children Who Are HIV Positive

Elelwani Ramugondo,[1] Anande Ferreira,[1] Donna Chung,[2] and Reinie Cordier[2]

[1]*Department of Health and Rehabilitation Sciences, Faculty of Health Sciences, University of Cape Town, Cape Town 7935, South Africa*
[2]*School of Occupational Therapy, Social Work and Speech Pathology, Faculty of Health Sciences, Curtin University, Perth 6012, Australia*

Correspondence should be addressed to Reinie Cordier; reinie.cordier@curtin.edu.au

Guest Editor: Diane Parham

Background/aim. In South Africa, contextual factors have been identified as barriers to outdoor, unstructured play. The human immunodeficiency virus (HIV) and resulting progressive HIV encephalopathy (PHE) is a pandemic in this area, associated with development delays that are not addressed by highly active antiretroviral treatment (HAART). This study aimed to describe the playfulness in children with HIV and PHE on HAART living in challenging socioeconomic areas in South Africa aged 6 months to 8 years and to evaluate the feasibility and preliminary effectiveness of a play-informed, caregiver-implemented, home-based intervention (PICIHBI) for improving play. *Methods.* A feasibility randomized control trial allowed for comparison of PICIHBI and conventional one-on-one occupational therapy interventions. Children were filmed playing pre-, mid-, and postintervention, using the Test of Playfulness (ToP) to assess playfulness. The PICIHBI comprised of 10 monthly sessions facilitated by an occupational therapist, involving group discussions with caregivers and periods of experiential play. *Results.* Twenty-four children with HIV and/or PHE were randomized into one of the two intervention groups. Overall, the group ($n = 24$) had a median score of 0 (lowest item score) on nine of 24 ToP items and only had a median score of 3 (highest score) on two items. Pre- to postintervention overall ToP scores improved marginally for the PICIHBI group ($n = 12$) and the conventional group ($n = 12$). Between-group differences were not significant. The PICIHBI group demonstrated a significant increase in one ToP item score at midassessment. No significant ToP item changes were found in the conventional group. *Conclusion.* Children with HIV were found to have the most difficulty on ToP items relating to the play elements of internal control and freedom from constraints of reality. The PICIHBI did not significantly improve children's play and was not more effective than the conventional intervention. Considerations for feasibility and effectiveness, including barriers to attendance, are discussed.

1. Introduction

Play is a primary childhood occupation and encompasses all aspects of a child's early years and development [1, 2]. Although play is not easily defined, overlapping perspectives have contributed to a widely accepted definition of play as a transaction between the individual and environment that is internally controlled, intrinsically motivated, and free from external constraints of reality and is framed by the play transaction [3–5]. The terms *play* and *playfulness* are occasionally used interchangeably; however, in this study, *play* refers to the transaction between the individual and environment and *playfulness* refers to an individual's tendency to engage in play. All play experiences are unique, as they do not involve the same set of play things, mates, or spaces, and a child brings their own interests, playfulness, and developmental skills to the play transaction. The environment is an important part of the transaction, as it can facilitate or inhibit play. Play and playfulness also occur in varying familial, cultural, social, and political contexts all of which impact on the extent to which children can be playful. Children's development is influenced by these contexts, so it is important to examine how play occurs in differing contexts and what interventions can optimise opportunities where environmental circumstances do not hinder children's play-related development.

In short, play is important for children as the context in which children develop physical, cognitive, emotional, and social skills. To play successfully, a child's own playfulness and developmental skills need to match the play task and environmental demands. This means that play is partially dependent on the achievement of certain developmental skills (e.g., gross motor skills) that a child may use to play [1]. A persistent mismatch between a child's developmental skill level, playfulness, and environment may lead to withdrawal from play opportunities. Deprivation of play can have a negative impact on a child's development [1], and playfulness has been positively linked to overall well-being [6]. Thus, occupational therapists may focus on either play as a means (using play to enhance developmental skills), play as an end (to enhance playfulness characteristics), or both, to assist children to become successful players.

For children infected with the human immunodeficiency virus (HIV), the negative impact of HIV on children's developmental milestones and areas of development needed to play (i.e., social and emotional development, behaviour, and motor and cognitive skills) are well documented [7, 8]. However, there is limited research on the play skills and aspects of playfulness which are most impacted for this population, as well as contextual factors that may contribute to lower levels of playfulness. Such information is essential in order to develop interventions that focus on using play as a means or an end to assist children in developing play and other developmental skills for this population.

HIV commonly invades the central nervous system (CNS) by means of vertical transmission. Replication of the virus within the CNS causes injury within the developing brain, leading to progressive HIV encephalopathy (PHE), associated with developmental delays [9–11]. An updated systematic review has found delays in various domains of development and executive functioning in children with HIV [8]. To date, there are no published results regarding the play patterns or development of playfulness amongst children with HIV.

In South Africa, HIV is a pandemic, with 7 million of the 55.9 million (12.5%) population estimated to be HIV positive [12]. Whilst increased use of antiretrovirals has extended people's lives, for many children, the extended family members are the primary carers of children whose parents have died of HIV-related causes. It is estimated in South Africa that there are 2.1 million children who are orphaned as a result of HIV-related parental deaths and 240,000 children are infected with HIV [13]. Therefore, many families in South Africa are affected by HIV in relation to caring arrangements, household income, and parenting and capacity.

Many children with PHE have been placed on highly active antiretroviral treatment (HAART), significantly reducing mortality and frequency of hospital admissions, allowing children to spend more time in play activities [8, 9]. However, the functioning and overall development of children within the South African context is impacted by concomitant illnesses and low socioeconomic circumstances [10, 11, 14]. For instance, low-income families may not deem play as a priority, due to concerns about daily survival needs [15]. Parental descriptions of play often include the use of toys and materials which they may not be able to afford, rather than using themselves as an active participant in play [15]. The latter is often influenced by a caregiver's working hours, which may reduce their availability to spend time engaging in play.

Another contextual factor relevant to South African children may be parental concerns about safety, which can contribute to limited opportunities for unstructured play outdoors [16]. The impact of xenophobia was found to further contribute to safety concerns and a shift from outdoor to indoor play in the Caribbean [17]. Conversely, South African children from a small community with low socioeconomic circumstances were found to engage in gross motor play, possibly because physical games do not often require equipment or materials [18]. These physical games can often have a social focus; therefore, children who are less skilful can be excluded, which can have a negative impact on playfulness.

Ferguson and Jelsma [14] and Whitehead et al. [10] highlight the need for early childhood intervention programs that address developmental concerns related to children with HIV from low socioeconomic circumstances. Occupational therapy interventions aiming to improve playfulness levels in these children must consider the contextual barriers to participation, elements of playfulness, and the manner in which the tools and knowledge are transferred to caregivers. Further, group-based interventions are important to consider where resources are limited as they increase the reach of an intervention.

This study addresses the need for early childhood intervention programs that address developmental concerns by aiming to investigate the play challenges of children with HIV and evaluating a newly developed play-informed, caregiver-implemented, home-based intervention (PICIHBI) for improving children's playfulness. This study forms part of a larger project investigating the effects of the PICIHBI on a range of developmental skills.

A feasibility randomized controlled trial (RCT) was used for this study in order to establish the viability of using the PICIHBI for improving the playfulness of children with HIV and PHE in South Africa. The aims of this study were therefore twofold and the study contained two components. The first aim and component of this study was to investigate the playfulness of children with HIV and PHE in South Africa. This first step was integral to testing the feasibility of the PICIHBI with this population as the PICIHBI gives careful consideration to playfulness elements and is intended to impart caregivers and children with strategies to alter play engagement within their homes. The second aim and component of the study was to evaluate the feasibility of a play-informed, caregiver-implemented, home-based intervention (PICIHBI) for improving children's playfulness, compared to conventional one-on-one occupational therapy.

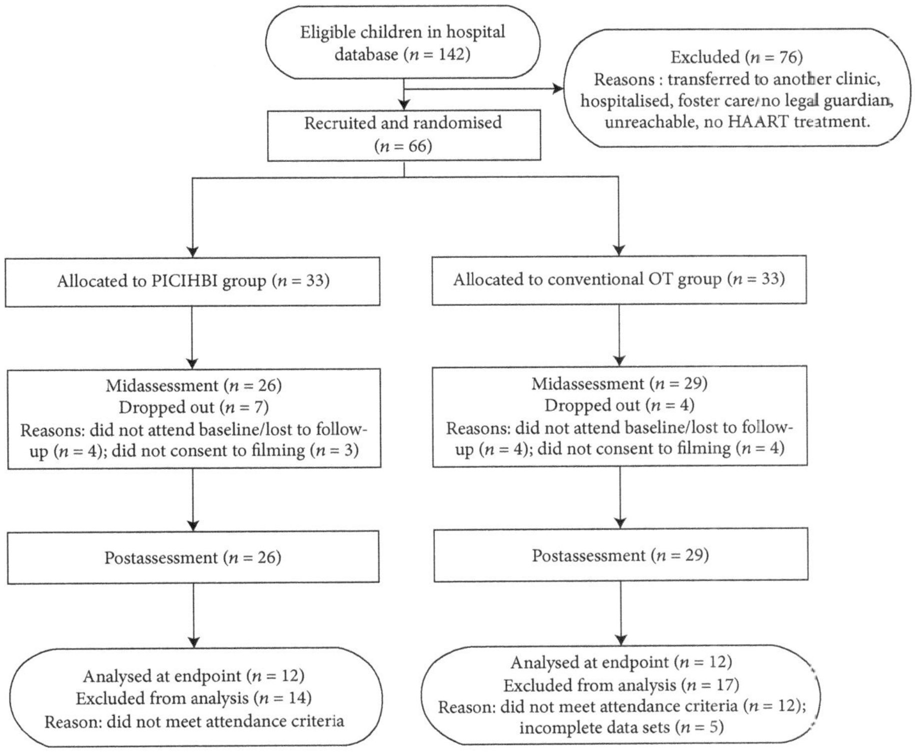

Figure 1: Participant flowchart.

2. Materials and Methods

The CONSORT statement guided the reporting of this feasibility RCT that used an assessor-blinded, block-randomized, parallel-group, pretest-posttest control-group design [19]. A feasibility RCT was used to further establish the nature of the playfulness difficulties of children with HIV, which was needed to evaluate the viability of the PICIHBI in addressing these play difficulties compared to conventional one-on-one occupational therapy. This study was needed prior to further adapting and definitively testing the preliminary effectiveness of the PICIHBI across a range of developmental skills in a larger multisite trial. Ethical approval was obtained from the University of Cape Town Human Research Ethics Committee for the larger study (HREC/REF: 560/2013) and this nested research project (HREC/REF:771/2014). The larger study is registered with the South African National Clinical Trial Registry through the National Health Research Ethics Council (trial number: DOH-27-0115-4892).

2.1. Participants. All children with HIV on HAART aged between 6 months and 8 years who attended the G26 outpatient paediatric antiretroviral (ARV) clinic at Groote Schuur Hospital on a monthly basis were eligible to participate in the larger study. The clinic database contained records for 142 children who met this criterion. Participants were all from low socioeconomic areas.

Attempts were made to contact families of the 142 children meeting the 6 months to 8 years age requirements contained within the hospital database. Translators assisted where needed. There were 76 children in the database who did not participate due to the following reasons: they had been transferred to a different clinic, they had been hospitalised, they were in foster care or did not have a legal guardian, they were unreachable, or they had not started HAART treatment at the time of recruitment. A total of 66 participants were randomized into the PICIHBI or conventional occupational therapy intervention groups.

After the intervention had concluded, data was available from 26 PICIHBI group participants, as four were lost to follow-up or did not attend a baseline assessment and three caregivers did not agree for their child to be filmed. Two participants in the conventional occupational therapy group were lost to follow-up or did not attend a baseline assessment and a further two caregivers did not agree for their child to be filmed, leaving a total of 29 conventional occupational therapy group participants with available data after the intervention period.

Only data from participants who attended more than 50% of the intervention sessions were included in the analysis, as it was thought that these participants would have engaged in a majority of sessions. Children with missing playfulness data from any assessment time point were also excluded upon completion of all three assessment blocks. All data sets in the PICIHBI group were complete; however, 14 participants were excluded when the minimum attendance criterion was applied. There were 5 incomplete data sets in the conventional occupational therapy group, and 17 participants did not attend the minimum 5 sessions. The final sample consisted of 24 participants, 12 participants in each intervention group. See Figure 1 for a participant flow chart.

2.2. Sample Size and Power. Sample size was calculated with GPower 3.1. A total sample of 32 participants, with 16 participants per group, was required to detect the difference between the means of the two groups at a power level of 80% and a significance level of 0.05. To allow for loss to follow-up and poor attendance, the recruited 66 participants were included as part of the initial sample.

2.3. Randomization. A researcher independent of the project completed the randomization process for the larger research project. Therefore, participants were first randomized into two blocks stratified by age (6 months–6 years and 11 months, and 7 years–8 years and 11 months) using *Research Randomizer* [20]. Randomization to treatment groups for this study was completed within each block using *Random Sequence Generator* [21]. This resulted in two intervention and two alternative treatment groups, stratified by age. As the age stratification was required for other studies in the larger project, and not this study, the groups were collapsed to create one intervention and one alternative treatment group for this study. Randomization occurred after participants had consented to participate, and participants were blinded to the allocation process. The researchers and assessors were blinded to the allocation sequence. There were two children in the sample who were siblings, so they were randomized to the same group (PICIHBI) to avoid contamination of the intervention.

2.4. Instruments

2.4.1. Background Information Questionnaire. A demographic and background information questionnaire was completed by caregivers. Information was collected regarding caregiver and child sociodemographics, medical and surgical history, developmental history, HAART treatment regimen and history, rehabilitative service history, schooling history, play engagement, and television habits. Caregivers were asked how they viewed their child's development, learning, and play skills in relation to their peers. This information was utilised to gain a sense of sample characteristics and an understanding of play engagement that may influence implementation of playfulness principles from the PICIHBI within the home.

2.4.2. Test of Playfulness (ToP). The tool used to measure children's playfulness was the ToP Version 4 [4]. The 29-item observational scale was designed to assess the extent (amount of time), intensity (degree of participation), and skill (ease of performance) of play behaviours of children and adolescents aged 6 months to 18 years. ToP items are operationalised according to the definition of play across four elements: intrinsic motivation, internal control, freedom from constraints of reality, and skills related to framing (reading and responding to cues). Items are ranked on a four-point scale and rated during a fifteen-minute observation of a child's free play. A raw item score of 0 is the lowest score and a score of 3 is the highest score, with higher scores indicating greater levels of playfulness. Some items may be rated "not applicable" if the child does not have adequate opportunity to demonstrate the particular playfulness skill during the 15-minute observation. The ToP is reported as clinically valid for children who are typically developing and children with developmental delay, across genders and cultural backgrounds [4, 22]. Accurate and positive construct validity (98% of respondents and 93% of test items conformed to the Rasch model) and interrater reliability (96% of raters conformed to Rasch model) are reported [4, 23]. The ToP has a moderate test-retest reliability (0.67 at $p < 0.01$) [4]. The ToP has also been used as an outcome measure in previous intervention studies involving children cerebral palsy, ADHD, and typically developing children [24–27].

2.4.3. Assessment Procedures. The background information questionnaire was provided to caregivers at baseline assessment, and children were filmed playing in the clinic's play area for 15 minutes. Children were allowed to choose other children enrolled in the study or adults (namely their caregivers) as playmates, or they could play alone. The children were familiar with each other as they attend monthly clinics together. Caregivers who acted as playmates were coached to follow the child's play to ensure children had adequate opportunity to display their own levels of playfulness. The presence or absence of playmates was replicated for each child during subsequent recordings to ensure consistency over the three assessment occasions. Videos were recorded by research assistants who were also instructed to follow the child's play. Children were filmed playing on three occasions: prior to intervention, midintervention, and postintervention.

The playroom was large enough for children to be able to engage in various types of play (e.g., solitary, parallel, or games with rules) and to initiate or join play. The same toys, play materials, and other objects were available for all children during all video recordings. The toys catered to gender differences and the broad age range. Some toys may have been unfamiliar to some children due to limited exposure, but attempts were made to ensure that toys were similar to those in the playroom that they would naturally engage with when they attended other clinic appointments. Each child was given 10 minutes to explore the toys in the room before the videotape was turned on for their 15-minute video footage that would be used for assessment data. After the child's 15-minute filmed play session, caregivers were asked if their child's play at the clinic reflected their play at home. Data were also collected on intervention session attendance rates and participant dropout rates for both intervention groups.

2.5. Interventions

2.5.1. Experimental Group: Play-Informed, Caregiver-Implemented, Home-Based Intervention (PICIHBI). The PICIHBI focused on the caregivers of children with HIV, aiming to equip them to playfully engage with their children and to improve children's playfulness. The PICIHBI gives careful consideration to playfulness elements and is intended to impart strategies to caregivers to alter their children's play engagement within their homes. The PICIHBI also used play to facilitate fine and gross motor development, visual perceptual development, prenumeracy and preliteracy skills, and self-care. It was developed by seven occupational therapists with experience in paediatric occupational therapy. The feasibility of the PICIHBI was guided by occupational therapists experienced in working with children who are HIV positive from low socioeconomic areas within South Africa's Western Cape. Manuals were created for each age group, including detailed outlines and activities for all sessions [7].

The PICIHBI was implemented in three groups based on participant age: 6 months to 2 years and 11 months, 3 years to 5 years and 11 months, and 6 years to 8 years and 11 months. Included in the data analysis for this study were 2, 7, and 3 participants from each group, respectively. This grouping ensured skills of focus were relevant to each developmental stage. The same occupational therapist facilitated all sessions for all groups, and a translator assisted when required. The intervention comprised of 10 monthly sessions per age group, and grading options for activities were provided to allow for individual skill differences amongst the children. While the goals of the PICIHBI were not individualised for each child, they were informed by the participant's baseline assessments and were developmentally appropriate for each subgroup.

Sessions lasted 90 minutes, completed in two 45-minute parts. The first 45 minutes consisted of group discussions with caregivers to introduce the focus skill or concept for the month. The second 45 minutes was experiential, allowing each caregiver the opportunity to attempt play activities with their child to improve the earlier introduced skill in a supported environment. The occupational therapist also modelled playful behaviour to caregivers during this time, relying on caregivers to reflect internally (i.e., integrating learning from the earlier group discussion with the playful model provided by the therapist) to become more playful themselves and to create a play milieu where the children themselves would be playful. The ToP items on which children received the lowest scores during the baseline assessment were incorporated as goals of the experiential activities so that caregivers could observe the occupational therapist model these skills.

Participants (caregivers) received a "Go Box" and an information handout at each session. The Go Box contained items relevant to play, self-care, learning, and development, and the handout contained play activity suggestions that would assist caregivers to incorporate target skills into their daily routine.

2.5.2. Alternative Intervention: Conventional One-on-One Occupational Therapy Intervention. Children were seen monthly, on an individual basis, by an occupational therapist who was not involved in the PICIHBI. Two different therapists were employed at different times during the research project to conduct this intervention arm. Sessions lasted 45 minutes, targeting occupational performance components relevant to the needs and assets of each child. The therapist carried out treatment sessions according to the needs identified through the baseline assessments of the larger research study and their own clinical observations. Caregivers were not the focus of the conventional one-on-one intervention; however, information on activities for the home were given to those who requested it or when deemed necessary by the occupational therapist.

2.6. Blinding. The researcher who scored the videos was not involved in the implementation of the interventions, was aware of the research purpose, but had no knowledge of participants' group allocation. Videos were scored after each assessment block, so the researcher was aware of the study phase when scoring. The occupational therapists running the interventions and the participants could not be blinded to group allocation.

2.7. Statistical Analysis. The ToP item scores of each participant were imported into the Rasch analysis Winsteps program (version 3.70.1). Rasch analysis was then completed to convert ordinal data into interval level scores. This process produced an interval level overall ToP measure score for each participant for each measurement time point. The measure scores that are generated are a function of the performance of the children within the sample against other children in the same sample. Prior to further data analysis, goodness-of-fit statistics was performed to determine infit and outfit statistics of each participant's ToP scores. This determined the goodness of fit between the ToP item scores, rater, and participants through t-test and mean square statistics [26]. All data conformed to the Rasch measurement model.

Analysis for the first aim and component of this study involved developing an understanding of the playfulness of children with HIV. Descriptive statistics including median and interquartile range scores were used to analyse children's ordinal-level ToP item scores at baseline to understand which items and elements of playfulness the children experienced as relatively easy or difficult.

Analysis for the second aim and component of the study involved both the overall ToP scores (interval level data) and raw ToP item scores (ordinal data) for the PICIHBI ($n = 12$) and comparison conventional ($n = 12$) groups at each assessment point. Between-group differences on ToP scores and demographic information were analysed using SPSS (version 19). t-Tests were used to compare continuous variables, and chi-squared tests were used to compare categorical variables between the groups. Nonparametric statistical tests were used with a combination of Friedman repeated measures and Wilcoxon Signed Rank Tests to compare within- and between-group differences on ToP items. Significance was set at $p < 0.05$. To account for the number of calculations used in this analysis, a post hoc Dunn-Bonferroni test was applied and adjusted p values reported. r-Effect size was used to calculate the effect sizes for nonparametric data. This effect size is calculated using the formula $r = Z/\sqrt{24}$. Cohen's guidelines were utilised to interpret effect sizes as small effect ≥ 0.1, medium effect ≥ 0.3, or large effect ≥ 0.5 [28].

3. Results

3.1. Participant Demographics. There were 24 participants in the sample, including 11 males and 13 females. The mean age of the PICIHBI group was 4.0 years and 4.7 years in the conventional group. The youngest participant was aged 10 months at baseline assessment and was part of the conventional group. Of the 24 children, two were reported by caregivers to have an additional diagnosis; however, the children's files indicated at least half of the participants in each group had additional diagnoses.

TABLE 1: Demographic information for PICIHBI and comparison conventional groups.

	PICIHBI group ($n = 12$)	Comparison group ($n = 12$)
Caregiver particulars		
Age of caregiver (years), mean	39.7	33.3
Sex M/F	0/12	0/12
Home language		
Xhosa	66.7%	83.3%
Afrikaans	17%	0%
Shona	8%	0%
French	8%	0%
English	0%	8%
Zulu	0%	8%
Primary caregiver		
Mother	58.3%	83.3%
Grandparent	25%	8%
Aunt	17%	0%
Other	0%	8%
Caregiver education level		
Grade 5	8.3%	8.3%
Grade 6	16.7%	0%
Grade 9	8.3%	8.3%
Grade 10	8.3%	41.7%
Grade 11	16.7%	8.3%
Year 12 (matriculation)	25.0%	33.3%
1 year post school	8.3%	0%
2 years post school	8.3%	0%
Number of adults in household, mean (SD)	2.83 (1.59)	3.58 (1.75)
Number of children in household, mean (SD)	3.25 (1.71)	2.17 (1.03)
Unemployment (%)	83.3%	75%
Child particulars		
Age, mean	4.0	4.7
Sex M/F	4/8	7/5
Gestation > 37 weeks (%)	66.7%	58.3%
Birth weight in kg, mean (SD)	1.83 (1.03)	2.45 (1.04)
Years on HAART, mean (SD)	5.33 (2.39)	4.50 (3.03)
First line of treatment (%)	100%	100%
Tuberculosis history (%)	83.3%	50%
Additional diagnoses		
None	37%	50%
Spastic diplegia	9%	0%
Failure to thrive	9%	8%

TABLE 1: Continued.

	PICIHBI group ($n = 12$)	Comparison group ($n = 12$)
Developmental delay	9%	25%
Other	27%	17%
Missing data	9%	—
Caregiver perceptions of child's learning development and play		
Developing far better than peers	0%	8%
Developing slightly better than peers	0%	8%
Development on par with their peers	67%	59%
Developing slightly slower than peers	25%	17%
Very concerned with child's development	8%	8%

All caregivers were female, and high levels of unemployment were reported across both groups. Xhosa was the language spoken at home by a majority of participants in both groups. Further information on caregiver and child demographics, including caregiver perceptions of their child's play, development, and learning, is provided in Table 1.

3.2. Intervention Attendance. Power dropped from 80% to 68% as 26 participants from the final sample were excluded due to withdrawal, loss to follow-up, and low attendance. Participants most commonly reported missing appointments due to lack of transport money. On average, the PICIHBI group attended 7.16 out of 10 assessments, while the conventional group participants attended 6.75.

3.3. Aim 1: Playfulness Profile of Children with HIV. Descriptive statistics using the median baseline ToP item scores for the total sample within this study ($n = 24$ children) demonstrated that the group had a median score of 0 (reflecting a low score/skill) for nine of the 24 ToP items where sufficient data were collected. These items were *mischief* (*E*), *pretends* (*E*), *unconventional use of objects* (*E*), *clowns* (*E*), *modifies* (*S*), *supports* (*S*), *initiates* (*S*), *giving cues* (*S*), and *responding to cues* (*S*). The group had a median score of 3 (reflecting a high score/skill) for two items *decides* (*E*) and *safety* (*E*) and a median score of 2.5 for the item *engaged* (*E*). Seven items did not have sufficient data to analyse. See Table 2 for all group median baseline ToP item scores and ToP item descriptions.

Mapping these items against the element of play/playfulness each item is associated with (i.e., intrinsic motivation, internal control, freedom from constraints of reality, or framing) [23], children were found to have the least difficulty with the element of intrinsic motivation. No items associated with intrinsic motivation had a median score of 0, and the item *engaged* (*E*) had a median score of 2.5.

Within the element of internal control, children were found to have least difficulty with items associated with the area of self-control. This was demonstrated with high scores

Table 2: Baseline ToP raw item scores for overall group ($n = 24$ children).

ToP item[a] and *description*	Baseline (Pre) Med	IQR
Engaged (E)[IM]: *is activity engaged*	2.5	1.0
Decides (E)[IC]: *what to do*	3.0*	1.0
Safety (E)[IC]: *maintains level of safety sufficient to play*	3.0*	0.0
Mischief (E)[FCR]: *engages in mischief or teasing*	0.0**	0.0
Process (E)[IM]: *engages in activity for the sheer pleasure*	2.0	2.0
Pretends (E)[FCR]: *to be someone else, to do something else*	0.0**	1.0
Unconventional (E)[FCR]: *incorporates objects in variable ways*	0.0**	1.0
Social play (E)[IC]: *engages in social play*	2.0	2.0
Clowns (E)[FCR]: *or jokes*	0.0**	0.0
Cues (E)[FR]: *gives readily understandable verbal/nonverbal cues*	1.0	2.0
Engaged (I)[IM]: *is activity engaged*	2.0	2.0
Social play (I)[IC]: *engages in social play*	1.0	0.0
Affect (I)[IM]: *demonstrates positive affect during play*	1.0	1.0
Object (I)[IC]: *interacts with objects*	2.0	1.0
Engaged (S)[FR]: *is activity engaged*	1.0	1.0
Modifies (S)[IC]: *activity to maintain challenge/make fun*	0.0**	0.0
Social play (S)[IC]: *engages in social play*	1.0	1.0
Supports (S)[IC]: *play of others*	0.0**	0.0
Initiate (S)[IC]: *play with others*	0.0**	1.0
Shares (S)[IC]: *toys, equipment, friends, and ideas*	1.0	1.0
Cues (S)[FR]: *gives readily understandable verbal/nonverbal cues*	0.0**	1.0
Responds (S)[FR]: *to others' cues*	0.0**	1.0
Objects (S)[IC]: *interacts with objects*	1.0	1.0
Transitions (S)[IC]: *from one play activity to another*	1.0	2.0

Notes: (E) = extent item (amount of time), (I) = intensity item (degree of participation), (S) = skill item (ease of performance). [a]Some ToP items were scored "not applicable" for some children; as a result, the following ToP items did not have enough data for analysis: Enters (S), Persists (I), Engages in playful mischief or teasing (S), Pretends (S), Creative (I), Negotiates (S), and Clowns or jokes (S). IQR = interquartile range. Item is associated with the following elements of play and playfulness: [IM]intrinsic motivation, [IC]internal control, [FCR]freedom from constraints of reality, [FR]skills related to framing. *Highest item score; **lowest item score.

on items *decides* (*E*) and *safety* (*E*). However, children demonstrated greatest difficulty within the area of shared control. This was demonstrated by low median scores of 0 on items *modifies* (*S*), *supports* (*S*), and *initiates* (*S*). In addition to the area of shared control within the element of internal control, children also had greatest difficulty in the element of freedom from constraints of reality. This was demonstrated by low median scores of 0 on items *pretends* (*E*), *unconventional use of objects* (*E*), and *clowns* (*E*). Children also demonstrated difficulty in the element of framing with low median scores of 0 for items *giving cues* (*S*) and *responding to cues* (*S*).

3.4. Aim 2: Preliminary Effectiveness of the PICIHBI for Improving Children's Play

3.4.1. ToP Overall Measure Scores. The mean ToP overall measure score was higher at baseline assessment for the PICIHBI group at 33.6 (SD = 17.3) than the comparison conventional group at 31.5 (SD = 23.2). However, the between-group differences in mean baseline ToP scores were not statistically significant ($p > 0.05$).

The PICIHBI group ToP measure score decreased at midintervention assessment to 28.0 (SD = 24.2), however, not to a degree of statistical significance ($p > 0.05$). The PICIHBI group ToP measure score improved from 33.6 (SD = 17.3) at baseline assessment to 35.0 (SD = 17.0) at postintervention assessment. This change was not statistically significant ($p > 0.05$).

The comparison conventional group ToP measure score increased from 31.5 (SD = 23.2) at baseline to 33.4 (SD = 23.9) midintervention assessment. This change was not statistically significant ($p > 0.05$). The group ToP measure score of the conventional group did not improve significantly from baseline assessment of 31.5 (SD = 23.2) to 38.7 (SD = 9.6) at postintervention assessment ($p > 0.05$). No statistically significant between-group differences were found between the PICIHBI group and comparison conventional intervention group at any time point ($p > 0.05$).

3.4.2. ToP Item Scores. Changes in ToP item scores for the PICIHBI group are presented in Table 3. Friedman's tests showed that the PICIHBI group demonstrated a

TABLE 3: Changes in PICIHBI group ToP item scores over time.

ToP item[#]	Descriptive statistics Baseline		Mid		Post		Friedman's Baseline-mid-post		Post hoc pairwise comparison Baseline to mid		Baseline to post		Mid to post	
	Med	IQR	Med	IQR	Med	IQR	χ^2	p	Z	p	Z	p	Z	p
Engaged (E)	2.5	1.0	1.0	1.8	2.0	1.0	9.06	0.01*	9.00	0.01*	1.29	0.26	2.28	0.13
Decides (E)	3.0	1.0	1.5	2.0	3.0	1.0	12.07	<0.01*	7.00	0.01*	0.20	0.66	8.00	0.01*
Safety (E)	3.0	0.0	3.0	0.0	3.0	0.0	2.00	0.37	1.00	0.32	—	—	1.00	0.32
Mischief (E)	0.0	0.0	0.0	0.0	0.0	0.0	2.00	0.37	1.00	0.32	1.00	0.32	—	—
Process (E)	2.0	1.0	1.0	2.5	2.5	2.0	3.80	0.15	0.00	1.00	1.60	0.25	3.60	0.06
Pretends (E)	0.0	1.0	0.0	0.8	0.0	1.5	1.83	0.40	1.29	0.26	0.20	0.66	1.00	0.32
Unconventional (E)	0.0	0.0	0.0	0.8	0.0	0.0	0.34	0.85	0.20	0.66	0.00	1.00	0.34	0.57
Social play (E)	2.0	2.0	1.0	0.0	1.0	1.0	6.42	0.04*	2.78	0.10	7.00	0.01*	0.00	1.00
Clowns (E)	0.0	0.0	0.0	0.0	0.0	0.0	1.00	0.61	1.00	0.32	1.00	0.32	0.00	1.00
Cues (E)	1.0	2.0	0.5	1.0	1.0	0.8	1.60	0.45	0.67	0.42	0.00	1.00	1.60	0.21
Engaged (I)	2.0	1.0	1.0	1.8	1.0	1.0	0.39	0.83	0.20	0.66	0.00	1.00	0.40	0.53
Social play (I)	1.0	1.0	1.0	1.0	1.0	2.0	0.61	0.74	0.00	1.00	0.67	0.42	0.15	0.71
Affect (I)	1.0	1.0	0.0	0.8	0.0	1.0	4.21	0.12	2.00	0.16	5.00	0.03*	0.15	0.76
Object (I)	2.0	1.0	1.0	1.0	2.0	1.0	2.24	0.33	2.67	0.10	0.00	1.00	1.00	0.32
Engaged (S)	1.0	1.0	1.0	2.0	1.0	0.0	0.44	0.81	0.15	0.71	0.50	0.48	0.15	0.71
Modifies (S)	0.0	0.0	0.0	1.0	0.0	1.0	2.00	0.37	2.00	0.16	1.00	0.32	0.34	0.57
Social play (S)	1.0	1.0	1.0	1.0	1.0	1.0	1.62	0.45	0.20	0.66	0.67	0.42	1.29	0.26
Supports (S)	0.0	1.5	0.0	1.0	0.0	1.0	0.13	0.94	0.00	1.00	0.00	1.00	0.20	0.66
Initiate (S)	0.0	0.3	0.5	1.0	1.0	1.0	2.24	0.33	1.80	0.18	1.80	0.18	0.15	0.76
Shares (S)	1.0	0.0	1.0	0.0	1.0	1.0	0.37	0.84	0.20	0.66	0.20	0.66	0.20	0.66
Cues (S)	0.5	1.8	0.5	1.0	1.0	0.0	1.43	0.49	0.15	0.71	0.15	0.71	1.60	0.21
Responds (S)	0.0	2.0	1.0	0.0	1.0	0.0	2.23	0.33	0.50	0.48	2.67	0.10	0.20	0.66
Objects (S)	1.0	1.0	1.0	1.0	1.0	0.8	3.50	0.18	2.67	0.10	0.15	0.71	2.68	0.10
Transitions (S)	1.0	2.0	1.0	2.0	1.0	1.0	9.06	0.01*	9.00	<0.01*	0.50	0.48	2.78	0.10

Notes: [#]Some ToP items were scored "not applicable" for some children; as a result, the following ToP items did not have enough data for analysis: Enters (S), Persists (I), Engages in playful mischief or teasing (S), Pretends (S), Creative (I), Negotiates (S), and Clowns or jokes (S); IQR = interquartile range; Friedman's two-way ANOVA; post hoc pairwise comparison tests. p: adjusted p value after post hoc Dunn-Bonferroni test; —: test did not run as the mean rank values were identical; $^*p < 0.05$.

significant change in scores on four of the ToP items across time: *engaged* (*E*): $\chi^2 = 9.1$, $p = 0.01$; *decides* (*E*): $\chi^2 = 12.8$, $p = 0.00$; *social play* (*E*): $\chi^2 = 6.4$, $p = 0.04$; and *transitions* (*S*): $\chi^2 = 9.1$, $p = 0.01$. Post hoc pairwise comparison tests show that the scores of the item *engaged* (*E*) decreased significantly from baseline assessment to midintervention assessment ($Z = 9.0$, $p = 0.01$). *Decides* (*E*) significantly decreased from baseline to midassessment ($Z = 7.0$, $p = 0.01$) and improved significantly from mid- to postintervention assessment ($Z = 8.0$, $p = 0.01$; returning to baseline assessment scores). *Social play* (*E*) decreased significantly from baseline to postintervention assessment ($Z = 7.0$, $p = 0.01$). *Transitions* (*S*) improved significantly from baseline to midintervention ($Z = 9.0$, $p = 0.01$; maintaining from mid- to postintervention assessment). No significant changes were found in the comparison conventional one-on-one occupational therapy group on any of the ToP items. Results for the conventional group are presented in Table 4.

Effect sizes for ToP item scores for the PICIHBI and comparison groups are presented in Table 5. For the PICIHBI group, a total number of 11 small, medium, or large effect sizes were found across the ToP items. There was a small effect size for change in *initiates* (*S*) from baseline to midintervention. There were also small effect sizes from baseline to postintervention for *process* (*E*), *initiates* (*S*), *cues* (*S*), and *responds* (*S*). Mid- to postintervention revealed a small effect size for *cues* (*S*), *cues* (*E*), and *object* (*I*); a medium effect size for *engaged* (*E*) and *process* (*E*); and a large effect size for *decides* (*E*) (see Table 5).

For the comparison group involving conventional one-on-one occupational therapy group intervention, 11 small or medium effect sizes were found across the ToP items. There were small effect sizes from baseline to midintervention for *process* (*E*) and *cues* (*S*). There were six notable effect sizes from mid- to postintervention; small effect sizes for *pretends* (*E*), *shares* (*E*), and *cues* (*S*); and medium effect sizes for *process* (*E*), *supports* (*S*), and *responds* (*S*). Mid- to postintervention revealed small effect sizes for *engaged* (*E*) and *supports* (*S*) and a medium effect size for *decides* (*E*) (see Table 5).

4. Discussion

This study aimed to develop a play profile of children with HIV living in low socioeconomic contexts in South Africa and to understand whether a play-informed, caregiver-implemented, home-based intervention (PICIHBI) was feasible and showed preliminary effectiveness for developing children's playfulness. A key finding from this study was that children with HIV obtained the lowest possible score on almost 40% of ToP items that had sufficient data for analysis. These low scores were particularly pronounced in items associated with the playfulness elements of internal control, freedom from constraints of reality (pretend play), and, to a lesser extent, skills related to framing.

Interestingly, the same level of difficulty was not found in ToP items reflecting intrinsic motivation. This was demonstrated by children's relatively high scores across these items, demonstrated by their ability to be actively and intensely *engaged* in play; their ability to engage in play for the *process*, rather than an external reward; and the extent of time they engaged in *social play* with another play partner. Similarly, children with HIV were found to have relatively high scores in ToP items reflecting aspects of the element internal control [29]. This was demonstrated by their ability to *decide* what game to play and maintain a level of *safety* sufficient to play and the degree to which they used *objects* in their play. A person-item map is produced during Rasch analysis to indicate the spread of item difficulty within a measure. It is therefore important to note that the Rasch modelling of ToP items indicate that items related to internal control are relatively easy items to obtain a high score on [23].

In contrast to children's relatively high scores on ToP items associated with the play element of intrinsic motivation, they had low scores on ToP items associated with the play element of framing and some ToP items related to internal control. This was demonstrated by children actively engaged in play but lacking the interpersonal skills to maintain play interactions with another, including their ability to *initiate* play and *support* the play of others and *share* toys, space, or equipment during play with another; the skill and intensity in which they engaged in *social play* with another person; and their ability to *give* and *respond to cues* (verbal and nonverbal) during a play interaction. Children were also found to have low scores on ToP items associated with the element of freedom of constraints of reality. This was demonstrated by the lack of skills demonstrated in pretend play. Difficulty in pretend play could have adverse effects on the current and future development of emotional understanding in children with HIV, as childhood developmental theory denotes that pretend play is central to the development of emotional attunement [30].

Collectively, these findings about the playfulness of children with HIV indicate that children are motivated and able to engage in play; however, they have difficulty in areas of play that are highly dependent on their ability to interact with others. This indicates that children with HIV may have difficulty in the area of empathy (including emotional attunement and perspective-taking skills) and social interaction skills. These findings are consistent with previous studies which found that children with other developmental difficulties also demonstrate low levels of playfulness in ToP items that require these skills [26, 31–36]. No studies could be located that investigated the play of children without HIV from the same communities to enable comparison.

It is important to note that a number of factors about the play of children with HIV living in low socioeconomic contexts remain unknown. There were some ToP items that had insufficient data to be included in the analysis. To address this issue, further research is needed to gain a more ecologically valid snapshot of children's play. This will likely require play observations across multiple settings, including the child's home and a familiar outdoor play space. It is also unknown how the levels of playfulness of children with HIV compare to control children from the same socioeconomic contexts, as well as the broader population of children with HIV living in South Africa. Therefore, further research is needed to determine if these findings can be replicated within

Table 4: Changes in conventional occupational therapy group ToP item scores over time.

ToP item#	Descriptive statistics: Baseline		Descriptive statistics: Mid		Descriptive statistics: Post		Friedman's Baseline-mid-post		Post hoc pairwise comparison: Baseline to mid		Post hoc pairwise comparison: Baseline to post		Post hoc pairwise comparison: Mid to post	
	Med	IQR	Med	IQR	Med	IQR	χ^2	p	χ^2	p	χ^2	p	χ^2	p
Engaged (E)	2.5	1.8	2.0	1.0	2.5	1.0	0.71	0.71	0.11	0.74	0.50	0.48	0.50	0.48
Decides (E)	3.0	1.8	2.5	1.0	3.0	0.8	2.37	0.31	0.15	0.71	1.29	0.26	2.00	0.18
Safety (E)	3.0	0.0	3.0	0.0	3.0	0.0	4.00	0.14	2.00	0.16	2.00	0.18	—	—
Mischief (E)	0.0	0.0	0.0	0.0	0.0	0.0	2.00	0.37	1.00	0.32	1.00	0.32	—	—
Process (E)	1.5	2.0	2.0	1.0	2.0	1.0	1.25	0.54	0.11	0.74	1.34	0.25	0.15	0.71
Pretends (E)	0.0	1.0	0.5	2.3	0.5	1.3	1.85	0.40	1.29	0.26	0.67	0.42	1.29	0.26
Unconventional (E)	0.0	1.0	0.0	0.0	0.0	0.0	3.50	0.18	1.80	0.18	1.80	0.18	1.00	0.32
Social play (E)	2.0	2.0	1.0	2.0	1.0	1.0	2.68	0.27	2.67	0.10	1.80	0.18	0.20	0.66
Clowns (E)	0.0	0.0	0.0	0.0	0.0	0.0	1.00	0.61	0.00	1.00	1.00	0.32	1.00	0.32
Cues (E)	1.0	1.8	0.5	2.0	1.0	1.0	0.16	0.92	0.11	0.74	0.00	1.00	0.11	0.74
Engaged (I)	2.0	1.8	2.0	2.0	2.0	1.5	0.38	0.83	0.11	0.74	0.15	0.71	0.40	0.53
Social play (I)	1.0	1.0	1.0	2.0	1.0	1.0	0.30	0.86	0.15	0.71	0.34	0.57	0.00	1.00
Affect (I)	0.0	1.8	0.0	1.0	1.0	1.0	0.06	0.97	0.00	1.00	0.00	1.00	0.15	0.71
Object (I)	2.0	1.0	2.0	2.0	2.0	0.0	0.21	0.90	0.00	1.00	0.67	0.42	0.00	1.00
Engaged (S)	1.0	1.0	1.0	1.0	1.0	0.0	1.27	0.53	0.00	1.00	0.50	0.48	1.29	0.26
Modifies (S)	0.0	0.3	0.0	1.0	0.0	1.0	0.30	0.86	0.00	1.00	0.20	0.66	0.20	0.66
Social play (S)	0.0	1.0	0.0	2.0	1.0	1.0	0.30	0.86	0.15	0.71	0.34	0.57	0.00	1.00
Supports (S)	0.0	0.0	0.0	0.3	0.5	1.3	3.50	0.18	2.00	0.16	3.00	0.09	0.20	0.66
Initiate (S)	0.0	1.0	0.0	0.0	0.0	2.0	1.29	0.53	0.20	0.66	0.34	0.57	0.34	0.57
Shares (S)	0.0	1.5	1.0	0.3	1.0	1.3	2.63	0.27	1.00	0.32	1.80	0.18	1.80	0.18
Cues (S)	0.0	1.0	1.0	2.0	1.0	2.0	0.62	0.74	0.50	0.48	0.20	0.66	0.00	1.00
Responds (S)	0.5	1.0	0.0	2.0	1.0	1.8	3.00	0.23	0.67	0.42	2.67	0.10	1.29	0.26
Objects (S)	1.5	1.0	1.0	1.0	1.0	0.0	3.16	0.21	0.50	0.48	2.78	0.10	1.00	0.32
Transitions (S)	1.5	2.0	1.5	1.3	1.5	1.0	0.71	0.71	0.11	0.74	0.15	0.70	0.00	1.00

Notes: #Some ToP items were scored "not applicable" for some children; as a result, the following ToP items did not have enough data for analysis: Enters (S), Persists (I), Engages in playful mischief or teasing (S), Pretends (S), Creative (I), Negotiates (S), and Clowns or jokes (S); IQR = interquartile range; Friedman's two-way ANOVA; post hoc pairwise comparison tests. p: adjusted p value after post hoc Dunn-Bonferroni test; —: test did not run as the mean rank values were identical; $p < 0.05$.

Table 5: Effect sizes of ToP item scores.

ToP item	PICIHBI group Baseline to mid		PICIHBI group Baseline to post		PICIHBI group Mid to post		Comparison group Baseline to mid		Comparison group Baseline to post		Comparison group Mid to post	
	Z	r	Z	r	Z	r	Z	r	Z	r	Z	r
Engaged (E)	−2.81**	−0.57	−1.27	−0.26	1.71	0.35+	−0.12	−0.02	0.00	0.00	1.10	0.22+
Decides (E)	−2.43*	−0.50	0.00	0.00	2.64**	0.54+	−0.17	−0.04	0.00	0.00	1.61	0.33+
Safety (E)	0.00	0.00	0.00	0.00	0.00	0.00	0.00	0.00	0.00	0.00	0.00	0.00
Mischief (E)	0.00	0.00	0.00	0.00	0.00	0.00	0.00	0.00	0.00	0.00	0.00	0.00
Process (E)	−0.59	−0.12	1.12	0.23+	2.00*	0.41+	0.73	0.15+	1.57	0.32+	0.00	0.00
Pretends (E)	0.00	0.00	0.00	0.00	0.00	0.00	−1.72	−0.35	1.19	0.24+	0.00	0.00
Unconventional (E)	0.00	0.00	0.00	0.00	0.00	0.00	0.00	0.00	0.00	0.00	0.00	0.00
Social play (E)	−2.13*	−0.43	−2.46*	−0.50	0.00	0.00	−1.73	−0.35	−1.66	−0.34	0.00	0.00
Clowns (E)	0.00	0.00	0.00	0.00	0.00	0.00	0.00	0.00	0.00	0.00	0.00	0.00
Cues (E)	−0.54	−0.11	0.00	0.00	0.92	0.19+	−0.06	−0.01	0.00	0.00	0.31	0.06
Engaged (I)	−0.97	−0.20	−0.54	−0.11	0.00	0.00	0.00	0.00	0.00	0.00	0.00	0.00
Social play (I)	0.00	0.00	0.00	0.00	0.00	0.00	0.00	0.00	0.00	0.00	0.00	0.00
Affect (I)	−1.51	−0.31	−2.24*	−0.46	0.00	0.00	0.00	0.00	0.30	0.06	0.26	0.05
Object (I)	−1.08	−0.22	0.00	0.00	0.75	0.15+	0.00	0.00	0.00	0.00	0.00	0.00
Engaged (S)	0.00	0.00	0.00	0.00	0.00	0.00	0.00	0.00	0.00	0.00	0.00	0.00
Modifies (S)	0.00	0.00	0.00	0.00	0.00	0.00	0.00	0.00	0.00	0.00	0.00	0.00
Social play (S)	0.00	0.00	0.00	0.00	0.00	0.00	0.00	0.00	0.27	0.06	0.11	0.02
Supports (S)	0.00	0.00	0.00	0.00	0.00	0.00	0.00	0.00	1.63	0.33+	0.71	0.14+
Initiate (S)	0.96	0.20+	1.34	0.27+	0.00	0.00	0.00	0.00	0.00	0.00	0.00	0.00
Shares (S)	0.00	0.00	0.00	0.00	0.00	0.00	0.28	0.08	1.34	0.27*	0.00	0.00
Cues (S)	0.00	0.00	0.63	0.13+	0.83	0.17+	0.58	0.12+	0.71	0.14+	0.00	0.00
Responds (S)	0.51	−0.10	1.00	0.20+	0.00	0.00	−0.97	−0.20	1.63	0.33+	0.34	0.07
Objects (S)	0.00	0.00	0.00	0.00	0.00	0.00	−0.72	−0.15	−1.35	−0.28	0.00	0.00
Transitions (S)	0.00	0.00	0.00	0.00	0.00	0.00	0.00	0.00	0.00	0.00	0.00	0.00

Notes: The r-effect size was used to calculate the effect sizes for nonparametric data. In this calculation, the effect size (i.e., r) is obtained by dividing the Wilcoxon Z score by the square root of the sample size; $r = Z/\sqrt{24}$. Cohen's guidelines for r are small effect ≥ 0.1, medium effect ≥ 0.3, or large effect ≥ 0.5; +: small, medium, and large effect sizes; $^{*}p < 0.05$, $^{**}p < 0.01$, $^{***}p < 0.001$.

a larger more representative sample and if children's play is significantly lower than control children without HIV. This is an important avenue of research to explore, as a high percentage of caregivers within this study considered their children's play skills to be on par with or better than those of their peers. Once established, this will allow for further adaptation and refinement of the PICIHBI to better address the specific play needs of children with HIV.

A second key finding from this study was that the PICIHBI did not significantly improve the play skills of children with HIV and was not significantly more effective than the comparison conventional one-on-one occupational therapy intervention. We postulate that there are likely many factors that have impacted the feasibility and therefore effectiveness of the PICIHBI. Firstly, the loss of participants through attrition and lack of attendance suggest that there are significant barriers that prohibit the majority of families from engaging in this intervention. These findings applied to both the PICIHBI and comparison intervention. The loss of power within this study may have prevented the detection of differences between groups, if there were in fact any differences to be detected. This study nonetheless demonstrated that the PICIHBI can achieve similar results to one-on-one conventional therapy which enables more efficient use of occupational therapists' time.

A major factor may have been the high levels of unemployment within both intervention groups. The difficulties associated with high unemployment and challenging socioeconomic circumstances were demonstrated within this study with participants reporting missing appointments due to lack of transport money. Furthermore, caregivers of children with HIV experience high levels of stress and require emotional support due to the impact of HIV on family life [10, 14]. Concerns related to basic survival will overshadow the need to further understand child development, and play engagement may not be deemed a priority [15]. These challenges of time and socioeconomic constraints were evident in this study, and while attempts were made to reduce the burden on caregivers by scheduling appointments on the same day as other appointments and reimbursement of transport costs, they did not prove adequate. These findings are consistent with another study based in South Africa that also reported a high attrition rate, despite similar attempts to ease the burden of clinic attendance [10]. These findings highlight the challenges of access to early childhood intervention programs for families of children with HIV living in low socioeconomic contexts. It signifies the critical importance of providing community outreach services which lessen the burden for attendance on caregivers. The use of outreach, community-based interventions may offer the best chance for early intervention and sustained attendance.

Another major factor that may have influenced participation in the study became evident in participants' demographic data, which indicated a perception amongst most caregivers that their children's play, development, and learning were at an equivalent or higher level to those of their peers. Further, caregivers did not appear well informed about their children's concomitant diagnoses. This perception and lack of understanding may have impacted caregiver "buy-in" to the interventions, likely contributing to having missed appointments. Maternal play beliefs have a profound influence on the types of play activities and the frequency of their child's play engagement [37]. In the context of this study, education of caregivers at clinic check-ups was required prior to offering intervention. A greater understanding regarding their child's medical conditions and developmental milestones may have altered caregiver perceptions of their child's overall developmental status and needs and therefore increased motivation to attend intervention sessions.

A finding of note for the design and delivery of interventions was issues around the participant's adherence to the intervention protocol. It was noted that children did not always attend the clinic for intervention sessions with the same caregiver, usually due to work commitments. This was particularly pertinent for the PICIHBI intervention which relied on the main caregiver attending all sessions. The modelling provided by the therapist during the experiential part of the sessions was critical to improving the play behaviours and playfulness of children. Future interventions should consider ways to consistently engage the same caregiver in intervention sessions or have a family-based approach, so information and skills are passed on to other family members, including extended family members, in an easy and understandable way. Again, primary caregivers may engage more easily with interventions provided closer to home through community clinics, with flexible appointment scheduling that is compatible with other work and family commitments.

Another important aspect to consider in future studies is the intervention dosage. The findings show that very few families recruited to the study received the intended dosage of both interventions studied. Increasing intervention dosage for these families is challenging against the context of aforementioned difficulties associated with environmental stressors. Behavioural learning research indicates little outcome from monthly learning sessions at the acquisition stage of learning. This could also explain the low change in playfulness scores. The exact solution to this challenge is unclear, but part of the solution should involve considering a location more convenient to the family, such as home or community settings.

The findings from this study support recommendations of the importance of providing long-term early childhood intervention programs for children with HIV living in challenging socioeconomic circumstances in South Africa [10, 14, 38, 39]. Preparing children for schooling through an early childhood play-based intervention will provide children with more opportunity to practice, learn, and develop through play [3, 23, 32]. As play is deemed the main occupation of childhood and described as a determinant of health and well-being [3], the play needs of children with HIV should be brought to the forefront in this area of research.

Consideration and attention to the specific elements of playfulness that are challenging for children with HIV could guide future interventions, and improvements in some ToP items could guide therapists to focus on certain playfulness skills, before moving to more advanced skills.

A challenge for this area of research will always be the retention of the sample when it demands high levels of attendance and commitment from participants with socioeconomic challenges and who are often experiencing high levels of stress.

4.1. Limitations. The high levels of attrition resulted in a small sample size, thus limiting the generalisability of the results. The loss of power in the study also potentially impacted the detection of differences between the two intervention groups. Even though it is unlikely, there is a possibility that the cluster randomization of two siblings to the same group may have had an effect on the analysis in a sample of this size. Multiple comparisons were made during data analysis, and we opted to adjust the *p* values using the post hoc Dunn-Bonferroni test. Such an adjustment may be too conservative in the case of this study and may have impacted the ability to detect significant differences. Also, baseline scores were not accounted for in the nonparametric tests, and this too may have impacted on the findings.

Furthermore, language barriers impacted the manner in which the therapists were able to engage with caregivers and children during both interventions. Therapists had to rely heavily on translators to convey information to caregivers and children, leaving open the potential for critical information to be lost.

While evaluating the effectiveness of the PICIHBI in relation to traditional occupational therapy was not a primary aim of this study, future studies of effectiveness might consider including a waitlisted control group to determine whether the PICIHBI is more effective than no intervention. Also, the PICIHBI was implemented in this study by a single therapist who was familiar with the intervention approach.

Only indoor play was filmed within this study. Concerns with safety appear to limit freedom and time spent engaging in outdoor play in most urban-based South African communities. A difference in playfulness levels may have been observed if the study was extended to observe outdoor play. Attempts were made for adequate space, toys, and materials available to the children; nonetheless, it was an unnatural play environment due to the observers and researchers filming the play. While the research assistant remained at a distance, the recording process may have made some children feel uncomfortable, thus negatively impacting on their play behaviours.

5. Conclusions

This study described the playfulness levels of 24 children with HIV and PHE from challenging socioeconomic contexts attending a clinic within South Africa. It is the first study to establish that children with HIV on HAART from low socioeconomic areas demonstrate low levels of playfulness, indicating that these children are at risk of occupational deprivation as they do not engage in play with ease. Though whether these challenges are unique to the population of children with HIV in this study or all children from the same low socioeconomic areas is unknown. Children with HIV obtained the lowest possible score on almost 40% of ToP items, demonstrating the need for play-focused early interventions. No significant differences were found between the PICIHBI and one-on-one conventional groups at baseline, mid-, and postassessments. Considerations of factors that reduce barriers to attendance and improve caregivers' access to intervention, such as community-based service delivery, are critical and could further contribute to improved playfulness levels for children with HIV and minimise developmental disruption for children.

Conflicts of Interest

The authors declare that there is no conflict of interest regarding the publication of this paper.

Acknowledgments

The authors would like to thank the children and their families who participated in this research. We would also like to thank Prof. Anita Bundy for her assistance with the use of the Test of Playfulness, Dr. Richard Parsons for his guidance with statistical analysis, and Pam Gretschel, Robyn Meissner, Jessica Ferguson, Caraleigh Otto, and Jesse Kum who all formed part of the larger research study and intervention planning process. This manuscript is based on the master's thesis written by Anande Uys [40].

References

[1] S. Rodger and J. Ziviani, "Play-based occupational therapy," *International Journal of Disability, Development and Education*, vol. 46, no. 3, pp. 337–365, 1999.

[2] B. Sutton-Smith, "Play theory: a personal journey and new thoughts," *American Journal of Play*, vol. 1, no. 1, pp. 80–123, 2008.

[3] L. D. Parham, "Play and occupational therapy," in *Play in Occupational Therapy for Children*, L. D. Parham and L. Fazio, Eds., pp. 3–39, Elsevier, St. Louis, MO, USA, 2nd edition, 2008.

[4] G. Skard and A. C. Bundy, "Test of playfulness," in *Play in Occupational Therapy for Children*, L. D. Parham and L. Fazio, Eds., pp. 71–93, Elsevier, St. Louis, MO, USA, 2nd edition, 2008.

[5] B. Sutton-Smith, *The Ambiguity of Play*, Harvard University Press, Cambridge, MA, USA, 1997.

[6] G. Gordon, "Well played: the origins and future of playfulness," *American Journal of Play*, vol. 6, no. 2, p. 234, 2014.

[7] R. J. Meissner, J. Ferguson, C. Otto, P. Gretschel, and E. Ramugondo, "A play-informed, caregiver-implemented, home-based intervention for HIV-positive children and their

families living in low-income conditions in South Africa," *World Federation of Occupational Therapists Bulletin*, vol. 73, no. 2, pp. 83–87, 2017.

[8] L. Sherr, N. Croome, K. Parra Castaneda, K. Bradshaw, and R. Herrero Romero, "Developmental challenges in HIV infected children—an updated systematic review," *Children and Youth Services Review*, vol. 45, pp. 74–89, 2014.

[9] C. A. Chiriboga, S. Fleishman, S. Champion, L. Gaye-Robinson, and E. J. Abrams, "Incidence and prevalence of HIV encephalopathy in children with HIV infection receiving highly active anti-retroviral therapy (HAART)," *The Journal of Pediatrics*, vol. 146, no. 3, pp. 402–407, 2005.

[10] N. Whitehead, J. Potterton, and A. Coovadia, "The neurodevelopment of HIV-infected infants on HAART compared to HIV-exposed but uninfected infants," *AIDS Care*, vol. 26, no. 4, pp. 497–504, 2014.

[11] S. Skeen, M. Tomlinson, A. Macedo, A. Miltz, N. Croome, and L. Sherr, "Child development in HIV-positive and HIV-affected children in South Africa and Malawi—what role for community organisations?," *Children and Youth Services Review*, vol. 45, pp. 90–97, 2014.

[12] Statistics South Africa, "Mid-Year estimates 2016," 2016, http://www.statssa.gov.za/?p=8176.

[13] UNAIDS, "HIV and AIDS estimates," 2015, http://www.unaids.org/en/regionscountries/countries/southafrica.

[14] G. Ferguson and J. Jelsma, "The prevalence of motor delay among HIV infected children living in Cape Town, South Africa," *International Journal of Rehabilitation Research*, vol. 32, no. 2, pp. 108–114, 2009.

[15] K. R. Ginsburg, and the Committee on Communications, and and the Committee on Psychosocial Aspects of Child and Family Health, "The importance of play in promoting healthy child development and maintaining strong parent-child bonds," *Pediatrics*, vol. 119, no. 1, pp. 182–191, 2007.

[16] D. G. Singer, J. L. Singer, H. D'Agnostino, and R. DeLong, "Children's pastimes and play in sixteen nations: is free-play declining?," *American Journal of Play*, vol. 1, no. 3, pp. 283–312, 2009.

[17] B. David, "The shift from outdoor to indoor play in the French Caribbean island of Guadeloupe: implications for childhood development," *Review of Human Factor Studies*, vol. 21, no. 1, 2015.

[18] M. Bartie, A. Dunnell, J. Kaplan et al., "The play experiences of preschool children from a low-socio-economic rural community in Worcester, South Africa," *Occupational Therapy International*, vol. 23, no. 2, 102 pages, 2016.

[19] K. F. Schulz, D. G. Altman, D. Moher, and the CONSORT Group, "CONSORT 2010 statement: updated guidelines for reporting parallel group randomised trials," *BMC Medicine*, vol. 8, no. 1, 2010.

[20] G. Urbaniak and S. Plous, *Research Randomizer (Version 4.0) [Computer Software]*, 2013, http://www.randomizer.org/.

[21] M. Haahr, "Random Sequence Generator," February 2009, https://www.random.org/sequences.

[22] D. Cameron, M. Leslie, R. Teplicky et al., "The clinical utility of the test of playfulness," *Canadian Journal of Occupational Therapy*, vol. 68, no. 2, pp. 104–111, 2001.

[23] A. C. Bundy, L. Nelson, M. Metzger, and K. Bingaman, "Validity and reliability of a test of playfulness," *The Occupational Therapy Journal of Research*, vol. 21, no. 4, pp. 276–292, 2001.

[24] S. Wilkes-Gillan, A. Bundy, R. Cordier, M. Lincoln, and Y.-W. Chen, "A randomised controlled trial of a play-based intervention to improve the social play skills of children with attention deficit hyperactivity disorder (ADHD)," *PLoS One*, vol. 11, no. 8, article e0160558, 2016.

[25] S. Wilkes, R. Cordier, A. Bundy, K. Docking, and N. Munro, "A play-based intervention for children with ADHD: a pilot study," *Australian Occupational Therapy Journal*, vol. 58, no. 4, pp. 231–240, 2011.

[26] A. M. Okimoto, A. Bundy, and J. Hanzlik, "Playfulness in children with and without disability: measurement and intervention," *The American Journal of Occupational Therapy*, vol. 54, no. 1, pp. 73–82, 2000.

[27] A. C. Bundy, T. Luckett, G. A. Naughton et al., "Playful interaction: occupational therapy for all children on the school playground," *The American Journal of Occupational Therapy*, vol. 62, no. 5, pp. 522–527, 2008.

[28] J. Cohen, *Statistical Power Analysis for the Behavioural Sciences*, Lawrence Earlbaum Associates, Hillsdale, NJ, USA, 2nd edition, 1988.

[29] R. Cordier, A. Bundy, C. Hocking, and S. Einfeld, "A model for play-based intervention for children with ADHD," *Australian Occupational Therapy Journal*, vol. 56, no. 5, pp. 332–340, 2009.

[30] K. Stagnitti, "Pretend play assessment," in *Play as Therapy: Assessment and Therapeutic Interventions*, K. Stagnitti and R. Cooper, Eds., pp. 87–101, Jessica Kingsley Publishers, London, UK, 2009.

[31] P. A. Mortenson and S. R. Harris, "Playfulness in children with traumatic brain injury: a preliminary study," *Physical & Occupational Therapy in Pediatrics*, vol. 26, no. 1-2, pp. 181–198, 2006.

[32] J. O'Brien, P. Coker, R. Lynn et al., "The impact of occupational therapy on a child's playfulness," *Occupational Therapy In Health Care*, vol. 12, no. 2-3, pp. 39–51, 2000.

[33] J. L. Pearton, E. Ramugondo, L. Cloete, and R. Cordier, "Playfulness and prenatal alcohol exposure: a comparative study," *Australian Occupational Therapy Journal*, vol. 61, no. 4, pp. 259–267, 2014.

[34] N. Skaines, S. Rodger, and A. Bundy, "Playfulness in children with autistic disorder and their typically developing peers," *British Journal of Occupational Therapy*, vol. 69, no. 11, pp. 505–512, 2006.

[35] S. Wilkes-Gillan, A. Bundy, R. Cordier, and M. Lincoln, "Evaluation of a pilot parent-delivered play-based intervention for children with attention deficit hyperactivity disorder," *The American Journal of Occupational Therapy*, vol. 68, no. 6, pp. 700–709, 2014.

[36] R. Cordier, A. Bundy, C. Hocking, and S. Einfeld, "Empathy in the play of children with attention deficit hyperactivity disorder," *OTJR: Occupation, Participation, Health*, vol. 30, no. 3, pp. 122–132, 2010.

[37] K. R. Fisher, K. Hirsh-Pasek, R. M. Golinkoff, and S. G. Gryfe, "Conceptual split? Parents' and experts' perceptions of play in the 21st century," *Journal of Applied Developmental Psychology*, vol. 29, no. 4, pp. 305–316, 2008.

[38] J. Potterton, N. Hilburn, and R. Strehlau, "Developmental status of preschool children receiving cART: a descriptive cohort study," *Child: Care, Health and Development*, vol. 42, no. 3, pp. 410–414, 2016.

4

Cognitive Rehabilitation of Adaptive Behavior in Children with Neurodevelopmental Disorders

Si-nae Ahn[1] **and Sujin Hwang**[2]

[1]*Department of Occupational Therapy, Cheongju University, 298 Daesung-ro, Cheongju-si, Republic of Korea*
[2]*Deparment of Physical Therapy, Division of Health Science, Baekseok University, 76 Munam-ro, Dongnam-gu, Cheonan-si, Chungnam, Republic of Korea*

Correspondence should be addressed to Sujin Hwang; sujin928@gmail.com

Academic Editor: Lynette Mackenzie

Objectives. Negative behavioral problems often occur following the onset of neurodevelopmental disorders and have an overall impact on the affected children, specifically in terms of their social developmental level. In children, social development behavior has been shown to spontaneously mature over time with the cognitive therapy intervention effects. This study performed a meta-analysis to provide a statistical synopsis of the available evidence of social development behavioral changes following cognitive therapy in children with neurodevelopmental disorders. *Methods.* Data was collected from two online search engines, including EBSCOhost and PubMed, from January 1, 2006, to August 31, 2016, using the terms "cognition," "cognitive function," and "disease including neurodevelopmental disorder with DSM-5." Two assessors searched the literature using independent inclusion criteria and evaluated the quality of results using the Jadad score. Six articles were chosen using the Comprehensive Meta-Analysis program (version 2.0). *Results.* Six articles reporting randomized controlled trial studies were included. The effective scores for improving adaptive behavior following cognitive therapy in children with neurodevelopmental disorder were 0.64. The effective score of adaptive behavior was significant in this study ($p < 0.05$). The results showed no significant statistical heterogeneity and publication bias. *Conclusions.* The findings of the meta-analysis suggest that cognitive interventions are effective at improving adaptive behavior associated with neurodevelopmental disorders.

1. Introduction

Neurodevelopmental disorders refer to developmental, cognitive function, motor function, verbal communication, social skill, and behavioral disorders. The growth and development of the central nervous system is affected by these disorders. The American Psychiatric Association categorizes ten neurodevelopmental disorders: intellectual disabilities, global developmental delay, communication disorders, autism spectrum disorder, attention-deficit/hyperactivity disorder, specific learning disorders, developmental coordination disorders, stereotypical movement disorders, tic disorders, and Tourette's syndrome [1].

Children affected by neurodevelopmental disorders often face difficulties in undergoing normal cognitive development, because of the occurrence of cognitive problems from an early stage of development [2]. As a result, affected children fail to achieve the expected developmental progress for their respective developmental ages. Neurodevelopmental disorders are also associated with poor social function and various other negative behavior aspects in school-age and adolescent children [3, 4]. Specifically, neurodevelopmental disorders are characterized by difficulties with social communication and interaction across contexts, as well as restricted and repetitive patterns of behavior aspects [5, 6].

There has been a marked increase in cognitive interventions that are aimed at improving the symptoms or features of neurodevelopmental disorders. However, there is no evidence to support the use of such cognitive therapies to treat symptoms of behavioral abnormalities associated with neurodevelopmental disorders. Several articles conclude that early and intensive interventions can lead to improvements in adaptive and communicative behaviors, as well as in social skills [7, 8].

Children with a neurodevelopmental disorder who receive occupational therapy during early childhood can perform a variety of tasks according to their respective cognitive abilities [9–11]. These studies have shown that children with neurodevelopmental disorders have a good prognosis with regard to their ability to participate in tasks when early cognitive treatments are received early. Specifically, cognitive therapy at the preschool level was found to improve the prognosis of behavioral outcomes in children with neurodevelopmental disorders [9].

According to Lucas et al., some occupational therapy interventions with a task-oriented framework are shown to likely improve overall motor outcomes in children with neurodevelopmental disorders but overall results are limited because of the low quality of available evidence [12]. Weston et al. studied meta-analytic and systematic appraisal of the literature investigating the effectiveness of cognitive behavioral therapy (CBT) when used with individuals who have autism spectrum disorder (ASD). Their results demonstrate that the CBT is an empirically validated treatment for use with people who have ASDs [13].

As mentioned previously, few studies have examined the effectiveness of certain types of cognitive interventions with neurodevelopmental disorders (Wright et al., 2013). Additionally, there is insufficient evidence to support the beneficial effects of cognitive therapy on individuals with neurodevelopment disorders, including disorders such as intellectual disabilities, global developmental delay (GDD), communication disorders, ASD, attention-deficit/hyperactivity disorder (ADHD), specific learning disorders, and developmental coordination disorder (DCD).

Adaptive behavior is viewed as what an individual does to effectively meet social/cultural standards of personal independence and social responsibility. Social skills represent behaviors which, in specific situations, predict important social outcomes for children and youth [14]. Adaptive behaviors are an essential part of occupational therapy in facilitating the development of growing children with neurodevelopmental disorders [14]. Therefore, there is a need to understand the best therapeutic method to support the utilization of adaptive behavioral strategies.

Meta-analysis is needed to determine whether or not cognitive therapy to positively change adaptive behavior was useful in children with neurodevelopmental disorders. Therefore, we conducted a comprehensive meta-analysis of the literature, which is aimed at investigating the effectiveness of cognitive therapy as a part of a comprehensive rehabilitation program focused on improving functional performance in individuals with neurodevelopmental disorders.

2. Method

2.1. Search Strategy. The search was performed in a stepwise manner between January 1, 2006, and August 31, 2016. A comprehensive search of electronic databases was completed on the following electronic sources using EBSCOhost and PubMed. The search keywords used were "disease including neurodevelopmental disorder with DSM-5" AND "cognition," and "disease including neurodevelopmental disorder with DSM-5" AND "cognitive function." The final search expression was as follows: "cognition" AND "Intellectual Disability," "cognitive function" AND "Intellectual Disability," "cognition" AND "Intellectual Developmental Disorder," "cognitive function" AND "Intellectual Developmental Disorder," "cognition" AND "Global Developmental Delay," "cognitive function" AND "Global Developmental Delay," "cognition" AND "Autism Spectrum Disorder," "cognitive function" AND "Autism Spectrum Disorder," "cognition" AND "Attention Deficit Hyperactivity Disorder," "cognitive function" AND "Attention Deficit Hyperactivity Disorder," "cognition" AND "Developmental Coordination Disorder," "cognitive function" AND "Developmental Coordination Disorder," "cognition" AND "Stereotypic Movement Disorder," "cognitive function" AND "Stereotypic Movement Disorder," "cognition" AND "Tic Disorders," "cognitive function" AND "Tic Disorders," "cognition" AND "Tourette Disorder," "cognitive function" AND "Tourette Disorder."

2.2. Filtering Procedure and Study Selection. This study searched for original articles that were published in academic journals, written in English, and met our inclusion and exclusion criteria. Using this method, a total of 3115 articles were identified in this study. Since it was not possible to automatically exclude animal trials in this search engine, this was done by hand. Abstracts of the remaining publications were scrutinized for eligibility by two independent assessors (i.e., the author Ahn and Hwang), using the inclusion criteria and exclusion criteria described below. Thus, a total of 80 articles were included in the full-text review by both assessors. The final list consisted of 6 studies (Figure 1).

2.3. Inclusion Criteria and Exclusion Criteria. First, titles and abstracts of studies were scanned for eligibility according to the following inclusion criteria: (a) population age range (i.e., children up to school-going ages under 13 years of age), (b) type of study design (i.e., randomized controlled trial), (c) targeting for neurodevelopmental disorder, (d) assessments of adaptive behavior, and (e) language in which article was written (English).

Secondly, titles and abstracts of studies were excluded based on the following criteria: (a) using medication treatment, (b) using injection, and (c) using acupuncture. Subsequently, the abstracts of the remaining subset were reviewed further.

2.4. Data Extraction. The following information was extracted: year of publication, first author, period, number of children with neurodevelopmental disorder in each group, diagnosis of a neurodevelopmental disorder, age of subjects enrolled, types of cognitive function intervention, and assessment tools of adaptive behavior. Data were extracted from eligible studies by two investigators acting independently,

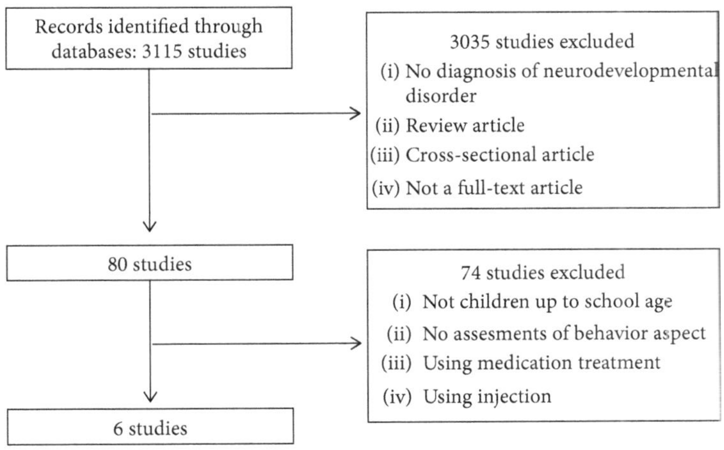

Figure 1: Study process.

and any disagreement was resolved by consulting with two reviewers (Ahn and Hwang).

2.5. Data Analysis. The Jadad score was used for analyzing the methodological quality of the meta-analysis and in evaluating and summarizing the 6 studies. Assessment of study quality was performed independently by two reviewers according to the Jadad scale [15]. The Jadad score is needed to ascertain the quality of clinical trials by using blind raters' assessment of the potential bias into the meta-analyses and other systematic reviews and peer review processes. The Jadad score evaluated methodologic quality by using a 5 score. The scores ranged from 0 to 5, based on randomization, blinding, allocation concealment, withdrawals, and dropouts. Studies with randomized controlled trials were considered to be of high quality if the methodological score was 3–5 points and of low quality if the methodological score was less than 3 points [15, 16].

To conduct a quantitative meta-analysis, this study performed calculations by computing the standardized difference of mean scores. This study completed all analyses using the Comprehensive Meta-Analysis program [17]. Effect size was calculated by the ratio of the mean difference between the experimental and control groups divided by the standard deviation of the control group. For example, in an evaluation with a treatment group and control group, the effect size is the difference in means between the two groups divided by the standard deviation of the control group. The effect size for cognitive therapy in children with neurodevelopmental disorder was determined using a standardized mean difference and 95% confidence intervals (CI) in a fixed-effect model, which indicates the mean improvement in standard scores of the experimental group relative to the control group. To estimate the effect size in this meta-analysis, we performed t-tests and F tests and calculated the means and standard deviations and exact p values.

In calculating the size of the overall effect, the sign of effect was deemed to be positive (+) when the experimental group demonstrated better effects than the control group following cognitive therapy in children with neurodevelopmental disorder and negative (−) if the converse was true. By convention, the effect size of the adaptive behavior following cognitive therapy was interpreted as large if the effect size was greater than 0.8, moderate if it was above 0.5, and small if it was above 0.2 [18]. In addition to estimating the effect size in numerical order, a forest plot was used to visually depict the estimated value of the studies' handling effect and the confidence interval of the effect size.

3. Results

3.1. General Characteristics of the Studies. The general characteristics of the six studies included in the meta-analysis are as follows. All of them were controlled trials. The methodologic quality of the primary data was assessed by using the Jadad score. This study found that 6 studies ranged from scores between 3 and 5, out of the maximum score of 5 points. The total number of participants in the studies was 544. The number of participants in each study ranged from 30 to 302. Participants in four of the studies were affected by ASD [19–22]; those in one study were diagnosed with GDD [23], and those in another singular study were diagnosed with ADHD [24]. As can be seen in Table 1, intervention of cognitive function in each of the studies included a comprehensive autism program [22], SENSE Theatre intervention [19], interpersonal synchrony [21], early start Denver model intervention [20], institutional-based therapy program [23], and visuospatial working memory training [24].

All studies used same assessment tools to evaluate adaptive behavior: Vineland Adaptive Behavior Scales [20, 22], Adaptive Behavior Assessment System [19], socially engaged imitation [21], Comprehensive Developmental Inventory for Infants and Toddlers [23], and Behavior Rating Inventory of Executive Function [24] for assessing behavior function (Table 1).

3.2. Effects of Cognitive Therapy on Adaptive Behavior. The effect sizes in this meta-analysis of studies investigating the efficacy of cognitive therapy in improving adaptive behavior

Table 1: Characteristic of included studies.

Study	Design	Jadad score	Participants	Intervention: Intervention/groups	Intervention: Session/time	Outcome measure	Outcome
Young et al. [22]	RCT	4	3–5-year-old students with autism spectrum disorder ($n = 302$)	(i) Comprehensive autism program ($n = 178$) (ii) Business as usual public schools ($n = 124$)	1 day per month/for 6 months	Vineland Adaptive Behavior Scales	Treatment effects were moderated by severity of ASD.
Corbett et al. [19]	RCT	3	8–14 years with autism spectrum disorder ($n = 30$)	(i) SENSE Theatre intervention ($n = 17$) (ii) Control ($n = 13$)	4 hours/10 sessions	Adaptive Behavior Assessment System	The theatre-based intervention was provided initial support for the efficacy.
Landa et al. [21]	RCT	3	Toddlers with autism spectrum disorder ($n = 48$)	(i) Interpersonal synchrony ($n = 24$) (ii) Noninterpersonal synchrony ($n = 24$)	2.5 hours per day/four days per week	Communication and Symbolic Behavior Scales Developmental Profile	A significant treatment effect was found for socially engaged imitation in the interpersonal synchrony group.
Dawson et al. [20]	RCT	3	18–30-month-old children with autism spectrum disorder ($n = 48$)	(i) Early start Denver model intervention group ($n = 24$) (ii) Assess-and-monitor group ($n = 23$)	2-hour sessions/twice per day/5 days per week/2 years	Vineland Adaptive Behavior Scales	The intervention for toddlers with ASD is for improving cognitive and adaptive behavior and reducing severity of ASD diagnosis.
Tang et al. [23]	RCT	3	Infants and toddlers with motor or global developmental delay ($n = 70$)	(i) Institutional-based therapy program (ITP) ($n = 35$) (ii) ITP plus a structured home activity program (HAPs) ($n = 35$)	(i) ITP for 45 minutes per session/12 weeks (ii) ITP 30 minutes with 15 minutes of HAPs per session/12 weeks	Comprehensive Developmental Inventory for Infants and Toddlers	Early intervention programs are helpful for these children.
van Dongen-Boomsma et al. [24]	RCT	5	5–7-year-old children with attention-deficit/hyperactivity disorder	(i) Visuospatial working memory group ($n = 26$) (ii) placebo group ($n = 21$)	15 minutes/5 days a week/25 sessions	Behavior Rating Inventory of Executive Function	No significant treatment effect on any of the primary or other secondary outcome measurements was found.

Study name	Statistics for each study						
	Std diff In means	Standard Error	Variance	Lower Limit	Upper Limit	Z value	p value
Young et al. (2016)	0.845	0.272	0.074	0.311	1.379	3.103	0.002
Corbelt al. (2016)	0.794	0.382	0.146	0.044	1.543	2.075	0.038
Landa et al. (2011)	0.470	0.293	0.086	−0.103	1.044	1.608	0.108
Dawson et al. (2010)	0.785	0.303	0.092	0.191	1.378	2.592	0.010
Tang et al. (2011)	0.822	0.249	0.062	0.334	1.310	3.303	0.001
van Dongen-Boomsma et al. (2014)	0.070	0.293	0.086	−0.505	0.645	0.238	0.812
	0.636	0.119	0.014	0.403	0.869	5.348	0.000

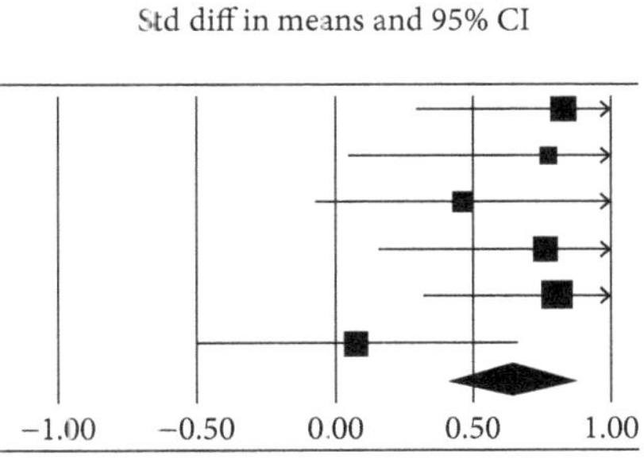

Figure 2: Forest plot showing individual effect sizes.

Table 2: Heterogeneity.

Model	Effect size	p value	Q value	p value
Fixed	0.64	0.00	5.60	0.35
Random	0.64	0.00		

ranged from −0.50 to 1.54. The overall effect size of 0.64 can be interpreted as moderate with a 95% CI (0.40, 0.87) ($p < 0.05$) (Figure 2).

3.3. Statistical Heterogeneity Test. The Cochran's Q value of 5.60 ($p = 0.35$) in our test of statistical heterogeneity indicates no significant heterogeneity. Both the fixed-effects and random-effects models showed an effect size of 0.64, providing further evidence of the lack of statistical heterogeneity among the studies included in the present meta-analysis (Table 2).

3.4. Publication Bias. Analysis of the funnel plot showed the six values to be distributed in every section, taking an asymmetric funnel shape, with more values falling on the right-hand side of the mean effect size plot. As a result, the results were considered reliable, as no significant publication bias was found (Figure 3).

4. Discussion

The current meta-analysis is aimed at providing a statistical synthesis of the effect on available evidence of adaptive behavior changed following cognitive therapy in children with a neurodevelopmental disorder. The overall effect size of applying cognitive therapy to address adaptive behavior with children with a neurodevelopmental disorder was found to be 0.64, a statistically significant result indicating that cognitive therapy has a moderate effect on improving adaptive behavior. No significant heterogeneity or publication bias was identified. It had adequate effect size for each study included in this meta-analysis, but the effect size by Liu et al. [25] is far from being close to an overall effect size 0.64. It may also have affected the results of a moderate effect size because few studies have utilized meta-analysis.

Based on the results of this research, it is proposed that an effective method of conducting cognitive therapy to improve adaptive behavior be developed. This meta-analysis is, so far, the first attempt to examine the empirical evidence regarding the effectiveness of cognitive therapy for adaptive behavior. The effect size of adaptive behavior with intervention of cognitive therapy found in the present investigation is larger than expected.

The results of the meta-analysis indicate that intervention of cognitive function is associated with a medium effect size, when compared with results found in the meta-analysis of the effectiveness of augmented gross motor performance in children with neurodevelopmental disorders [12]. Therefore, cognitive therapy can be used as a method of acquiring a suitable adaptive behavior to be used along with occupational therapy in a rehabilitative setting. Our research used the selected studies used in cognitive therapy to improve adaptive behavior. We are cautiously asserting that cognitive therapy is more effective than therapy of motor performance alone to improve adaptive behavior.

Intervention of cognitive function in each of the studies included a comprehensive autism program, which is used to teach communication and social behavior skills [22]. In one study, a theatre intervention was used to improve social relationships and adaptive behaviors through video modeling and concentration training by having participants visually trace from an opposite screen [19]. Interpersonal synchrony is a supplementary curriculum for social initiation, and socially synchronized engagement in toddlers is overlaid on an existing group-based comprehensive intervention [20, 21, 23, 24].

The main limitation of this meta-analysis is that many studies did not meet the inclusion criteria and therefore were excluded from the final analysis. The findings of this study have limited generalizability. Nevertheless, it has been suggested that the interpretation of the results of the meta-analysis may be valid when it is based on a data set of at least 5 studies [26]. In addition, several factors may also affect the efficacy of adaptive behavior, including such individual characteristics as types of disease, degree of cognitive and physical function, and the method of cognitive therapy. This first meta-analysis suggests that cognitive therapy improves adaptive behavior in children with neurodevelopmental disorders. A moderate effect size of cognitive therapy was identified as improving adaptive behavior in children with neurodevelopmental disorders. The results

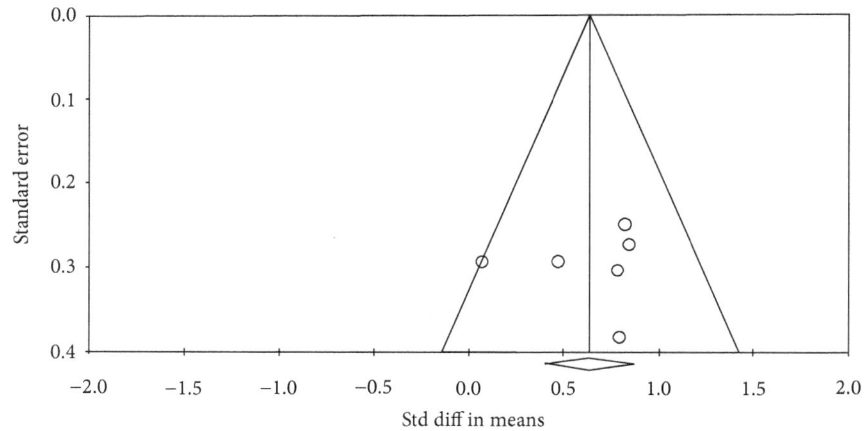

FIGURE 3: Funnel plot for publication.

suggest that cognitive therapy is an effective clinical intervention that occupational therapists can use for children with neurodevelopmental disorders.

Conflicts of Interest

The authors declare no conflict of interest.

References

[1] American Psychiatric Association, *Diagnostic and Statistical Manual of Mental Disorders*, American Psychiatric Association, Washington, DC, USA, 2013.

[2] E. G. Spratt, S. L. Friedenberg, C. C. Swenson et al., "The effects of early neglect on cognitive, language, and behavioral functioning in childhood," *Psychology*, vol. 3, no. 2, pp. 175–182, 2012.

[3] R. A. Barkley, K. R. Murphy, T. O'Connell, D. Anderson, and D. F. Connor, "Effects of two doses of alcohol on simulator driving performance in adults with attention-deficit/hyperactivity disorder," *Neuropsychology*, vol. 20, no. 1, pp. 77–87, 2006.

[4] K. P. Feder and A. Majnemer, "Handwriting development, competency, and intervention," *Developmental Medicine & Child Neurology*, vol. 49, no. 4, pp. 312–317, 2007.

[5] F. R. Volkmar, R. Paul, A. Klin, and D. J. Cohen, *Handbook of Autism and Pervasive Developmental Disorders, Diagnosis, Development, Neurobiology, and Behavior*, vol. 1, John Wiley & Sons, Hoboken, NJ, USA, 2005.

[6] L. D. Wiggins, S. E. Levy, J. Daniels et al., "Autism spectrum disorder symptoms among children enrolled in the Study to Explore Early Development (SEED)," *Journal of Autism and Developmental Disorders*, vol. 45, no. 10, pp. 3183–3194, 2015.

[7] B. Reichow, E. E. Barton, B. A. Boyd, and K. Hume, "Early intensive behavioral intervention (EIBI) for young children with autism spectrum disorders (ASD)," *Cochrane Database of Systematic Reviews*, no. 10, article CD009260, 2012.

[8] L. W. Williams, J. L. Matson, J. Jang, J. S. Beighley, R. D. Rieske, and H. L. Adams, "Challenging behaviors in toddlers diagnosed with autism spectrum disorders with the *DSM-IV-TR* and the proposed *DSM-5* criteria," *Research in Autism Spectrum Disorders*, vol. 7, no. 8, pp. 966–972, 2013.

[9] C. S. H. Aarnoudse-Moens, N. Weisglas-Kuperus, J. B. van Goudoever, and J. Oosterlaan, "Meta-analysis of neurobehavioral outcomes in very preterm and/or very low birth weight children," *Pediatrics*, vol. 124, no. 2, pp. 717–728, 2009.

[10] C. H. Blauw-Hospers and M. Hadders-Algra, "A systematic review of the effects of early intervention on motor development," *Developmental Medicine & Child Neurology*, vol. 47, no. 6, pp. 421–432, 2005.

[11] J. Orton, A. Spittle, L. Doyle, P. Anderson, and R. Boyd, "Do early intervention programmes improve cognitive and motor outcomes for preterm infants after discharge? A systematic review," *Developmental Medicine & Child Neurology*, vol. 51, no. 11, pp. 851–859, 2009.

[12] B. R. Lucas, E. J. Elliott, S. Coggan et al., "Interventions to improve gross motor performance in children with neurodevelopmental disorders: a meta-analysis," *BMC Pediatrics*, vol. 16, no. 1, p. 193, 2016.

[13] L. Weston, J. Hodgekins, and P. E. Langdon, "Effectiveness of cognitive behavioural therapy with people who have autistic spectrum disorders: a systematic review and meta-analysis," *Clinical Psychology Review*, vol. 49, pp. 41–54, 2016.

[14] F. M. Gresham and S. N. Elliott, "The relationship between adaptive behavior and social skills: issues in definition and assessment," *The Journal of Special Education*, vol. 21, no. 1, pp. 167–181, 1987.

[15] A. R. Jadad, R. A. Moore, D. Carroll et al., "Assessing the quality of reports of randomized clinical trials: is blinding necessary?," *Controlled Clinical Trials*, vol. 17, no. 1, pp. 1–12, 1996.

[16] A. M. Wilson, P. M. O'Byrne, and K. Parameswaran, "Leukotriene receptor antagonists for allergic rhinitis: a systematic review and meta-analysis," *The American Journal of Medicine*, vol. 116, no. 5, pp. 338–344, 2004.

[17] M. Borenstein, L. Hedges, J. Higgins, and H. Rothstein, *Comprehensive Meta-Analysis Version 2*, Biostat, Englewood, NJ, USA, 2005.

[18] J. Cohen, *Statistical Power Analysis for the Social Sciences*, L. Erlbaum Associates, Hillsdale, NJ, USA, 1988.

[19] B. A. Corbett, A. P. Key, L. Qualls et al., "Improvement in social competence using a randomized trial of a theatre intervention for children with autism spectrum disorder," *Journal of Autism and Developmental Disorders*, vol. 46, no. 2, pp. 658–672, 2016.

[20] G. Dawson, S. Rogers, J. Munson et al., "Randomized, controlled trial of an intervention for toddlers with autism: the Early Start Denver Model," *Pediatrics*, vol. 125, no. 1, pp. e17–e23, 2010.

[21] R. J. Landa, K. C. Holman, A. H. O'Neill, and E. A. Stuart, "Intervention targeting development of socially synchronous engagement in toddlers with autism spectrum disorder: a randomized controlled trial," *Journal of Child Psychology and Psychiatry*, vol. 52, no. 1, pp. 13–21, 2011.

[22] H. E. Young, R. A. Falco, and M. Hanita, "Randomized, controlled trial of a comprehensive program for young students with autism spectrum disorder," *Journal of Autism and Developmental Disorders*, vol. 46, no. 2, pp. 544–560, 2016.

[23] M. H. Tang, C. K. Lin, W. H. Lin, C. H. Chen, S. W. Tsai, and Y. Y. Chang, "The effect of adding a home program to weekly institutional-based therapy for children with undefined developmental delay: a pilot randomized clinical trial," *Journal of the Chinese Medical Association*, vol. 74, no. 6, pp. 259–266, 2011.

[24] M. van Dongen-Boomsma, M. A. Vollebregt, J. K. Buitelaar, and D. Slaats-Willemse, "Working memory training in young children with ADHD: a randomized placebo-controlled trial," *Journal of Child Psychology and Psychiatry*, vol. 55, no. 8, pp. 886–896, 2014.

[25] K. P. Liu, C. C. Chan, T. M. Lee, and C. W. Hui-Chan, "Mental imagery for promoting relearning for people after stroke: a randomized controlled trial," *Archives of Physical Medicine and Rehabilitation*, vol. 85, no. 9, pp. 1403–1408, 2004.

[26] L. V. Hedges and J. L. Vevea, "Fixed- and random-effects models in meta-analysis," *Psychological Methods*, vol. 3, no. 4, pp. 486–504, 1998.

5

Developing and Sustaining Recovery-Orientation in Mental Health Practice: Experiences of Occupational Therapists

Alexandra Nugent, Nicola Hancock, and Anne Honey

The University of Sydney, Cumberland Campus, 74 East St., Lidcombe, NSW 2141, Australia

Correspondence should be addressed to Nicola Hancock; nicola.hancock@sydney.edu.au

Academic Editor: Claudia Hilton

Background/Aim. Internationally, mental health policy requires clinicians to shift from a medical to a recovery-oriented approach. However, there is a significant lag in the translation of policy into practice. Occupational therapists have been identified as ideally situated to be recovery-oriented yet limited research exploring how they do this exists. This study aimed to explore Australian occupational therapists' experiences of developing and sustaining recovery-orientation in mental health practice. *Methods.* Semistructured, in-depth interviews were conducted with twelve occupational therapists working across different mental health service types. Participants identified themselves as being recovery-oriented. Data were analysed using constant comparative analysis. *Results.* Occupational therapists described recovery-oriented practice as an active, ongoing, and intentional process of seeking out knowledge, finding fit between understandings of recovery-oriented practice and their professional identity, holding hope, and developing confidence through clinical reasoning. Human and systemic aspects of therapists' workplace environment influenced this process. *Conclusions.* Being a recovery-oriented occupational therapist requires more than merely accepting a specific framework. It requires commitment and ongoing work to develop and sustain recovery-orientation. Occupational therapists are called to extend current leadership activity beyond their workplace and to advocate for broader systemic change.

1. Introduction

In contrast to a medical understanding of mental health recovery as "cure," recovery as defined by people with lived experience of mental illness refers to an individual's ongoing and nonlinear journey towards creating and living "a meaningful and contributing life in a community of choice with or without the presence of mental health issues" [1]. With this definition of recovery, people using mental health services, or "consumers," are necessarily active and leading agents in their own recovery [2, 3]. Therefore, recovery cannot be done to, or for, consumers by service providers [4]. Rather, services are called on to adopt recovery-oriented practice to better support consumers as they take the lead in their unique recovery journeys [5–7].

Recovery-oriented practice involves being consumer-focused, facilitating choice and opportunity, and holding and promoting hope for each consumer's future [8]. Recovery journeys are driven by the consumers and their choices, goals, and rights [9]. This requires movement away from medically oriented care in which absence of symptoms is the primary outcome measured and medication is the focus of treatment [9]. Recovery-oriented practice instead strives to enable consumers to reclaim and develop new meaning in their lives [8, 10].

Occupational therapists have repeatedly been identified as ideally placed to facilitate a shift towards recovery-oriented practice due to the congruence between occupational therapy theory and recovery-oriented principles [11–14]. Autonomy, choice, strong therapeutic partnerships, and enablement are central components of both client-centred occupational therapy [15] and recovery-oriented practice.

Current policies and guidelines across the English-speaking world, including Australia, require the adoption of recovery-oriented practice in mental health service delivery [16–20]. Further, recent outcome studies indicate that recovery-oriented practice may lead to better consumer engagement in treatment and quality of life [21] and that aspects of recovery-oriented practice such as choice and therapeutic alliance are strongly linked to positive recovery outcomes [22]. Yet, commentators in the field have consistently identified a lag in the implementation of recovery-oriented practice in mental health services (e.g., [23]). In fact, services have been described as "simply repackaging old wine in the new bottle of recovery language" [24].

Research that, with the exception of nursing, does not distinguish between professional backgrounds has identified a range of challenges in operationalising recovery-oriented practice (e.g., [25, 26]). These include a lack of clarity regarding what recovery-oriented practice entails [7, 8, 27], staff scepticism [27, 28], and incongruence between recovery and workplace priorities [7, 25–27]. Facilitators of recovery-oriented practice are less commonly reported but include developing a workplace culture that values innovation and clinicians having a willingness to test the boundaries set by restrictive organisations [25, 27, 29]. Various guidelines are available which explain what recovery-orientation looks like in practice (e.g., [9]). However, missing from the literature are (1) a nuanced understanding of how recovery-oriented clinicians actually go about sustaining their recovery-orientation within the context of the identified barriers and facilitators and (2) a specific investigation of recovery-orientation amongst occupational therapists despite assertions that they are uniquely placed to be recovery-oriented.

The aim of the current study was to explore Australian occupational therapists' experiences of developing and sustaining recovery-orientation in mental health practice.

2. Methods

2.1. Study Design. A detailed and contextualised understanding of the experiences of occupational therapists is required to aid in the operationalisation of recovery-oriented approaches. Therefore, a qualitative design was needed [30]. Grounded theory data collection and analysis techniques were used to ensure methodological rigour and inductively explore and understand participants' experiences. The techniques used were purposive and theoretical sampling, concurrent data collection and analysis, and constant comparative analysis [31]. These are described below. Ethical approval for this research was obtained from the University of Sydney Human Research Ethics Committee.

2.2. Initial Sampling and Recruitment. Participants were purposively sampled based on their direct experience with, and thus insight into, the research topic. Australian occupational therapists working in any mental health service who identified themselves as adopting recovery-oriented practice were eligible to participate. Participants were recruited through an email sent to members by the Mental Health Interest Group in the NSW Division of Occupational Therapy Australia. All participants provided written informed consent.

2.3. Data Collection and Analysis. Data collection and analysis were conducted concurrently to allow the researchers to pursue lines of inquiry informed by their ongoing analyses [30]. Data were collected through in-depth, semistructured interviews to foster a deep understanding of participants' unique experiences [30]. An interview guide was designed to encourage participants to raise important issues within the research topic and allow the interviewer to flexibly follow up on these issues [32]. Participants were asked about what being recovery-oriented meant for their own practice and how they sustained their recovery-orientation in their unique context. Because preliminary analysis of each interview occurred before engaging with the next participant [31], questions could be modified in response to emerging ideas. For example, after four interviews, risk management was identified as an important concept. Risk was discussed with subsequent participants to deepen the researchers' understanding. Interviews lasted 40–60 minutes and were audio recorded and transcribed verbatim.

Constant comparative analysis was used throughout the study [31]. Each section of data was coded with one or more words or phrases that described its underlying meaning. For example, the statements "not all managers have an understanding of what recovery-oriented practice might look like" and "it's hard if you have to be the one to convince your boss" were coded "lack of understanding from seniors." These initial codes were compared with each other and with new data as they were collected. Conceptually similar codes were grouped to form categories [31]. The broad category "workplace attitudes and culture," for example, was created by comparing the initial code "lack of understanding from seniors" with other initial codes such as "negative team attitudes." Methodological rigour was enhanced through frequent reflective discussions between authors about the codes and their relationships. This enabled consensus to be reached on the interpretation of data.

After analysis of twelve interviews, it became apparent that while no new codes were emerging, two potentially important concepts were underdeveloped: the fit between occupational therapy and recovery-oriented principles and the ongoing development (as opposed to simply maintenance) of recovery-orientation. Therefore, in accordance with theoretical sampling, further data collection was required. Examination of transcripts revealed that some participants had not been asked to expand on these issues as they had emerged in later interviews. Thus, follow-up interviews were conducted with a purposively selected subset of existing participants using a new interview guide designed to address these topics. Participants whose interviews had not covered these topics in detail were selected to obtain coverage of the topic across different service settings and levels of seniority [33]. After five follow-up interviews, new data were no longer revealing new concepts and all categories were well covered. Data collection therefore ceased, with no recruitment of new participants being required [30]. Participant characteristics are provided in Table 1.

In the final stage of constant comparative analysis, the relationships between categories were confirmed, and a framework was developed to explain the experiences of occupational therapists developing and sustaining recovery-orientation in mental health practice.

Table 1: Participant demographics.

Participant	Years since graduation	Current role			Current setting				
		OT-specific	Generic	Clinical supervisor	Acute/inpatient	Community	Forensic	Youth/early psychosis	NGO[†]
Addison[‡]	6	x				x		x	
Anna	14	x			x		x		
Jessica	16	x		x		x			
Chloe[‡]	<1		x						x
Ava[‡]	<1	x				x			
Chris[‡]	10		x	x					
Pat	22		x	x		x		x	
Amelia[‡]	19		x	x		x		x	
Jordan	13	x		x	x		x		
Charlotte	11		x	x		x			
Jamie	<1	x			x	x		x	
Casey	8	x		x	x		x		

[†]Nongovernmental Organisation.
‡ denotes those who participated in follow-up interviews.

3. Results

Participants described developing and sustaining recovery-oriented practice as an active and ongoing process. It was not a static, singular decision to be recovery-oriented or not. Neither was it a destination that participants had reached or hoped to reach. Rather, participants relayed stories of continued growth and a process or journey of striving towards recovery-oriented practice. This journey was shaped by participants' environments and they described both working within and attempting to modify or change their environments to enhance their capacity to work in a more recovery-oriented manner.

3.1. A Journey of Actively Striving towards Recovery-Oriented Practice. Participants described a need to continuously develop and strengthen their recovery-orientation. In order to do this, they detailed an active and ongoing process consisting of four components: intentionally seeking out knowledge, working to find fit or synergy between recovery-oriented practice principles and their professional identity and roles, maintaining hope, and developing confidence in defending recovery-oriented practices by strengthening their clinical reasoning skills.

3.1.1. Seeking Out Knowledge. All participants emphasised the importance of having a clear conceptualisation of recovery and recovery-oriented practice. Cultivating this was an intentional and active process. Participant understandings were constantly developing in response to new experiences and knowledge. They all highlighted a need to seek out opportunities to develop their knowledge, including learning directly from people with lived experience of mental illness. Casey highlighted the importance of taking time to "actually hear first-hand people's perspectives." In addition, participants described seeking out and reading recovery-based literature and personal narratives, attending recovery-focused training and conferences, and seeking advice from other recovery-oriented clinicians. Charlotte advised: "Do the course! Start doing workshops... things that are recovery-focused... you've got to have an understanding of what it means... It took me a lot of conscious effort."

3.1.2. Finding Fit. As participants learnt more and more about recovery and recovery-oriented practice, they described simultaneously integrating their developing conceptualisations with their personal and professional identities. All participants described a strong compatibility or synergy between recovery-oriented principles and occupational therapy philosophies. They talked about aspects such as person-centredness, supporting engagement in meaningful activity, empowerment of the individual, and taking a holistic and contextualised approach as being key and common facets of both recovery-oriented practice and occupational therapy. For example, Pat said, "I think naturally [occupational therapists are] attuned to being... holistic in our approach... the importance of meaningful activity ... how the environment plays a part in people's recovery... people developing meaningful roles... It's ingrained in us in our training." Similarly, Jamie felt that recovery-oriented practice "ties in really well with OT... finding out what is meaningful to them and framing our engagement with them around that," while Chris described the core business of occupational therapy as being "to facilitate them to have the life that they want, where they want."

Four participants suggested that recovery-orientation was more compatible with occupational therapy than other health professions. For example, Chris believed that occupational therapy was "a lot more about a person's roles and their overall functioning and how their entire life is, rather than 'you have this exact symptom, this is how you fix it.'" Because of this synergy, some participants saw the shift to recovery-oriented practice as an opportunity for the profession: "What's exciting about... recovery-orientated practice [is that it] supports a lot of what occupational therapists do... It might get to a point where... OTs find it easier to practice [and other professions] value the role of OT more" (Casey).

While two participants saw the alignment between occupational therapy and recovery as a straightforward "marriage made in heaven" (Charlotte), most also identified areas of potential misfit or challenge: "I still find 'recovery' a hard concept... trying to figure out what it means for me personally [and] professionally... What service it is that I want to be involved in providing... That was the first battle" (Ava).

Therapists described grappling to find fit between recovery and elements of their occupational therapy learning and identity. At times they needed to actively change their ways of thinking and "unlearn" old, medically oriented understandings and practices. Charlotte explained, "It took me a while... to move away from [a] deficit focus... When I went to uni it... looked at people's deficits... A lot of the assessments we still use are deficit-focused." Participants also wrestled with relinquishing the role of expert clinician to offer choice and hand control over to the consumer. For example, Chris thought that health professionals were trained to use their clinical expertise and to expect consumers to "kneel at the feet of clinicians." Likewise, Addison described her struggle with "trying to drop the therapist and the 'solving problems' part," adding that "sometimes it's not about solving the problem... it's about walking the journey."

Finally, while being not identified by participants as a challenge, a number appeared to define recovery through an occupational therapy or clinically based framework, emphasising independence and function as desired outcomes. For example, Amelia described recovery as being about consumers becoming "independent and able to look after themselves... in the community," and Chloe stated that having "that end goal of independence where possible is probably the tick we [OTs] have in our box compared to others."

3.1.3. Maintaining Hope. Having knowledge of recovery and recovery-oriented practice and being able to find fit between emerging recovery knowledge and occupational therapy were not enough for participants to practice in a recovery-oriented manner. They also stressed the importance of having and maintaining hope and holding a genuine belief in recovery.

Casey explained, "You have to [have] hope that... recovery is possible... It would become an awful place to work if you thought that was as good as it gets for people."

A belief that people can recover drove participants' recovery-orientation. Jessica, for example, described needing to have "a really strong belief that, [for] every single consumer that I work with... this is not your life. It will get better than this." Being witness to people recovering and seeing consumers benefiting from a recovery-oriented approach helped to ignite participants' hope and encouraged them to further pursue this approach to practice.

> *I was [initially] a bit nervous... these people have been through the mental health service for such a long period of time, so how much change are we going to be able to achieve? It really has amazed me... If you're working under a recovery model it is possible to make change. (Pat)*

In order to actively nurture this hope, some therapists sought connections with people recovering from mental illness outside of their immediate workplaces. For example, because Jessica's work primarily involved contact with people in acute phases of illness, she volunteered at the Hearing Voices Network in order to "spend time with people who are recovered and that maintains my hope." Casey also described observing people living their lives beyond the immediate workplace as critical because "if you look at the bigger picture, you can be... more hopeful."

3.1.4. Developing Confidence through Clinical Reasoning. To apply their knowledge and adopt practices they believed in, participants also described needing to develop confidence in their ability to make sound clinical decisions and to justify recovery-oriented practices when they conflicted with practice-as-normal. They particularly highlighted the practices around positive risk taking, a central mantra of recovery-oriented practice. Participants repeatedly talked about the confidence they needed to support and advocate for each consumer's right to choose to take positive risks. For example, Chris noted that being able to help consumers to take risks with treatments that might benefit their recovery "only comes with the confidence that your clinical skills and your clinical reasoning and decision making... are all good enough." Similarly, Jessica explained that because "the support network isn't really there yet to help us make those 'risky decisions'... you have to have really, really strong clinical reasoning and understanding of recovery to be able to justify why you made those decisions."

As they gained more experience and developed sound clinical reasoning skills, clinicians described becoming more comfortable and confident with advocating for recovery-oriented practice. Chris summed this up by saying that "the more of a new grad you are, the less comfortable you feel implementing recovery practices because it involves risk... The less experienced you are, the more frightening that is."

3.2. Working on and Working within the Environment. The journey of striving towards recovery-oriented practice was inextricably linked to and influenced by participants' work environments. Participants reported navigating, utilising, and, at times, struggling with both human and structural aspects of their environments in order to develop and sustain their recovery-orientation to practice.

3.2.1. Human Aspects. The human environment of the workplace, consisting of coworkers, supervisors or leaders, and peer workers, both positively and negatively influenced participants' ability to develop and sustain recovery-orientation. Most participants reported currently or previously experiencing negative coworker attitudes towards recovery. Medical orientation, poor communication, and a general lack of hope thwarted participants' recovery-oriented growth and discouraged their belief in recovery-oriented practice. Ava, describing a previous workplace, said the following:

> *[Negative attitudes] can really give you a negative point of view of your professional development and your career. Like... there's no point in trying to improve or change things because these people have been around longer than you and have kind of been damaged by being burnt out or not knowing the latest evidence or concepts.*

Casey explained how some staff attitudes in a forensic context made it difficult to be recovery-oriented: "they still want to see people punished and that can be really awful... they want to contain these people in these settings. That's a real challenge."

In contrast, working with a team of like-minded, recovery-oriented coworkers was perceived as highly beneficial. "You need to be strongly supported by a really good and caring team of people... in an environment where you never feel afraid to ask a question or... to get people to check that your reasoning is sound" (Chris). In these supportive environments, participants described pursuing and using the advice and support of recovery-oriented colleagues, more senior clinicians, and supervisors. Amelia described how her recovery-oriented colleagues helped and inspired her: "Sharing of that knowledge and supporting each other... That's what makes you come in and try, even though you've been butting your head." Addison used her sessions with her recovery-focused supervisor to "chat through... how I best could approach some situations."

While colleagues were an important part of the human environment, decision-makers or "people at the top" who supported recovery-oriented initiatives were seen as central to a supportive workplace. Describing the benefit of recovery-focused management or decision-makers, Jordan explained that their "support flows down into the frontline staff... It's reassuring and supportive." Casey concurred:

> *There is a hierarchy and if your consultant is recovery-orientated it makes a world of difference... they still direct treatments and they can push for recovery-orientated practices and have more authority than any other clinician... So, having them on board with recovery is the biggest enabler of all.*

Participants also repeatedly highlighted the benefit of having people with lived experience working in their service. Peer workers were viewed as valuable assets. In Chris's workplace, for example, peer workers "are getting more involved with actually improving the [recovery focus of the] service." Participants actively used their peer workers as sounding boards for their ideas and peer workers sometimes challenged clinicians' decision-making, prompting participants to critically reflect on their recovery-oriented principles and take action accordingly. Participants described peer workers as inspiring hope in consumers and clinicians alike. As Chloe reported, their presence "really helps with that understanding and that recovery-base and providing people hope that you can recover."

Importantly, participants did not see their relationship with the human environment of their workplace as a one-way transaction. Therapists also described taking action to enrich their workplace culture through leadership and example. As a supervisor, Casey said that "you have to be recovery-orientated yourself... be aware of what recovery is and bring that into the conversation... be aware of what tools are available... [to] guide people to be recovery-orientated."

Amelia suggested that, to influence the human environment, "you can use the language, you can talk about the frameworks, you can lead by example." She saw this leadership as an obligation for occupational therapists because of the synergy between the profession's philosophies and recovery-oriented approaches: "We are the ones that need to be leading the recovery-orientated approach within health services and if we're not there is something that is really wrong."

3.2.2. Structural Aspects. The structural elements of participants' work environments presented challenges to their journey of striving towards recovery-orientation. These structural aspects were both workplace specific and generic to the mental health system more broadly. Structural challenges included the biomedical outcome-driven and risk-averse nature of the mental health system, restrictive environments, and time limitations.

First, participants described a clinical outcome-driven system that did not recognise or place value on recovery-based practices or outcomes. As Ava said, "Meeting your KPIs [key performance indicators] as an OT does not necessarily mean giving them holistic care. But if you don't meet your KPIs then to your employer you're not doing your job."

Second, legislative and policy requirements, such as the Mental Health Act 2007 (NSW), lead to practices that restrict consumers' choice such as involuntary admission to hospital and compulsory treatment under community treatment orders (CTOs). Participants viewed these as restrictive, coercive, risk-averse, and therefore incompatible with recovery-oriented practice. Chris highlighted the challenge:

> *How do we actually implement [recovery-oriented practice] when we are dealing with CTOs and scheduling people... [and] having to dictate to people that they have to do these things under their forensic order... How do we... marry all those things up?*

Some environments, such as acute inpatient and forensic services, were described as particularly restrictive as they reduced opportunities for consumer choice and created greater power differentials between consumers and hospital staff. Jordan, for example, described the built environment of the hospital and its swipe-card access and exit for staff as reinforcing a "don't mess with authority" message.

Finally, participants across all service settings highlighted time limitations impacting negatively their ability to sustain recovery-orientation. For community-based participants, time restraints related to caseload size. Pat explained how care coordinators with "extraordinary numbers of consumers" had difficulty getting beyond "putting out fires." This made it difficult for them to focus on recovery. Anna described how, in acute settings, rapid consumer turnover created time constraints: "You really have no time to build up that [rapport]. They load up the patient with tablets and off [they] go." In contrast, participants in forensic settings described the difficulty of maintaining hope and progress towards recovery goals with patients who remained in inpatient settings for many years: "People want to set recovery goals and work towards them but then feel let down by the system, so we're not actually supporting their recovery. The length of time is too much" (Casey).

Despite these challenges, all participants continued to strive towards recovery-oriented practice because "engagement with [consumers] becomes much more meaningful" (Jamie), and as Jessica said, "for me, it's pleasurable to work in a recovery-orientated way."

4. Discussion

This study is, to our knowledge, the first to explore the ways in which occupational therapists go about developing and sustaining recovery-orientation in mental health practice. While it confirms previous findings on challenges and facilitators to recovery-oriented practice, it adds to the existing literature by outlining the ongoing, active, and intentional journey of striving to be recovery-oriented. Rather than simply putting their recovery-oriented beliefs into action, all participants, irrespective of workplace setting, described this as a process or journey that involved a combination of actively seeking out knowledge, finding fit, maintaining hope, developing confidence through clinical reasoning, and working on and within the environment.

A number of parallels can be drawn between the occupational therapists' ongoing journey of developing and sustaining recovery-orientation and some aspects of the mental health recovery journey described by consumers. First, both are individually driven [2]. Second, rather than being a singular event, both are characterised as a continual process with no fixed end-point or final destination [3]. Third, each process can be facilitated or hindered by the human and structural elements within the environment [6]. For example, just as participants in this study highlighted the importance of the support and guidance they gave to and received from colleagues, consumers have repeatedly identified the value of giving and receiving peer support from others travelling a similar journey [5]. Fourth, for therapists, strengthening their knowledge, hope, and confidence was essential in cultivating their recovery-oriented practice. Similarly, consumers have described an ongoing need to learn about themselves and make sense of their experiences in order to progress along their recovery journey [2]. Both describe needing hope and a belief that recovery can occur to inspire their ongoing efforts [3]. While consumers describe benefiting from the support of recovery-focused professionals, our participants valued the contributions of recovery-focused consumers to their practice. Perhaps recognition by both occupational therapists and consumers of the parallel journeys being undertaken could facilitate a consciously reciprocal alliance, each mutually supporting the other in their continual efforts and progress.

Participants in this study all described good synergy between principles of recovery-orientation and their occupational therapy professional identity. In this regard, clinicians' experiences are in keeping with perspectives previously expressed by occupational therapy scholars [11, 12, 14], adding credence to this argument. The overwhelming majority of participants in this study, however, described a need to actively find fit, suggesting that the common perception of occupational therapy and recovery-oriented practice as unproblematically synergistic may be an oversimplification. Participants described needing to unlearn aspects of their training and struggling to relinquish their expert role to better embrace principles such as choice and dignity of risk. Indeed, Lal [34] has warned against an oversimplistic assumption that there is perfect symmetry between occupational therapy philosophies and recovery-oriented practice.

Interestingly, while participants' conceptualisations of recovery were mostly consistent with consumer definitions [1], a number included an additional element: independent functioning. This is somewhat in contrast to consumer definitions of recovery in which independence may or may not be an individual's goal. Further, previous research has identified that sense of self and connecting with others, rather than independent functioning, were aspects of occupational engagement that consumers described as most meaningful [35]. The discrepancy is likely due to participants viewing recovery-oriented practice through a traditional occupational therapy lens that prioritises independent function. Similarly, it is meaningful engagement in activities that has been described as critical for recovery rather than the outcomes or products of activities which occupational therapists may be inclined to focus on [13]. Recognising these discipline based values and being wary of inadvertently superimposing them on consumers are important for occupational therapists in developing and sustaining their recovery-oriented practice [13, 34, 36].

Despite the perceived congruence between occupational therapy and recovery compared to other disciplines, participants experienced environmental barriers to and facilitators of recovery-oriented practice that were consistent with findings in previous multidisciplinary research. These included human aspects such as coworker attitudes towards recovery [8, 27, 28] and structural elements such as restrictive contexts [25] and dominance of systemic priorities [26]. Most participants in this study, however, did not merely recognise the environmental influences on their practice; they also described working to exert influence by doing things like using recovery-oriented language and leading by example, defending their practices with strong clinical reasoning, and supporting recovery-orientation in their supervision of others.

However, it is clear that changes at a systemic level are also needed. For example, health services should consider review and modification of KPIs to better align with recovery-oriented principles. Examples of recovery-oriented KPIs might include the percentage of consumers with a wellness or recovery action plan, scores of consumer satisfaction with service, measures of hopefulness, or percentage of consumers with self-identified goals. Health services can also better support therapists to use strategies they have identified to enhance their recovery-orientation. Our research supports the inclusion of peer workers in services and the creation of opportunities for therapists, particularly those working in restrictive or acute environments, to meet and learn from consumers who are further along their recovery journeys. For example, provision of consumer-facilitated training or rotating work positions that enable all therapists to experience working with consumers at varying stages of recovery might facilitate therapists' belief in and hope for recovery and thus their recovery-oriented practice. Because our results suggest that different practice contexts may present unique challenges, a one-size-fits-all, whole of system approach alone may be inadequate in supporting the realisation of recovery-oriented reform. Rather, engagement and troubleshooting at a context-specific level may prove essential to facilitating practice change.

Occupational therapists have been criticised for being "complicit in perpetrating oppressive institutional practices" and falling victim to organisational red tape rather than advocating for consumers [36]. The active strategies described by our participants suggest that occupational therapists may be beginning to take on a leadership role in helping shift mental health practice towards a more recovery-oriented approach as they have been called to do [12–14]. However, participants' spheres of influence appeared to remain at the immediate workplace level. They tried to work creatively within the existing systemic constraints rather than describing advocacy for change at this broader level. The next step for occupational therapy as a profession is to extend our leadership beyond our immediate workplaces and facilitate systemic transformation towards a more recovery-oriented mental health system. This can occur at all levels within the profession. Occupational therapists working directly with consumers can, for example, pursue opportunities to sit in on decision-making committees or panels with influence as well as advocating for consumers to be included on these. University educators can enhance the capacity of new graduates by focusing upon intervention at a systemic, rather than just an individual, level. Occupational therapy associations can also play a role through their advocacy and policy-based activities and provision of continuing professional education focused on facilitating system change.

4.1. Limitations. As with any qualitative research, the findings of this study are not universally applicable and should be interpreted with reference to the sample characteristics. All participants worked in New South Wales or Victoria, Australia. While the process of developing and sustaining recovery-oriented practice is likely to be relevant for occupational therapists in other geographical locations, as evidenced by the congruence of the findings with international literature, systemic and cultural differences warrant further research. Additionally, participants' experiences were diverse, and participants themselves identified contextual issues such as training, experience, practice context, and roles as influencing these. Research on larger samples would allow a more robust comparison of therapists' experiences and identification of issues that might be especially pertinent to particular groups. The aim to examine how occupational therapists develop and sustain recovery-orientation required targeted recruitment of therapists who identified themselves as being recovery-oriented. Future research exploring the experiences of those who feel unable or are unwilling to adopt recovery-oriented practice will be beneficial in further understanding the lag between policy and practice.

5. Conclusion

This small exploratory study describes how occupational therapists consciously and actively develop and sustain recovery-orientation in their mental health practice. It adds to previous multidisciplinary research by (a) illuminating active strategies, which may well be similarly relevant to other health professionals, and (b) highlighting specific tensions between occupational therapy and recovery-oriented practice frameworks and philosophies. This work provides guidance for therapists regarding the ongoing work needed to realise and maintain their own recovery-oriented practice, as well as challenging occupational therapists to extend their influence to broader system-level reform.

Competing Interests

The authors declare that there are no competing interests regarding the publication of this paper.

References

[1] Australian Health Ministers' Advisory Council, *A National Framework for Recovery-Oriented Mental Health Services: Guide for Practitioners and Providers*, Department of Health and Ageing, Canberra, Australia, 2013.

[2] J. Repper and R. Perkins, *Social Inclusion and Recovery: A Model for Mental Health Practice*, Baillière Tindall, Edinburgh, UK, 2003.

[3] M. Leamy, V. Bird, C. Le Boutillier, J. Williams, and M. Slade, "Conceptual framework for personal recovery in mental health: systematic review and narrative synthesis," *British Journal of Psychiatry*, vol. 199, no. 6, pp. 445–452, 2011.

[4] J. Williams, M. Leamy, V. Bird et al., "Measures of the recovery orientation of mental health services: systematic review," *Social Psychiatry and Psychiatric Epidemiology*, vol. 47, no. 11, pp. 1827–1835, 2012.

[5] M. A. Mancini, E. R. Hardiman, and H. A. Lawson, "Making sense of it all: consumer providers' theories about factors facilitating and impeding recovery from psychiatric disabilities," *Psychiatric Rehabilitation Journal*, vol. 29, no. 1, pp. 48–55, 2005.

[6] B. Happell, "Determining the effectiveness of mental health services from a consumer perspective: part 1: enhancing recovery," *International Journal of Mental Health Nursing*, vol. 17, no. 2, pp. 116–122, 2008.

[7] C. Le Boutillier, A. Chevalier, V. Lawrence et al., "Staff understanding of recovery-orientated mental health practice: a systematic review and narrative synthesis," *Implementation Science*, vol. 10, no. 1, article no. 87, 2015.

[8] C. Le Boutillier, M. Leamy, V. J. Bird, L. Davidson, J. Williams, and M. Slade, "What does recovery mean in practice? A qualitative analysis of international recovery-oriented practice guidance," *Psychiatric Services*, vol. 62, no. 12, pp. 1470–1476, 2011.

[9] M. Slade, *100 Ways to Support Recovery: A Guide for Mental Health Professionals*, Rethink, London, UK, 2009.

[10] Australian Health Ministers' Advisory Council, *A National Framework for Recovery-Oriented Mental Health Services: Policy and Theory*, Department of Health and Ageing, Canberra, Australia, 2013.

[11] M. Kelly, S. Lamont, and S. Brunero, "An occupational perspective of the recovery journey in mental health," *British Journal of Occupational Therapy*, vol. 73, no. 3, pp. 129–135, 2010.

[12] K. L. Rebeiro Gruhl, "Reflections on ... the recovery paradigm: should occupational-therapists be interested?" *The Canadian Journal of Occupational Therapy*, vol. 72, no. 2, pp. 96–102, 2005.

[13] D. J. Sutton, C. S. Hocking, and L. A. Smythe, "A phenomenological study of occupational engagement in recovery from mental illness," *Canadian Journal of Occupational Therapy*, vol. 79, no. 3, pp. 142–150, 2012.

[14] C. Lloyd, S. Tse, and H. Bassett, "Mental health recovery and occupational therapy in Australia and New Zealand," *International Journal of Therapy & Rehabilitation*, vol. 11, no. 2, pp. 64–70, 2004.

[15] M. Law, S. Baptiste, and J. Mills, "Client-centred practice: what does it mean and does it make a difference?" *Canadian Journal of Occupational Therapy*, vol. 62, no. 5, pp. 250–257, 1995.

[16] New Freedom Commission on Mental Health, *Achieving the Promise: Transforming Mental Health Care in America. Executive Summary*, New Freedom Commission on Mental Health, Rockville, Md, USA, 2003.

[17] Her Majesty's Government, *No Health without Mental Health: A Cross-Government Mental Health Outcomes Strategy for People of All Ages*, Department of Health, London, UK, 2011.

[18] Council of Australian Governments, *The Roadmap for National Mental Health Reform 2012–2022*, Council of Australian Governments, Canberra, Australia, 2012.

[19] Department of Health and Ageing, *Fourth National Mental Health Plan: An Agenda for Collaborative Government Action in Mental Health 2009–14*, Commonwealth Department of Health and Aged Care, Canberra, Australia, 2009.

[20] World Health Organization, *Comprehensive Mental Health Action Plan 2013–2020*, World Health Organisation, Geneva, Switzerland, 2013.

[21] G. H. Gudjonsson, C. S. V. Savona, T. Green, and R. Terry, "The recovery approach to the care of mentally disordered patients. Does it predict treatment engagement and positive social behaviour beyond quality of life?" *Personality and Individual Differences*, vol. 51, no. 8, pp. 899–903, 2011.

[22] V. Stanhope, S. Barrenger, M. Salzer, and S. Marcus, "Examining the relationship between choice, therapeutic alliance and outcomes in mental health services," *Journal of Personalized Medicine*, vol. 3, no. 3, pp. 191–202, 2013.

[23] M. Slade, N. Adams, and M. O'Hagan, "Recovery: past progress and future challenges," *International Review of Psychiatry*, vol. 24, no. 1, pp. 1–4, 2012.

[24] L. Davidson, M. J. O'Connell, J. Tondora, M. Lawless, and A. C. Evans, "Recovery in serious mental illness: a new wine or just a new bottle?" *Professional Psychology: Research & Practice*, vol. 36, no. 5, pp. 480–487, 2005.

[25] S.-P. Chen, T. Krupa, R. Lysaght, E. McCay, and M. Piat, "The development of recovery competencies for in-patient mental health providers working with people with serious mental Illness," *Administration and Policy in Mental Health and Mental Health Services Research*, vol. 40, no. 2, pp. 96–116, 2013.

[26] C. Le Boutillier, M. Slade, V. Lawrence et al., "Competing priorities: staff perspectives on supporting recovery," *Administration and Policy in Mental Health and Mental Health Services Research*, vol. 42, no. 4, pp. 429–438, 2015.

[27] M. Piat and S. Lal, "Service providers' experiences and perspectives on recovery-oriented mental health system reform," *Psychiatric rehabilitation journal*, vol. 35, no. 4, pp. 289–296, 2012.

[28] S. A. Kidd, K. J. McKenzie, and G. Virdee, "Mental health reform at a systems level: widening the lens on recovery-oriented care," *Canadian Journal of Psychiatry*, vol. 59, no. 5, pp. 243–249, 2014.

[29] M. Slade, M. Amering, M. Farkas et al., "Uses and abuses of recovery: implementing recovery-oriented practices in mental health systems," *World Psychiatry*, vol. 13, no. 1, pp. 12–20, 2014.

[30] S. J. Tracy, *Qualitative Research Methods: Collecting Evidence, Crafting Analysis, Communicating Impact*, Wiley, Hoboken, NJ, USA, 2012.

[31] K. Charmaz, *Constructing Grounded Theory*, SAGE, London, UK, 2014.

[32] B. DiCicco-Bloom and B. F. Crabtree, "The qualitative research interview," *Medical Education*, vol. 40, no. 4, pp. 314–321, 2006.

[33] T. Harris, "Grounded theory," *Nursing Standard*, vol. 29, no. 35, pp. 32–39, 2015.

[34] S. Lal, "Prescribing recovery as the new mantra for mental health: does one prescription serve all?" *The Canadian Journal of Occupational Therapy*, vol. 77, no. 2, pp. 82–89, 2010.

[35] N. Hancock, A. Honey, and A. C. Bundy, "Sources of meaning derived from occupational engagement for people recovering from mental illness," *British Journal of Occupational Therapy*, vol. 78, no. 8, pp. 508–515, 2015.

[36] K. W. Hammell, "Client-centred practice: ethical obligation or professional obfuscation?" *British Journal of Occupational Therapy*, vol. 70, no. 6, pp. 264–266, 2007.

6

Exploring Cultural Competence amongst OT Students

Pragashnie Govender, December M. Mpanza, Tarryn Carey, Kwenzile Jiyane, Bicolé Andrews, and Sam Mashele

Discipline of Occupational Therapy, School of Health Sciences, University of KwaZulu-Natal, Westville Campus, Westville, South Africa

Correspondence should be addressed to Pragashnie Govender; naidoopg@ukzn.ac.za

Academic Editor: Kathleen M. Matuska

Occupational therapy relies primarily on communication between the therapist and client for effective intervention. Adequate communication may be influenced by language and cultural differences between the therapist and client. Cultural competence in relation to language and culture is thus a vital part in practice. Limited research exists on cultural competence in occupational therapy students. This study thus aimed to explore the cultural competence of final year students and their perceptions of their own cultural competence, with respect to language and culture in their practice as students. An explorative qualitative study design was utilised with a nonprobability purposeful sample of 21 final year undergraduate students at a tertiary institute in South Africa. Three focus groups were conducted, comprising between 6 and 8 students in each group. Thematic analysis using inductive reasoning was undertaken in order to analyse the students' experiences and understanding of cultural competence. Findings of the study suggest that cultural competence, in relation to language and culture, influences the occupational therapy intervention process. It was shown to both positively and negatively influence intervention through supporting or hindering rapport building, client centeredness, and effective intervention.

1. Introduction

The concept of cultural competence, which in this study relates to the understanding of the influence of different languages and cultures, forms an essential component in the practice of any health care profession. Clear communication is necessary, between the clinician and client, for exchange of vital information for effective intervention [1]. Occupational therapy is one such profession which relies primarily on the interchange of communication between the therapist and client. Clients are viewed as unique beings, where their difficulties are as a result of a combination of factors and where the management of the client may rely on an understanding of the client's culture and family, including continued communication and/or support with the client and family [2]. Communication difficulties resulting from language and cultural differences between the therapist and client can thus have a significant impact on cultural competence and the occupational therapy intervention process. This is of concern in the South African context, given the country's multicultural population and eleven official languages. According to Penn [3], more than 80% of interactions between physicians and patients in South Africa take place across linguistic and cultural differences and therefore directly influence the patient-therapist relationship and quality of care. It is thus imperative that health practitioners and occupational therapists in general bridge these gaps in language and cultural differences in practice to gain a sense of cultural competence. To the authors' knowledge there has been only one other study conducted on cultural competence amongst student occupational therapists within South Africa [4] and one other study on cultural competence on professional South African occupational therapists [5]; thus limited evidence exists on how therapists in South Africa view language and culture as influencing practice and how students perceive and negotiate cultural competence in practice.

2. Literature Review

Occupational therapy is a diverse profession which relies on a functional relationship with the client whilst examining the

Cultural destructiveness	Characterised by the purposeful destruction of a culture such as undervaluing the role of traditional medicines due to prejudice
Cultural incapacity	Characterised by individuals or organisations who do not intentionally seek to be culturally destructive but lack the capacity to help minority clients or communities
Cultural blindness	Characterised by the belief that colour or culture makes no difference and that all people are the same; cultural strengths are ignored and assimilation is encouraged
Cultural precompetence	Exemplified by the realisation of agency or individual weakness in serving minorities and attempts to improve some aspect of service relative to a specific population
Cultural competence	The acceptance and respect for cultural differences with continuous expansion of cultural knowledge
Cultural proficiency	Holding culture in high regard and promoting competency in others. The difference between the competence and proficiency stages is the extent to which the therapist regards cultural differences and similarities

FIGURE 1: Cultural competence continuum [12, 13].

physiological, psychological, and environmental components that are unique to that person [1]. Intervention is thus more effective when the therapist can communicate with the patient about treatment [1]. Effective communication results when all participants in the communication process understand the content of what is being communicated [6]. A therapist speaking a different language to their client would thus have difficulty in fully grasping the client's cultural context without fully understanding the client's language first. Language is also a primary purveyor of culture. A study conducted by Levin [7] found that there was a link between language and culture. If language becomes a barrier between the practitioner and client, then the difference in their cultures could become a barrier as well. In situations such as these, cultural sensitivity needs to be applied. Moore [8] emphasised that to be culturally sensitive, one needs to be willing to consider the cultural background of the client and have at least the basic knowledge of the client's culture or beliefs within the society they practice. The Occupational Therapy Association of South Africa (OTASA) Code of Ethics and Professional Conduct [9] indicates that "occupational therapy services shall not allow prejudice or discrimination towards a patient/client based on race, culture, language, age, sexual orientation, disability, socioeconomic status." Ulrey and Amason [10] suggest that health care providers may not be aware of the client's cultural values, beliefs, and attitudes and learn as they experience it within the field of practice to become culturally competent.

Cultural competence is defined as "the process by which individuals and systems respond respectfully and effectively to people of all cultures, languages, classes, races and ethnic backgrounds in a way that recognizes, affirms, and values the worth of the individual and protects and preserves the dignity of each." [11]. It is thus imperative for students to be sufficiently exposed to different cultures and languages to build cultural competence which can be a lifelong learning process. Cultural competence, according to Cross [12], is described in six stages through which an individual develops along a continuum from cultural destructiveness to cultural proficiency. The stages are further defined as per Wittman and Velde's [13] definition of each stage (Figure 1).

Therapists in any of the first three stages, that is, destructiveness, incapacity, or blindness, may be considered to be culturally incompetent [13]. Evidence indicates that lack of cultural competence in the therapist can impact on therapeutic outcomes, treatment implementation, compliance, and follow-up [14]. Cheung et al. [15] conducted a study assessing perceptions of cultural competence amongst 51 occupational therapy students in England, in which they found a majority of students having reported limited awareness of and exposure to other cultures and insufficient training in cultural competence.

Cultural competence requires the health care practitioner to understand his/her own cultural values before understanding other cultures, their communication, behaviour, and the impact of their culture on the individual's health care beliefs. Language and cultural barriers are a common concern in clinical practice both in South Africa and internationally. With communication difficulties between the patient and the health care provider, there is often the use of interpreters either trained or untrained which could result in treatment being effective or ineffective.

A study conducted in the western United States explored the perspectives of 495 primary care physicians and their use of various methods to bridge language and cultural barriers between themselves and their clients [16]. In this study, authors found that in a place of cultural and ethnic diversity where physicians had access to the services of trained interpreters, a significantly higher quality of patient-physician communication and care occurred. Health care providers are exposed to diverse cultures and experience challenges to providing culturally and linguistically appropriate care to result in cultural competence. Occupational therapy as a profession thus needs to focus on providing culturally and linguistically appropriate care in order to provide holistic and culturally competent intervention.

3. Material and Methods

An explorative qualitative study design was utilised to explore occupational therapy undergraduate students' perceptions of cultural competence in relation to language and culture and the influence on their practice in the province of KwaZulu-Natal in South Africa. Nonprobability purposive sampling was used to select the study population of 24 final year undergraduate occupational therapy students from the school of health sciences at a tertiary institution in the province. From this sample, 21 participants agreed to participation in the study. The target population was comprised of a diverse group of students that speak different home languages and who hail from variable cultural backgrounds. Occupational therapy final year students were selected as they would have had at least three years of exposure to various service learning sites as part of their occupational therapy undergraduate training at the time. These service learning sites that the undergraduate students are exposed to during training are multicultural settings comprising hospitals, clinics, community sites, rehabilitation facilities, geriatric homes, and schools, serving a culturally and linguistically diverse population.

Three focus groups comprising a maximum of eight students were conducted spanning approximately one hour. Participants were divided into engineered heterogeneous focus groups to ensure cultural diversity. Questions posed to the groups included the following:

(i) The experience of students working with clients of a similar and divergent language and culture compared to their own.

(ii) The student's opinions on the influence they believed language and culture have on occupational therapy practice/intervention.

(iii) The opinion of students on the positive and negative aspects that language and culture have on their OT practice and how they dealt with this in practice.

(iv) Student's understanding of the term cultural competence.

(v) Student's opinions of their preparedness to deal with clients of varied cultures and language backgrounds.

(vi) Student's learnings of language and cultural influences in their practice and how they have negotiated this in OT practice.

Students responded to these questions and shared their fieldwork experiences of the past three years. Furthermore, probes were used to elicit deep reflection of their personal experiences rather than actual observations during fieldwork.

Audio voice recordings of each focus group, with participant consent, occurred and data were transcribed verbatim by authors. Transcriptions of the focus groups were proof-read by all authors prior to being analysed, to ensure investigator triangulation of results. Qualitative data collected from the focus groups were then thematically analysed using inductive reasoning. The process of thematic analysis involved the use of four levels of coding, including initial codes, creation of subcategories, categories, and themes. Trustworthiness was achieved through examination and comparison of data collected to existing bodies of knowledge on the topic (credibility). Transferability was achieved through the authors' documentation and justification of the methodological approach and the critical processes and procedures that helped them to construct and create meaning associated with the study. Dependability was achieved through regular peer briefings which ensure analytical triangulation. These strategies allowed for validation and congruency of research findings by all team members. To ensure confirmability steps were taken by the authors to ensure that the study findings are representative of the experiences of the participants' rather than being influenced by the researchers [17]. Four of the authors were final year occupational therapy students at the time of the study. Therefore, steps were taken to reduce bias; these included bracketing through reflexive journaling prior to and during data collection and triangulation during the data analysis process.

Ethical clearance was obtained from the University of KwaZulu-Natal Research Ethics Committee (Ethical Approval number SHSEC 007/16). Additionally, consent to access students in this study was obtained via gatekeeper permission from the registrar of the institution. Prior to consent from participants, an information document stating participant's rights, ethics, aims, and procedures of the study was forwarded to the participants. Those that volunteered to participate signed informed consent and were assured of confidentiality and no physical or emotional risk to them and that that they could withdraw from the study at any time.

4. Findings

Demographic Profile of OT Students. Of the 21 students that participated in the study, 19 (90%) were female and two (10%) were male. The median age of the participants was 20 years. In terms of home language, 11 (52%) participants were English-speaking, eight (38%) spoke isiZulu, one (5%) spoke SiSwati, and one (5%) was Sepedi-speaking. Of the participants, 10 (48%) spoke English as a second language, 4 (19%) spoke Afrikaans as a second language, one (5%) spoke Hindi as a second language, and six (28%) identified themselves as having no second language. Identified cultures and language of participants are highlighted in Figures 2 and 3, respectively.

Seven themes emerged, of which many were common to the content of the reflexive journals of student authors. These included "culture as an influence on intervention," "culture and language on client centeredness," and "is it lost in translation." Refer to an overview of themes presented in Figure 4 and described in detail below.

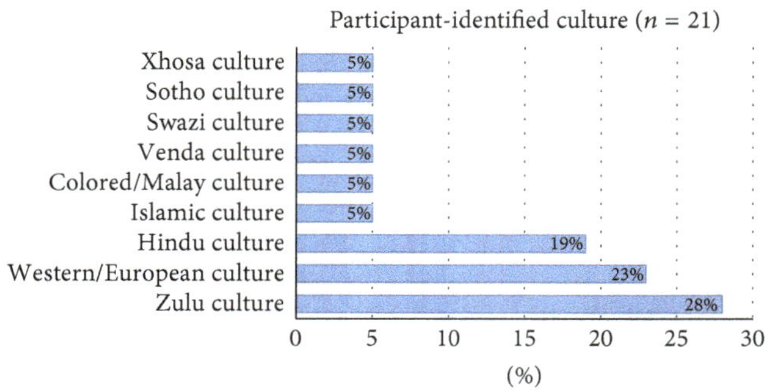

FIGURE 2: Participants identified culture (n = 21).

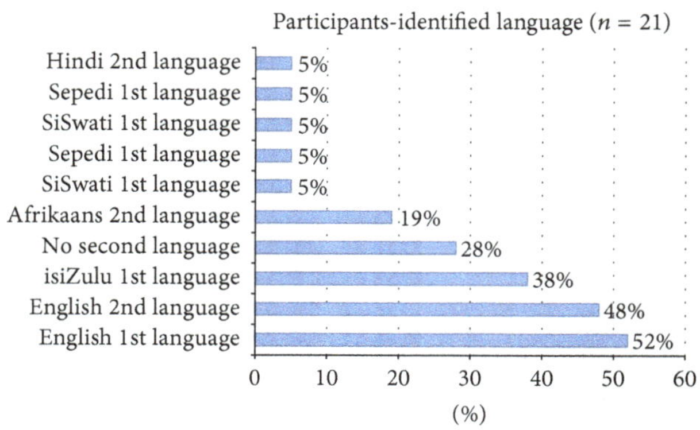

FIGURE 3: Participants identified language (n = 21).

Theme 1 (culture as an influence on intervention). Participants described culture as *"a mixture of beliefs,"* one's traditions, values, and interests. *It is "how we explain things, how we make sense of the world and everything...around us"* (Thami). This description was similar to the views expressed in the reflexive journal of four student authors which were documented prior to commencing data collection. As students, participants indicated that they had been exposed to diverse cultures both in the lectures and during service learning which had broadened their cultural knowledge and understanding: *"When I got a Zulu patient, I got to learn more about my culture, about how they...do their practices instead of how I do at home"* (Maggie). Sadie expressed that *"Even though they are the same colour as me does not mean they are the same culture."* Ashrena added that *"It gives you the opportunity to go back and learn about them and that's just increasing your knowledge into different cultures."*

Culture was further identified by participants to influence intervention both positively and negatively. *"There is some sort of emotional attachment...with people of the same culture"* (Thami) and *"They sort of take advantage of the fact that they are similar"* (Ashrena). Four student authors shared the same view; they identified culture to have a strong influence in the OT intervention.

Participants indicated that they acknowledge that culture itself is evolving. It is *"very dynamic, it changes and it differs"* (Fatima) from individual to individual and as they have grown and evolved, so has their perceptions of culture: *"...culture is changing as it goes...changing all the time"* (Sadie).

Theme 2 (the language debate). Participants understood language as the way in which they communicate and understand; it is the words and gestures used to get a message across. As Thami indicated *"...that one has a problem...I was like my goodness, the kid barely speaks...and then somebody one day was just like, oh ya, she's not from here."*

Participants, furthermore, found themselves frustrated by the linguistic barriers experienced. *"It's frustrating, not just frustrating for you, it is also frustrating for the person because they want to understand what you telling them...So it's a mutual frustration"* (Fatima).

Contrastingly, language for some participants had a positive impact on intervention; it assisted in building rapport with clients and had even resulted in participants learning a new language in order to connect to their clients. *"...It almost brought us together that all of us were talking different languages because we were all like trying to find a base that we could work from"* (Ashley). Sadie added *"working with a different language is it forces you to try and learn that language."*

Theme 3 (culture and language on client centeredness). Some participants viewed cultural and linguistic understanding within the South African context as aiding client-therapist rapport and understanding of their client's context within practice for more client directed therapy: *"Activities that we choose at the end of the day some of them have to be client centred and the only way you gonna know what your patient likes or doesn't like is if you actually communicate with them. So to make your therapy more client directed rather than therapist directed"* (Zandile).

However, majority of participants including the student authors viewed language and culture as detrimental to client centeredness when disregarded in intervention: *"I'm not familiar with games others (cultures) do. So that affects my plan of my treatment and it tends not to be client-centred but more of therapist-centred"* (Prince). Participant's further expressed that clients found comfort in familiarity which positively influenced client centeredness: *"The patient sort of gelled more with someone of the same culture as themselves... a familiarity thing"* (Thami). On the other hand, differences between the client's need and the therapists goals would result in the therapist's disregard of client centeredness: *"Because they (the client) are in need of something from you as a therapist and so they just accept whatever you may come with"* (Prince). The client's cultural and health beliefs were also perceived by participants as affecting client centeredness as one student reflects on an interaction with a client: *"...that man from Ubhumbulu sent a lightning bolt and I had a stroke so I need to go to Inyanga* (*Inyanga* is a traditional healer using cultural practices to speak to ancestors) *to cure"* (Thami). The participant was thus concerned that this cultural practice will affect interventions and acceptance of the therapeutic management offered.

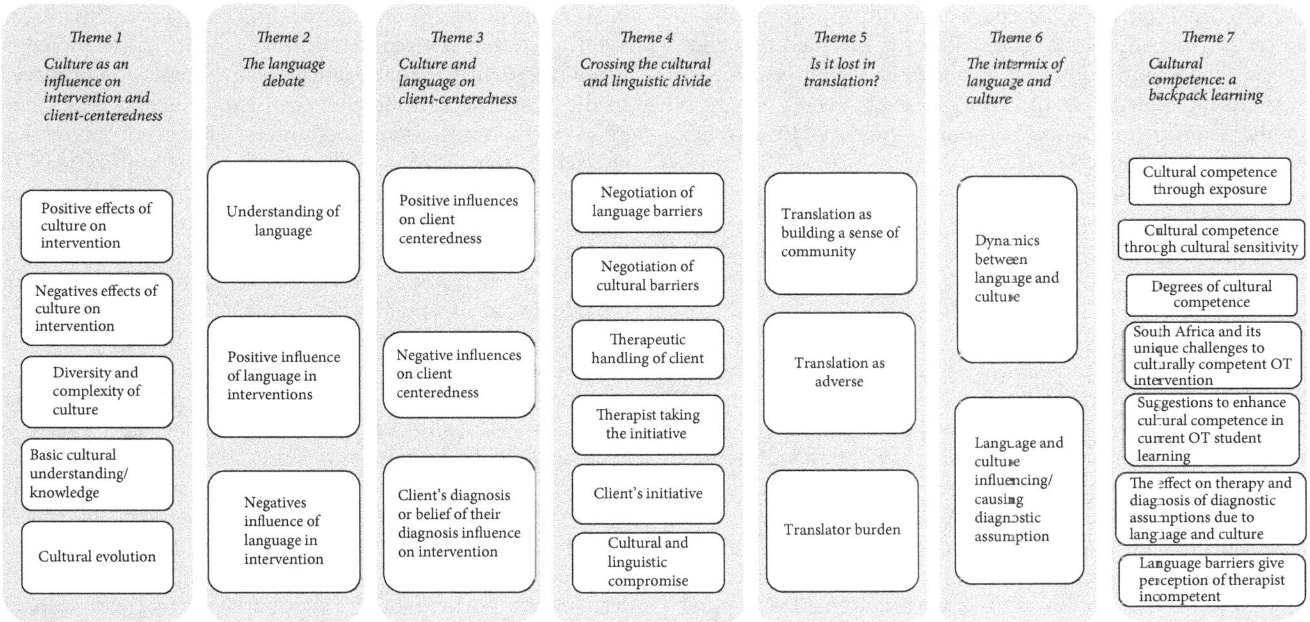

FIGURE 4: Themes and subthemes.

Theme 4 (crossing the cultural and linguistic divide). Participants made use of various strategies to negotiate language and cultural barriers which included translators, demonstration, effective handling of the client, learning written phrases, using digital applications for translation, researching language and culture, engaging with colleagues, and increasing intervention time to compensate for language barriers. Participants expressed the following:

> *A lot of it is done through body language um obviously if you get a translator that is amazing, on community I got another one of the students to write down the different instructions for me.* (Ashley)

> *I've learned (about) culture from my classmates.* (Ashley)

> *I'll go use the internet as a resource, books and other people of that culture so I just research about that.* (Sadie)

A small percentage of participants stated that research alone was not enough to bridge the cultural and linguistic gap: As Sipho indicated, *"Like do some research on it...you always get told that and then you go to Google and find a book and there's never any information about it and how it impacts therapy."*

Majority of participants, however, viewed themselves as personally responsible for taking the initiative to learn the culture and language and meet the client halfway:

> *It's up to me if I want to go deep or I want to be superficial.* (Sthabile)

> *You bring yourself down to their level, there's no 'my language' 'my culture' all of that, that's the thing, I don't think it's up to the client, I don't think it's up to the OT, I think it's up to both of you to try get there cause if one of you is not willing then it's not gonna work.* (Ashley)

Theme 5 (is it lost in translation?). Participants and two student authors highlighted the influence of translators in therapy in their attempt to be culturally competent. Translators were mostly seen to have a negative impact when attempting to build a therapeutic rapport with clients as well as resulting in therapists' exclusion which negatively influences therapeutic use of self in therapy.

> *You losing the intervention you doing coz they (the translator) then end up almost taking over.* (Sipho)

> *...the caregiver just always looks towards the translator and they actually never build that connection with you...* (Shanon)

> *Sometimes as a therapist you happen to go out of the loop which a therapist should never be.* (Fatima)

The burden placed on the translator, as viewed by the participants, was a further negative to translation:

> *...they say the long things...I'm not gonna remember everything, so I take the short cut and end up not giving the full message.* (Maggie)

> *It is difficult especially when they have their own client to treat, and they are taking the time out of all the stuff that they need to do.* (Sipho)

Theme 6 (the intermix of language and culture). Throughout the focus group discussions, participants revealed that they view language and culture as synonymous with each other or as having a dynamic influence on each other: *"There is definitely a link between language and culture even though they are 2 separate things"* (Sadie).

Participants found that they could bridge the cultural gap with language: *"To communicate with patients in their language it helps you understand their context and once you understand their context you're able to go deeper into their culture"* (Thando).

Theme 7 (cultural competence: a backpack of learning). Opinions of students varied on what it meant to be culturally competent, with majority of participants perceiving themselves as culturally incompetent, but with a willingness to engage in lifelong learning and growing towards the ideal of cultural competence: *"I don't know if you can ever be fully culturally competent but I feel like you can aspire towards cultural competence by using cultural sensitivity...it is something you should always work towards"* (Ashley). Penny indicated *"I don't even think that I am competence (competent) in all areas in my own culture."*

However, participants still displayed cultural awareness, growth, and sensitivity due to exposure to and learning of different languages and cultures: *"I am definitely cultural sensitive...I don't just barge in with who I am and what I bring"* (Sadie). Ashrena added *"As you grow with the degree and learn about more culture and you become more emotionally attached to other cultures as well."*

Majority of students felt that they had been provided with appropriate information and exposure to cultures and language during their training but some students including student authors still viewed this as insufficient: *"We get into the OT course and then we experience all these cultural forms and diversity, but it's not deep enough, we don't know deep enough"* (Sthabile). Phindile felt that this process is complex, *"...for the course teaching us about being competent, it's not that simple or easy."*

Cultural competence in occupational therapy practice specific to the South African context was found to challenge students: *"I also think with the tests we have...they are like not adapted for everyone...they don't incorporate everyone there is in South Africa"* (Prince). Sarah added *"It has been tough working with such a diverse population."*

5. Discussion

The findings of this study indicate that the student cohort who formed the study sample have been exposed to varied cultures through their undergraduate training. Cultural differences were found to negatively affect intervention, where, in some cases, clients refused intervention due to the cultural difference thus causing frustration for both the participants and their clients. These findings are aligned to other findings from a study by Mabuza et al. [18] on community placement areas of South African Universities, in which he demonstrated that, in some instances due to cultural or religious norms, treatment was often refused. Additionally, a study conducted by Levin [19] identified that cultural misinterpretation occurred, so did negative attitudes between the therapist and client, in some therapist-client encounters. However, culture was viewed by participants as having positive implications on intervention where it had improved rapport, intervention, and therapist's cultural knowledge, through exposure to various cultures. Consequently, this was influenced most often by the therapist's initiative in the interventions and in establishing rapport with clients that they encountered.

Language is considered to provide the means by which humans communicate, and communication plays a pivotal role in the health profession in developing trust and cooperation between the practitioner and client [20]. This is in keeping with findings of this study which highlighted that when trying to speak the client's language, participants noted positive changes in the client-therapist rapport building. It forced participants to learn a language to improve their intervention. Language was still, however, the greatest concern of the participants as this barrier negatively impacts intervention and their ability to be culturally competent. Participants found therapeutic opportunities were missed and the intervention provided was superficial or even incorrect. The findings are consistent with those of Ong et al. [21] and Schlemmer and Mash [22] who found that patient care and clinical outcomes suffered due to the language barrier. It is noteworthy to the authors to note the lack of distinction between language and culture in the study where students viewed both of these concepts as one entity or as one influencing the other. This corresponds with the literature that highlights that language is a primary purveyor of culture and the connection between language and culture is extensively rooted [20].

Occupational therapists view clients holistically, taking into account their linguistic and cultural context in order to create a client centred intervention. Majority of participants showed that when communicating effectively they were able to provide client centred intervention which was similarly found in a study conducted on occupational therapy students in the University of Free State in South Africa [4]. It is of a concern that some participants struggling with linguistic and cultural understanding were unable to provide the client centred therapy they felt their clients deserved. Furthermore, failure to consider a client's identified problems was noted by a few participants resulting in inaccurate history taking and misinterpretation of diagnosis which has also been well documented in the literature [23, 24]. This disregard for client centeredness, in most of the cases reported, would result in the acceptance of the student's cultural incompetence by the client due to client desperation and need for their help. It is thus important that practitioners find a way to cross the linguistic and cultural divide to meet the needs of the people with whom they work [7]. Whilst therapists try to bridge the cultural divide, they may consider that clients often "warm up" to therapists of similar culture which positively influences client centeredness as noted in this study. This could be essential where rapport is difficult to build. Furthermore, in bridging the gap between language and culture, cultural brokering which serves as a mediator is said to be valuable [25]. Responses from participants revealed the use of this technique as well as various other measures to bridge the gap of a cultural or linguistic divide, which included use of translators, use of research, and use of body language. Using translation was found to be useful in intervention for some, however, majority reported that it resulted in dilution of the information and therapist exclusion from the intervention process. Other studies [11, 26] also found that the use of translators affected rapport and accuracy of data being translated making it superficial, thus, impeding on assessment and intervention outcomes. The most notable finding was in the ability of students to take the initiative to learn the language of their clients for improved therapeutic outcomes. This is similar to a study by Tjale and De Villiers [27] that highlighted that self-empowerment in terms of culture and language was a factor that enables the health practitioner to provide effective intervention, as this encourages client's willingness to participate and influences positive rapport with clients.

Overall this cohort of students showed cultural sensitivity and understood cultures as diverse, forever evolving, complex, and specific to each individual. This alone showed a high level of precultural competence according to Cross [12] cultural competence model. Students however viewed themselves as generally culturally incompetent. Cheung et al. [15] study found that the majority of students reported having limited exposure to other cultures and insufficient training in cultural competence.

Two similar studies [4, 5], from a South African perceptive, also showed that students felt they did not have enough exposure to cultural issues in both university-based education and fieldwork. Students in these studies did not feel sufficiently equipped with respect to cultural competence as a result of the occupational therapy curricula at their institutions. These findings are in contrast to the findings of this study as participants suggested they had felt prepared through exposure and training at this particular institution. Wohl [28] suggested that health practitioners may not fully know all their client's cultural customs and attitudes; they become equipped through experience as they become exposed. These findings [28] support the participant's responses that cultural competence may not be fully obtained but enhanced through exposure to various cultures and that it is a continuous learning journey of collecting knowledge as they experience it, carrying this knowledge into all their practice, as expressed by one participant *"it's like a little backpack you carry with you everywhere"*.

6. Conclusion

In this study, the authors aimed to explore the perspectives of final year occupational therapy students on the issue of cultural competence. Whilst occupational therapy students are exposed to diverse languages and cultures in various fieldwork placements within their undergraduate training, students still viewed themselves as being culturally incompetent. Instead, students displayed cultural sensitivity, due to the belief that culture and its many subcultures are too diverse and evolving to ever reach an ideal state of cultural competence. Cultural incompetence related to language barriers and misunderstanding of the client's culture have been viewed as negatively influencing the intervention process specifically in rapport building, accurate assessments, and client centred activity choices. The negative influence of cultural incompetence could be exacerbated when attending to difficult clients. However, clients of similar culture to their therapists often build rapport easily; therefore, situations where therapists of similar culture act as mediators can be considered a step closer to client centeredness intervention. The authors found that participants use the term language and culture interchangeably indicating a strong perceived link between language and culture as influencing their ability to achieve cultural competence and client centred intervention. Participants thus viewed it as essential to take responsibility or initiative to deal with linguistic and cultural barriers to achieve cultural sensitivity and strive towards cultural competence. Negotiation of barriers was found to include body language, use of translators, research on the Internet, and learning from others. Participants were thus found to show cultural awareness and cultural sensitivity on a precultural competence level in this study. As a way forward further studies can address how cultural competence is enacted in daily practice of occupational therapists; there may also be the need for adaptations to existing OT curricula on cultural competence in more formal ways to ensure a more comprehensive understanding of the concept by exploring terms such as cultural awareness, cultural sensitivity, and cultural knowledge. Finally, we encourage the occupational therapy community to engage in critical debate on whether a state of cultural competence may ever be possible within occupational therapy practice and how this may contribute to the professions identity.

7. Limitations of the Study

The study was limited to one cohort of students in a particular context and the authors did not assess or observe actual behaviours of the students within the framework of cultural competence. Thus, participants may have recalled and expressed their experiences differently to their actual behaviour or attitudes.

Conflicts of Interest

The authors declare that there are no conflicts of interest regarding the publication of this paper.

References

[1] B. Richardson and B. Smith, "Communication in occupational therapy during diagnosis & treatment using the case study of an injured violinist," http://mathcs.ups.edu/~bryans/Current/Journal_Spring_2009/BRichardson_2009.pdf, 2009.

[2] J. M. Lum, A. P. Williams, S. Rappolt, M. D. Landry, R. Deber, and M. Verrier, "Meeting the challenge of diversity: results

from the 2003 survey of occupational therapists in Ontario," *Occupational Therapy Now*, vol. 6, no. 4, pp. 13–17, 2004.

[3] C. Penn, "Factors affecting he success of mediated medical interviews in South Africa," *Current Allergy & Clinical Immunology*, vol. 20, no. 2, pp. 66–71, 2007.

[4] E. J. van Rensburg, T. van der Merwe, and M. Nel, "Cultural competence among occupational therapy students at the University of the Free State, South Africa," *Acta Academica*, vol. 44, no. 3, pp. 119–155, 2012.

[5] A. E. Leendertz, *Cultural competency: perceptions of South African trained occupational therapists [Ph.D. thesis]*, 2013.

[6] S. M. Lee, *A Review of Language and Other Communication Barriers in Health Care*, US Department of Health and Human Services, Portland, Ore, USA, 2003.

[7] M. E. Levin, "Language as a barrier to care for Xhosa-speaking patients at a South African paediatric teaching hospital," *South African Medical Journal*, vol. 96, no. 10, pp. 1076–1079, 2006.

[8] S. E. Moore, "Cultural sensitivity treatment and research issues with black adolescent drug users," *Child & Adolescent Social Work Journal*, vol. 9, no. 3, pp. 249–260, 1992.

[9] Occupational Therapy Association of South Africa, *Code of Ethics and Professional Conduct*, OTASA, Cape Town, South Africa, 2005, http://coteceurope.eu/COTEC%20Docs/Publications/Reference_list.pdf.

[10] K. L. Ulrey and P. Amason, "Intercultural communication between patients and health care providers: An exploration of intercultural communication effectiveness, cultural sensitivity, stress, and anxiety," *Health Communication*, vol. 13, no. 4, pp. 449–463, 2001.

[11] R. Murden, A. Norman, J. Ross, E. Sturdivant, M. Kedia, and S. Shah, "Occupational therapy students' perceptions of their cultural awareness and competency," *Occupational Therapy International*, vol. 15, no. 3, pp. 191–203, 2008.

[12] T. L. Cross, "Towards a culturally competent system of care: a monograph on effective services for minority children who are severely emotionally disturbed," https://eric.ed.gov/?id=ED330171, 1989.

[13] P. Wittman and B. P. Velde, "Attaining cultural competence, critical thinking, and intellectual development: A challenge for occupational therapists," *American Journal of Occupational Therapy*, vol. 56, no. 4, pp. 454–456, 2002.

[14] J. P. Muñoz, "Culturally responsive caring in occupational therapy," *Occupational Therapy International*, vol. 14, no. 4, pp. 256–280, 2007.

[15] Y. Cheung, S. Shah, and S. Muncer, "An exploratory investigation of undergraduate students' perceptions of cultural awareness," *The British Journal of Occupational Therapy*, vol. 65, no. 12, pp. 543–550, 2002.

[16] J. Hornberger, H. Itakura, and S. R. Wilson, "Bridging language and cultural barriers between physicians and patients," *Public Health Reports*, vol. 112, no. 5, pp. 410–417, 1997.

[17] A. K. Shenton, "Strategies for ensuring trustworthiness in qualitative research projects," *Education for Information*, vol. 22, no. 2, pp. 63–75, 2004.

[18] L. H. Mabuza, P. Diab, S. Reid et al., "Communities' views, attitudes and recommendations on community-based education of undergraduate health sciences students in South Africa: a qualitative study," *African Journal of Primary Health Care and Family Medicine*, vol. 5, no. 1, article 456, 2013.

[19] M. E. Levin, "Impact of language and culture on the quality of medical communication and care," *Current Allergy and Clinical Immunology*, vol. 20, no. 2, article 54, 2007.

[20] A. Bischoff, P. A. Bovier, R. Isah, G. Françoise, E. Ariel, and L. Louis, "Language barriers between nurses and asylum seekers: their impact on symptom reporting and referral," *Social Science and Medicine*, vol. 57, no. 3, pp. 503–512, 2003.

[21] L. M. Ong, J. C. De Haes, A. M. Hoos, and F. B. Lammes, "Doctor-patient communication: a review of the literature," *Social Science & Medicine*, vol. 40, no. 7, pp. 903–918, 1995.

[22] A. Schlemmer and B. Mash, "The effects of a language barrier in a South African district hospital," *South African Medical Journal*, vol. 96, no. 10, pp. 1084–1087, 2006.

[23] C. Watson, "Why warriors lie down and die: towards an understanding of why the Aboriginal people of Arnhem Land face the greatest crisis in health and education since European contact: R. Trudgen," *Australian Journal of Rural Health*, vol. 9, no. 3, pp. 141-142, 2001.

[24] G. Flores, "Culture and the patient-physician relationship: achieving cultural competency in health care," *Journal of Pediatrics*, vol. 136, no. 1, pp. 14–23, 2000.

[25] K. Singleton and E. Krause, "Understanding cultural and linguistic barriers to health literacy," *The Online Journal of Issues in Nursing*, vol. 14, no. 3, 2009.

[26] O. Carrasquillo, E. J. Orav, T. A. Brennan, and H. R. Burstin, "Impact of language barriers on patient satisfaction in an emergency department," *Journal of General Internal Medicine*, vol. 14, no. 2, pp. 82–87, 1999.

[27] A. Tjale and L. De Villiers, *Cultural Issues in Health and Health Care: A Resource Book for Southern Africa*, Juta and Company, 2004.

[28] J. Wohl, "Integration of cultural awareness into psychotherapy," *American Journal of Psychotherapy*, vol. 43, no. 3, pp. 343–355, 1989.

7

Patient and Therapist Experiences of the SaeboFlex

Larissa Andriske,[1] Debbie Verikios,[1] and Danielle Hitch[2]

[1] *Barwon Health, Geelong, VIC, Australia*
[2] *Deakin University, Geelong, VIC, Australia*

Correspondence should be addressed to Danielle Hitch; dani.hitch@deakin.edu.au

Academic Editor: Patricia Belchior

Objective. The aim of this pilot study was to explore the experiences of both patients and therapists of using the SaeboFlex. *Method.* A mixed methods approach was adopted. Patients completed a questionnaire which included the Psychosocial Impacts of Assistive Devices Scale (PIADS) (Version 3.0) and 6 qualitative questions. Therapists completed 2 qualitative questionnaires, which collected data on the regimen adopted for the SaeboFlex and reflections on their practice with this device. *Results.* The SaeboFlex had a mostly positive impact on both the psychosocial experience of patients and their ability to do, be, and become. Intervention regimens were broadly similar between therapists, and both patients and therapists stated that the SaeboFlex increased motivation for therapy. *Conclusion.* This study has added to our tentative understanding of the SaeboFlex, but more rigorous research is required to build a robust evidence base.

1. Introduction

The SaeboFlex is a dynamic custom fabricated wrist, hand, and finger orthosis (WHFO). As a purely mechanical spring assisted device, the SaeboFlex enables people with decreased wrist, hand, and finger function to participate more actively in both rehabilitation and daily occupations. The SaeboFlex is considered particularly suitable for patients with insufficient wrist and finger extension to participate in repetitive task oriented therapy, including those who have experienced stroke, spinal cord injury, and acquired brain injury [1].

The SaeboFlex has been on the market for several years, and a small body of evidence has now emerged about its effectiveness. A pre-post study with people experiencing chronic poststroke hemiparesis followed up participants who engaged in a total of 30 hours of training with the device. Improvements were found in shoulder and elbow movement, wrist extension, and muscle tone [2]. A further series of case studies were completed with people following severe stroke, who used the SaeboFlex for just 1 week for a total of 3 hours [3]. Small gains were found in reaching and grasping, and the subject found to make the greatest gain had a primary problem of weakness. The two conference abstracts have also reported pre-post studies with people following stroke. The first reported significant increases in grip strength and wrist extension following a 6-week program involving use for 90 minutes per day [4]. The other reported improvements in active shoulder flexion and abduction, decreased muscle tone, and improved motor recovery and grip strength [5]. This study also used an occupational therapy outcome measure focusing on meaningful activities and found that 80% of the participants achieved their personal functional goals after the 5 months of the program.

Most recently, a clinical case series study focused on the feasibility of SaeboFlex upper-limb training in acute stroke rehabilitation [6]. A sample of 8 patients with less than 3 months after stroke were recruited and participated in a 12-week individualized training program (of up to 3 × 45-minute sessions per day). Clinically significant improvements were found in the majority of participants for upper-limb function, although one participant experienced shoulder complications. The authors concluded that the SaeboFlex has the potential to improve participation and independence in activities of daily living but did not recommend further research.

There have also been two descriptive accounts of the experiences of therapists with the SaeboFlex [7, 8], which were generally very positive. However, the experience of patients in using this device has not been the subject of research to date, nor has the use of the device with people other than those who have had a stroke. The aim of this pilot study was therefore to explore the experiences of both patients and therapists of using the SaeboFlex, as a first step towards understanding how it can be successfully translated into regular practice.

This pilot study focused on specific aspects of the patient and therapist experience of the SaeboFlex, which were identified as crucial to its uptake and sustainability as a part of therapy. The research questions addressed were the following:

(1) What impact did the SaeboFlex have on the psychosocial experience of patients undergoing neurological rehabilitation?

(2) What perceived impact did the SaeboFlex have on the patient's ability to do, be, become, and belong?

(3) How did the therapists utilize the SaeboFlex in practice?

(4) What were the therapist's reflections on his/her experience of using the SaeboFlex with his/her patients?

2. Method

This pilot study was conducted using a mixed methods approach, with both quantitative and qualitative data collected from patients and therapists. Ethics approval was sought and provided by both the health service in which the study was based and the university which provided research support.

2.1. Procedure. Several different methods of data collection were used, incorporating both standardized and nonstandardized methods. The inclusion criteria for patient participants were (1) patients with a neurological condition resulting in hemiparesis and (2) patients whose treatment has included use of the SaeboFlex within the Occupational Therapy Program between January 2012 and December 2013. Patients with mental health or cognitive issues which impacted on their ability to give informed consent were excluded from the study.

At the conclusion of their program with the SaeboFlex, patients were invited to participate and, if agreeable, given a single questionnaire to complete either individually or with the help of a carer. The questionnaire began with the Psychosocial Impacts of Assistive Devices Scale (PIADS) (Version 3.0), which addressed the first research question. The PIADS has been standardized and measures quality of life outcomes around the use of assistive technology via a 26-item self-rating scale [9]. There are 3 subscales (competence, adaptability, and self-esteem), with each item rated from *−3 (maximal negative impact)* to *+3 (maximal positive impact).* The PIADS has been shown to have good construct validity, test-retest stability, reliability and internal consistency, and acceptable concurrent validity [10–12]. Following the PIADS, patients were asked 6 open-ended questions seeking their comments on how the SaeboFlex supported their ability to do, be, become, and belong. These dimensions originated in Wilcock's [13]. Occupational Perspective of Health, although the updated definitions formulated by Hitch et al. [14] were provided on this questionnaire for the patient's reference. Single questions were devoted specifically to each dimension, while a further question asked the patient to comment on whether the SaeboFlex had affected his/her personal experience and a final question asked for any further comments. Please see the Appendix for the full list of qualitative questions posed.

All occupational therapists (known as therapists from this point on) working at the health service who had utilized the SaeboFlex were eligible to take part in this study. At the conclusion of their work with a patient using the SaeboFlex, therapists were invited to participate and, if agreeable, were asked to provide qualitative data regarding their experience of the device. The questionnaires included space to record the patients' medical and social history, the regimen of use adopted for the SaeboFlex, the patients functional goals reflections on clinical reasoning, opinion on usefulness in practice, and positive and negative experiences. While all this data has contributed to quality assurance activities at the service, only data related to the regimen adopted, clinician perceptions of utility, and experience of the device are reported here. These data were collected separately to keep the reflective data confidential, as occupational therapy students contributed to the extraction of medical and social history data from the patients file onto the first form. Analysis only commenced once all forms of data had been collected.

2.2. Data Analysis. Given the pilot nature of this study, all quantitative data from patients were analyzed descriptively by frequencies, means, and standard deviations. All qualitative data were transferred to a separate Microsoft Word document. Responses specifically related to the dimensions of occupation (doing, being, becoming, and belonging) were coded in relation to these dimensions; for example, responses which alluded to the patients aspirations were included in data related to becoming. These data were then analyzed thematically, and direct quotes have been extracted to illustrate each theme in the words of the patients.

Qualitative data from therapists around the utilization of the SaeboFlex were analyzed quantitatively using the first 7 sections of the TIDieR template for intervention description [15]. This template aims to encourage the complete description of published interventions, as a means to improving replicability in the longer term. The final 3 sections of this template (Tailoring, Modifications, and How Well) relate to highly variable factors, which cannot be adequately reported in a pilot study. Content analysis was used to quantify the responses required, with regimen features applied to three or more patients reported. Qualitative data from therapists related to the use of the device with their patients were analyzed thematically, with themes allowed to emerge from the data.

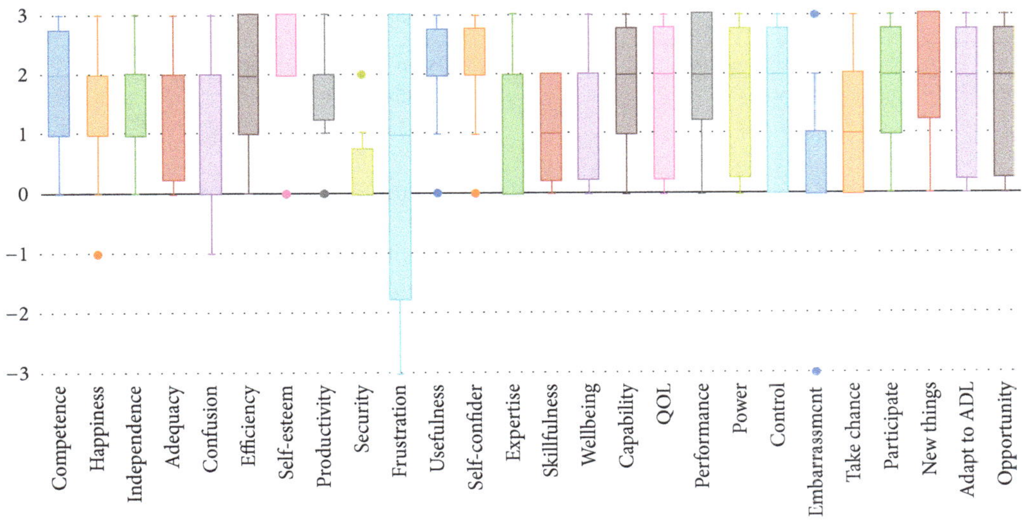

FIGURE 1: Box-and-whisker plot of PIADS ratings for the SaeboFlex from all participants.

3. Results

3.1. Sample. Eleven patient participants were recruited and completed both sections of the questionnaire. Seven participants (64%) were male, with around half of them (54%) being in their 60s. While the mean age was 60.2 (SD = 17.89), the youngest participant was in their mid-20s and the oldest participant was in their early 90s. While we had hoped to recruit participants with a range of diagnoses, all participants had experienced a stroke (with one also diagnosed with a brain tumor).

Five therapist participants were recruited, all of whom completed reflective responses for their work with clients (resulting in 11 records). Eight SaeboFlex intervention regimens were submitted for analysis. All patients were also using other treatment modalities along with the Saebo, including e-stim, wrist bracing, splinting, and/or casting, although the time after injury for each of the participants when using the SaeboFlex was variable. All were presenting with moderate to severe spasticity in their wrist and fingers, and none of them had any functional grasp or release movements in their upper limbs. All of these therapists were employed by a large regional health service and worked across both subacute and community services.

3.2. Patients

3.2.1. Psychosocial Experience. As displayed in Figure 1, the patients experienced mostly positive psychosocial experiences as a result of using the SaeboFlex. The box and whisker chart displays the interquartile ranges (boxes), maximums and minimums (whiskers), and outliers (dots) from all responses. The only item which elicited more than one negative response was "frustration," and qualitative comments associated with this item identified the customized fitting process as the source of this response.

3.2.2. Perceptions of Doing, Being, Becoming, and Belonging

(1) Doing. The majority ($n = 10$) of the patients noted they were able to do more when using the SaeboFlex, citing improvements in range of movement, strength, grip, and control; *"the more practice I had the more my ability to progress towards independence."* However, the amount of progress varied amongst the patients, some of whom were in the acute phase and some were up to several years after stroke; *"Still not able to use my hand functionally, but have noticed increased strength, increased control of movement."*

(2) Being. Individual confidence and motivation were the 2 main aspects of being identified by the patients ($n = 8$), with the SaeboFlex found to be supportive of both. Successful doing was a key factor in the building of confidence, which was also generalized by the patients to other activities of daily living; *"it definitely build my confidence to attempt to try other things because I knew that my brain was remembering the movement."* While some patients ($n = 4$) reported fluctuating motivation through their time using the SaeboFlex, the majority acknowledged that its use had contributed to maintaining their engagement in the rehabilitation process; *"It gave me a positive mind set and was the start of the hardest thing I have done in my life."*

(3) Becoming. Hope was a very strong theme in the data related to the occupational dimension of becoming ($n = 8$), with patients consistently highlighting a lack of self-belief in their abilities at the beginning of their use of the SaeboFlex; *"it helped me use my hand even though I thought I never would."* The realization that a return to function was possible was very powerful for some of the patients; *"My hand moved, I couldn't believe it! I finally could see a shining light and I was going to get some movement back in my arm and hand with hard work and encouragement."* This sense of hope also encouraged further aspiration, as patients looked forward to achieving

Table 1: SaeboFlex regimens.

Regimen	Overall length of use	Session time and frequency	Repetitions
1	2 months	45 mins, 1-2 daily	20–40
2	3 months	45 mins, 2-3 daily	45–100
3	1 week	Daily	Not recorded
4	4 months	20 mins, 1-2 daily	50–150
5	3 months	45 mins, 1-2 daily	50–100
6	3 months	20 mins, 2 daily	Not recorded
7	1.5 months	45 mins, 1-2 daily	80–120
8	1.5 months	45 mins, not recorded	Not recorded

future goals as a result of their use of the SaeboFlex; *"I'm hoping to get to the stage where I can open jars that are too hard for my wife."*

(4) Belonging. The majority of patients ($n = 9$) stated that the SaeboFlex did not impact on their sense of belonging to any appreciable degree. Their rehabilitation using this device was perceived as a very personal and individual experience, although two patients could see a link between their gains in doing and participation in social activities; *"I feel using the SaeboFlex will help me be more independent and less reliant on my family and friends."*

3.3. Occupational Therapists

3.3.1. Use of SaeboFlex in Practice. The consistent rationales cited for using the SaeboFlex were to (1) improve upper-limb functional performance, (2) improve active range of movement, (3) improve grip strength, and (4) provide a means for ongoing home based rehabilitation. The main material used was the SaeboFlex orthosis in combination with specific sized balls for use in rehabilitation exercises. The therapist was the only person providing the intervention, and the SaeboFlex was used individually in all cases. In this study, the SaeboFlex was used within both the clinical setting and the home environment. For home programs, equipment was provided on loan to the patients from the health service, with some patients going on to seek funding to purchase the SaeboFlex for ongoing use. As shown in Table 1, there was some variation in regard to when and how much the SaeboFlex was used. The shortest duration of SaeboFlex use was one week, although many regimens lasted 2-3 months. Sessions were either 20 or 45 minutes long, and all were performed at least once on a daily basis. Repetitions (i.e., each instance of grasp and release) tended to increase over time ranging from 20 to 150 per session.

3.3.2. Use of SaeboFlex in Practice. Themes elicited from data related to therapist experiences in using this device were benefits and barriers. The main benefit of using the SaeboFlex highlighted was the supportive impact it had on patient motivation; *"A few short sessions with SaeboFlex was enough to 'light a fire' to get him (to) increase the use of his left upper limb."* This was consistently identified by all therapists and appeared to be related to the rapid improvements observed in patient function: *"Quick results, quick translation into increased hand function."* This also elicited positive emotional responses, with several therapists describing the excitement they, the patients, and their families felt in response to these improvements.

The SaeboFlex also enabled therapists and patients to focus on the upper limb more intensely, *"Provided an opportunity to attend to left upper limb for extended periods."* However, unexpected and more generalized benefits of this intervention were also reported around improved standing tolerance, better transition to other treatment modalities, decreased neglect, and better mental state; *"It was immediately motivating and improved her mood...she was very determined during therapy and she persisted in using the SaeboFlex."* The flexibility possible in treatment activities was also highlighted as a benefit by therapists, who stated they enjoyed the challenge of finding new things for their patients to do; *"Ability to increase use of SaeboFlex is inspiring for clients who want a challenge."*

The main barrier experienced in using the SaeboFlex with patients was the need to have assistance in donning and doffing the orthosis. While some patients were able to do this independently, others were reliant on carers which impacted on their ability to use it at home; *"He was alone during the day and couldn't complete by himself."* The intensity of the regimens was also seen as a potential barrier if the patient found the repetitions boring or it overtook his/her occupational balance; *"As a therapy have been mindful not to overload patient with too much to do at home so that he doesn't have time to do other things and gets burnt out or disinterested."* Finally, a few therapists noted that the device is fairly expensive and may be beyond the means of many clients to use on an ongoing basis.

4. Discussion

This pilot study has achieved its aim of exploring the experiences of both patients and therapists of using the SaeboFlex, by answering all four of the research questions posed. The SaeboFlex was found to have a mostly positive impact on the psychosocial experience of patients undergoing neurological rehabilitation, although two patients expressed frustration around the fitting procedures required. Patients' perceptions of a device impact on their quality of life and wellbeing is crucial to their engagement with this form of therapy [12], so this could indicate potential for sustained use of the SaeboFlex during rehabilitation. The generally positive perception of the SaeboFlex was also found in qualitative comments from patients, who reported they were able to achieve greater function with this device and experience increased confidence and motivation. The strong theme of hope was striking in this study and supports other findings that mastery is a hope promoting factor for people recovering from stroke [16]. The lack of relationship between SaeboFlex use and belonging may be related to individual patient goals, with several patients noting that they perceive their recovery from an individual perspective.

The intervention regimens used by therapists in this study were broadly similar, with variations likely to be the results of programs being individualized to meet personal needs. Similar to Stuck et al. [6], the device was not used to the maximum recommended level (2 × 45 minutes daily) but many benefits were still observed and reported. Therapists were also able to identify barriers to using the SaeboFlex with their patients, which indicates an appropriately critical approach to its translation to practice. There were synergies between the patient and therapist experience around motivation and the motivating impact of visible results, although none of the patients specifically mentioned difficulties around donning and doffing the device.

The value of gathering perspectives from multiple stakeholders includes the possibility of highlighting different aspects of the use of the SaeboFlex, and the collection of both patient and therapist qualitative data was a strength of this pilot study. However, there were also several limitations which limit the generalizability of these findings. The sample included was quite small (for both patients and therapists), and all were recruited from a single geographical area. Without a control group, the magnitude of the improvements and benefits reported cannot be objectively measured. The variation in regimens prescribed is also a confounding factor and mitigates against the formulation of robust clinical practice guidelines at this point.

5. Conclusion

This pilot study has found that both patients and therapists perceive many benefits and some barriers to using the SaeboFlex as part of neurological upper-limb rehabilitation. While this study has added to our tentative understanding around how this device could successfully translate into regular practice, far more research is required to build a robust evidence base. Future studies should include data from both patients and therapists to gain a comprehensive understanding of how best to utilize the SaeboFlex and would benefit from being conducted with larger samples which include people who have experienced a range of diagnoses.

Appendix

Qualitative Questions for Patients

(i) Do you have any further comments you would like to make on any of these ways in which the SaeboFlex has affected you?

(ii) Do you think the SaeboFlex helped you to do the things you wanted to do? If yes, how?

(iii) Do you think the SaeboFlex helped you to be more skilled or build your capacities? If yes, how?

(iv) Do you think the SaeboFlex changed your hopes and aspirations – you view of what you might become? If so, how?

(v) Do you think using the SaeboFlex helped you to belong – to participate in relationships with others and in your community? If so, how?

(vi) Do you have any other comments you'd like to make about the SaeboFlex, or the way it was used in your rehabilitation?

Competing Interests

The authors declare that there is no conflict of interests regarding the publication of this paper.

References

[1] H. B. Hoffman and G. L. Blakey, "New design of dynamic orthoses for neurological conditions," *NeuroRehabilitation*, vol. 28, no. 1, pp. 55–61, 2011.

[2] J. F. Farrell, H. B. Hoffman, J. L. Snyder, C. A. Giuliani, and R. W. Bohannon, "Orthotic aided training of the paretic upper limb in chronic stroke: results of a phase 1 trial," *NeuroRehabilitation*, vol. 22, no. 2, pp. 99–103, 2007.

[3] S. Davenport, "Recovery within grasp? A report on a preliminary study investigating the short and medium term effects of the SaeboFlex (Functional Tone Management System) on chronic post stroke patients with residual upper limb deficit," *Synapse*, pp. 12–15, 2005.

[4] J. G. Barry, S. Saabye, D. Baker, J. Fogarty, and K. Beck, "Effects of the saeboflex® orthosis and a home exercise program on upper extremity recovery in individuals with chronic," *Journal of Neurologic Physical Therapy*, vol. 30, no. 4, p. 207, 2006.

[5] A. Gollega, S. Renton, and S. Dezall, "SAEBOFLEX—innovative technique to improve arm function following acquired brain injury," *Stroke: Journal of the American Heart Association*, vol. 43, pp. e115–e162, 2012.

[6] R. A. Stuck, L. M. Marshall, and R. Sivakumar, "Feasibility of SaeboFlex upper-limb training in acute stroke rehabilitation: a clinical case series," *Occupational Therapy International*, vol. 21, no. 3, pp. 108–114, 2014.

[7] J. Bomia, N. Helmkamp, and S. Lyons, "Stroke rehabilitation evolves. New strategies, improved outcomes," *Rehab Management*, vol. 20, no. 10, 2007.

[8] C. Ghan, "Dynamic therapy: OTs study success of stroke rehab tool," *The Touchstone*, 2009.

[9] A. M. Cook and J. M. Polgar, *Cook and Husseys' Assistive Technologies*, Mosby, 4th edition, 2013.

[10] L. Demers, M. Monette, Y. Lapierre, D. L. Arnold, and C. Wolfson, "Reliability, validity and applicability of the Quebec user evaluation of satisfaction with assistive technology

(QUEST 2.0) for adults with multiple sclerosis," *Disability and Rehabilitation*, vol. 24, no. 1–3, pp. 21–30, 2002.

[11] H. Day and J. Jutai, "Measuring the psychosocial impact of assistive devices; The PIADS," *Canadian Journal of Rehabilitation*, vol. 9, no. 2, pp. 159–168, 1996.

[12] H. Day, J. Jutai, and K. A. Campbell, "Development of a scale to measure the psychosocial impact of assistive devices: lessons learned and the road ahead," *Disability & Rehabilitation*, vol. 24, no. 1–3, pp. 31–37, 2002.

[13] A. A. Wilcock, *The Occupational Perspective of Health*, SLACK, 2nd edition, 2006.

[14] D. Hitch, G. Pépin, and K. Stagnitti, "In the footsteps of Wilcock, Part one: the evolution of doing, being, becoming, and belonging," *Occupational Therapy in Health Care*, vol. 28, no. 3, pp. 231–246, 2014.

[15] T. C. Hoffmann, P. P. Glasziou, I. Boutron et al., "Better reporting of interventions: template for intervention description and replication (TIDieR) checklist and guide," *BMJ*, vol. 348, Article ID g1687, 2014.

[16] A. Soundy, B. Stubbs, P. Freeman, P. Coffee, and C. Roskell, "Factors influencing patients' hope in stroke and spinal cord injury: a narrative review," *International Journal of Therapy & Rehabilitation*, vol. 21, no. 5, pp. 210–218, 2014.

Massage and Storytelling Reduce Aggression and Improve Academic Performance in Children Attending Elementary School

Lia Lopes Gonçalves, Mariana Callil Voos, Maria Helena Morgani de Almeida, and Fátima Aparecida Caromano

Department of Physical Therapy, Speech Therapy and Occupational Therapy Rehabilitation Sciences Post Graduation Program, Medical School, University of São Paulo, São Paulo, SP, Brazil

Correspondence should be addressed to Mariana Callil Voos; ftmarivoos@gmail.com and Fátima Aparecida Caromano; caromano@usp.br

Academic Editor: Claudia Hilton

Background. Aggressive behaviors must be addressed in elementary schools. Massage and storytelling can be strategies to deal with aggression because both involve experience exchange and social interaction. Both can decrease stress and anxiety and increase self-esteem. *Objective.* To evaluate the effect of two interventions (massage and storytelling) on aggressive behaviors and academic performance of elementary school children. *Method.* Three groups ($n = 35$ children in each group) of the second grade participated (aged 6.5–8.1 years). One group received ten extra classes of massage (MG), another group received extra classes of storytelling (SG), and the control group received extra classes of random subjects (CG). Extra classes lasted for 50 minutes, once a week. Aggressive behaviors were recorded on diaries, by the teachers and the coordinator. The frequency of aggressive behaviors and the academic performance of MG, SG, and CG were observed for six months and the groups were compared. *Findings.* ANOVAs evidenced that MG and SG, but not CG, showed a reduction in aggressive behaviors registered by the teachers and coordinator, after the intervention. Academic performance of MG and SC improved after the intervention ($p < 0.05$).

1. Introduction

Aggressive behavior for elementary school children is expressed as physical or verbal aggression [1–3]. Aggressive behaviors may be related to personal characteristics (e.g., lack of coping strategies, anxiety, depression, low intelligence coefficient, and attention deficits) and/or environmental factors (e.g., school performance pressures and competitions, peer relationship, and family issues) [1, 4, 5]. Aggressive behaviors in elementary schools instigate teacher-student conflicts and peer rejection and represent the primary reason for suspensions and expulsions. Children showing aggressive behaviors are more likely to face difficulties in learning and establishing positive relationships with teachers and classmates [1, 4].

Aggression in children aged up to three years is associated with difficulty communicating their needs to their parents, caregivers, and other children. For older children, between the ages of four and eight, such behaviors are related to difficulty learning appropriate, nonaggressive ways of communicating when faced with a difficult situation [3, 6, 7]. Other factors that may be associated with aggressive behaviors are family difficulties; learning disorders, such as dyslexia; neurological or behavioral disorders, for example, attention deficit/hyperactivity disorder and/or oppositional defiant disorder; emotional trauma, such as domestic violence or sexual abuse; and exposure to violent television shows and movies [8].

Studies about aggression usually focus on the children and their families, and little attention is given to school environment contingencies. Preventive actions against aggressive behaviors must be based on multidisciplinary approaches discussing values, lifestyle, and citizenship. Health promotion in schools is a current concern. An effective school health program can be one of the most cost effective investments a nation can make to simultaneously improve education and health [9].

School health programs aim to improve students' quality of life by promoting education and health and by offering disease prevention and coping with vulnerabilities that may compromise development [9]. Increased attention has been placed on the promotion of students' social and emotional competence to overcome poor academic motivation, dropouts, bullying/aggression, and mental health problems [4–6, 10, 11].

School engagement depends on several factors, such as behavioral engagement (participation in academic and nonacademic activities at school with positive conduct), emotional, and cognitive engagement [6]. Actions can address behavioral engagement in various ways, focusing on participation in academics (homework) and school-related extracurricular activities and motivating positive conduct (e.g., following classroom rules, cooperating with peers during classes) [12, 13].

Children's lack of behavioral engagement is associated with increased academic failure in elementary, middle, and high school (e.g., [13]). Negative developmental pathways of child-reported behavioral engagement have been associated with increased internalizing (e.g., anxiety and depression) and externalizing (e.g., aggression, delinquency, and drug abuse) behaviors [4, 14]. The cause of aggressive behaviors may be due to self-defense, being placed in a stressful situation, lack of routine, extreme frustration or anger, inadequate speech development, overstimulation or exhaustion, lack of adult supervision, and mirroring the aggressive behaviors of other children [1, 2, 15].

Massage can be practiced at school as a strategy to minimize aggressive behaviors [16, 17]. Touching and being touched are key actions in human development that increase body awareness, relax muscles, and promote physical, motor, neurological, and intellectual development. Touch enables the generation of mental images, emotions, and feelings and produces metabolic and physiological changes, especially in the immune, endocrine, neuromuscular, and cardiac systems [18, 19].

Currently, research about the benefits of massage in children focuses on attention, learning, immune function, bonding, self-esteem, body perception, and social/emotional/motor behavior [16–19]. The findings support massage as a resource of physical, emotional, and social health promotion. However, these studies are methodologically limited and rarely carried out at schools [17, 19].

Another strategy that can improve social behavior is storytelling. It encourages written and oral communication, promotes better bonding between teachers and children, and facilitates the comprehension, control, and expression of thoughts and feelings. Storytelling can be a recreational, educational, instructional, and emotional strategy to work with children. It broadens the social, cultural, and intellectual repertoires and helps to reduce stress and anxiety [20]. Storytelling promotes joy and confidence, as it instills virtues in children and makes them aware of their culture and other cultures. It enhances verbal proficiency and improves attention, concentration, creativity, imagination, and memory [21].

Both massage and storytelling promote confidence, relaxation, well-being, empowerment, and socialization. Both can improve attention and concentration and optimize respect, self-caring, affection, and perception. Based on these facts, this study aimed to evaluate the effect of massage and storytelling in aggressive behaviors at school and academic performance of elementary school children.

2. Method

2.1. Participants. This study was approved by the Research Ethics Committee of the Medical School of University of São Paulo (process number 11369). Students from the second grade of a public elementary school of São Paulo (n = 105), aged 6.5 to 8.1 years (mean age 7.4, SD 0.4), 56 boys and 49 girls, participated. Fifty-two were declared as mulatto, 22 as black, and 31 as white, according to the enrollment file, filled by parents. Three classes of students were attending the second year of elementary school in a public school in the city of São Paulo. The classrooms were randomly assigned to have 10 classes of massage (MG), storytelling (SG), or a random extra class of a curricular discipline (CG). All parents were informed about the study and gave informed consent prior to participation.

The school enrolled children between 3 and 14 years old. School time lasted for four hours and a half per day (Monday to Friday). Four hours were spent with regular classes and they had a 30-minute break. They practiced sports in the physical education classes, three times a week for 45 minutes. Experts in arts and music also gave 45 minutes classes in the regular curriculum, once a week each class. Children belonged to low-income families and lived near the school. Students received daily snacks in break time and powdered milk to take home monthly, school supplies, and uniforms. Only children who attended at least 85% of classes received the powdered milk to take home, which is part of a Brazilian program to reduce school evasion. In the present study, no children evaded school during data collection.

A typical school year in Brazil includes classes from March to June, one month winter holidays in July, and classes from August to November. Children may also have one or two weeks in February and December, but mostly for adaptation (February) and finalization (December) activities.

2.2. Massage Group. The teacher of MG was trained by the researcher for 4 hours, prior to the beginning of the massage classes. During the massage classes, children were randomly assigned in pairs. Each child sat facing his or her assigned partner, and massage techniques were demonstrated by the teacher. Children wore cotton T-shirts and performed the massage maneuvers on each other, on shoulders, arms, hands, and scalp. Classes lasted for 50 minutes, weekly, always in the same day of the week. After the first class, every day, before the snack break, children were asked to practice the massage with randomly determined pairs, for 10 minutes, being 5 minutes to give and 5 to receive massage.

2.3. Storytelling Group. The teacher of SG was trained by the researcher for 4 hours, before giving the storytelling classes. A list of fifteen books was selected, based on the age of participating children. The books approached the themes friendship, family, reflecting about relationships, expressing feelings, respecting differences, working cooperatively, imagination and creativity, health, empathy, environment, culture, science, philosophy, history, and geography.

The weekly storytelling classes lasted for 50 minutes and were always scheduled on the same day of the week. Every week, students chose one book from three offered by the teacher. Children sat in circle, on cushions, and the teacher told the story. Children could ask questions and make comments during the class. Every day, before the snack break, children were asked to retell the story of the week to a randomly determined pair, for 10 minutes, being 5 minutes to listen and 5 to tell the story.

2.4. Control Group. Students chose one of the regular disciplines (Portuguese, History, Geography, Mathematics, Physical and Biological Sciences, Physical Education, Arts, and Music) to have a 50-minute extra class. A teacher gave the class and children were free to ask questions and comments. The extra class was given weekly, always in the same day of the week. After the first class, every day, before the snack break, children were asked to recall the subject of the week with a randomly determined pair, for 10 minutes, being 5 minutes to listen and 5 to explain the subject.

2.5. Aggressive Behaviors Registering. Prior to the interventions, the teachers of the three participating groups and the coordinator were trained for eight hours by another researcher (not the same who gave instructions about massage and storytelling classes) to register on a diary the episodes of verbal or physical aggression, based on the observation of students and on parents' complaints. The records were performed for four months: two months before and two months after the interventions. The teachers were instructed to write one or two paragraphs reporting each observed incident. They had twenty minutes to perform this task daily. The teachers were not informed about the hypothesis/aims of the present study.

After that, an examiner, blind to the teachers, groups, interventions, and objectives of the study, read the diaries and filled the chart of aggressive behaviors, with tic marcs. Examples of aggressive behaviors were provided for this examiner as follows.

Examples of Aggressive Behaviors, Given to the Teachers Prior to Data Collection

Verbal Aggression

- Gossiping
- Mimicking
- Name calling
- Posting rumors/ embarrassing information
- Sending hurtful e-mails
- Teasing
- Threatening
- Yelling

Physical Aggression

- Biting
- Hitting
- Kicking
- Pulling one's hair
- Punching
- Pushing
- Spitting

Other Types of Aggression

- Breaking one's objects
- Posting embarrassing pictures or videos
- Taking one's objects

2.6. Academic Performance. Considering all curricular disciplines given (Portuguese, History, Geography, Mathematics, Physical and Biological Sciences, Physical Education, Arts, and Music), a mean grade was calculated for each child and then, for each group. The performance on disciplines was evaluated by exams in the last week of April (before intervention) and September (after intervention). The means of the three groups were compared before and after the intervention.

2.7. Data Analysis. The numbers of registers of aggressive behaviors made by the teachers and the coordinator and the mean grades of the groups showed normal distributions and were compared by analyses of variance (ANOVA for repeated measures and post hoc Tukey tests). Alfa was set as < 0.05. We selected the periods of observation April/May and September/October and the period of intervention June/August. We believed that children would be less influenced by the beginning and the end of the school year in these periods. In the beginning of school year (February/March), children may need some time to know each other and to adapt to the routine and group. In the end, they may be worried about the final exams (November/December). The research protocol is represented in Figure 1.

3. Results

3.1. Teachers and Coordinator's Observations. Analyses of variance compared the number of episodes of aggressive behaviors registered by the teachers and the coordinator on their diaries during the period before and after the interventions. We found a significant interaction between groups and periods, with $F_{2,117} = 23.49$; $p < 0.001$; effect size = 0.287. The post hoc Tukey test showed that the number

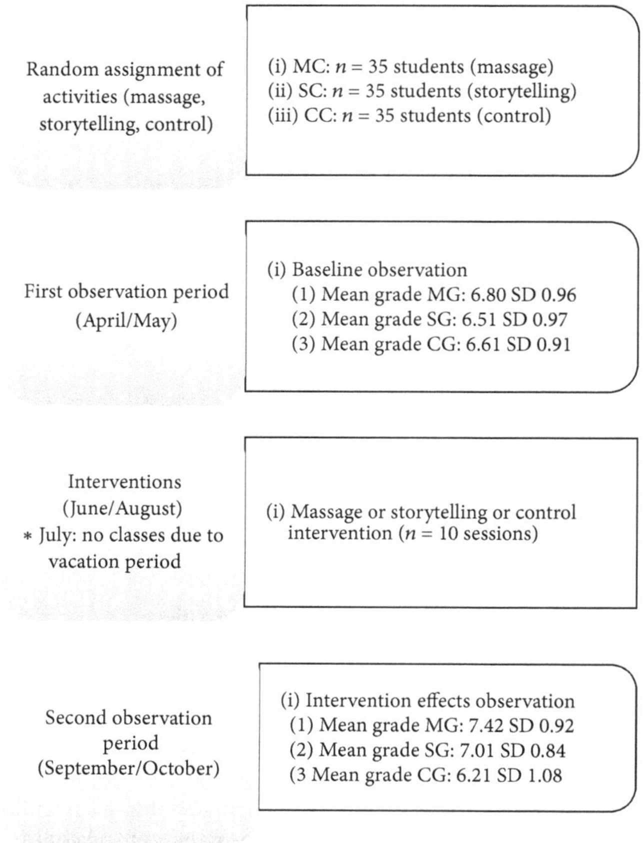

FIGURE 1: Research protocol.

of episodes of aggressive behaviors was significantly lower in MG ($p < 0.001$) and SG ($p = 0.002$) compared to the CG after the interventions (Figure 2).

Both teacher and coordination's records showed a reduction in the number of aggressive behaviors after the intervention and the teacher's records reached statistical significance (MG: 1.5 registers per student before the intervention to 0.5 registers per student after the intervention; SG: 1.4 registers per student before the intervention to 0.8 registers per student after the intervention).

3.2. Academic Performance. Analyses of variance compared the mean grades of each group during the period before and after the interventions. We found a significant interaction between groups and periods, with $F2,117 = 10.19$; $p < 0.001$; $\eta = 0.149$. The post hoc Tukey test showed that the mean grade was significantly higher in the MG ($p = 0.038$) and SG ($p = 0.045$) compared to the CG after the interventions (Figure 3).

The mean grade of MG was 6.8 before the intervention and 7.4 after the intervention. This group had the highest mean grade in the period studied, exceeding the expectation of school. The mean grade of the SG increased from 6.5, before the intervention, to 7.0, after the intervention.

4. Discussion

This study showed that classes of massage and storytelling reduced the number of aggressive behaviors and improved academic performance in 6–8-year-old-students attending elementary school. After the intervention period, we found a reduction in the number of types of verbal/physical aggression, meetings with the coordination due to inappropriate behavior, and parental complaints in the MG and SG groups.

The interventions of massage and storytelling provided benefits for children, as observed in the study by Powell and Potter [16], who showed that fifteen meetings in six months, with relaxation, yoga, and interactive games, reduced helplessness and aggression. Aggressive behaviors can be addressed in 6–8-year-old children by interventions that emphasize a positive model, of respect and affection [4]. Conversely, punishments and authoritarian relationships between children, teachers, and caregivers may not have such beneficial effects [6]. Besides, activities based on adults' expectancies may lead to aggression, as a form of resistance to frustration and academic failure.

Diversified educational interventions have implemented teaching and learning and have showed beneficial results. Approaches that promote the reflection and the understanding about new contents and experiences usually facilitate teaching and learning processes. Teachers can promote a higher interaction with and between the students. When students adopt a more active and protagonist posture, they can also detect and verbalize their needs and difficulties, as well as their possibilities and availabilities. Relationships at school can become a positive model of interaction and modify other relationships. Students can become more confident to express how they feel and to show more empathic and helpful behaviors.

4.1. The Beneficial Effects of Massage. Massage reduced the number of aggressive behaviors and improved academic performance in 6–8-year-old students attending elementary school. Massage affects the interaction with colleagues, extending friends networks. It increases the confidence to deal with vulnerabilities [16, 17, 19]. Touching and being touched involve acceptance and trust, exchange of physical experiences, and awareness of others. Opposite, cultures with rules and prohibitions may affect people's physical contact behavior and its benefits. Massage allows the experience of physically interacting with another person in the situation of being cared. Children experienced the situation of being the caregiver and providing something positive for someone else [17, 19].

Children aged 6–8 years are transitioning to the concrete operational stage, according to Piaget's theory of cognitive development [22]. This stage is characterized by the elimination of egocentrism, which is the inability to understand a perspective other than one's own. During this stage, the child acquires the ability to view things from another individual's perspective, even if they think that perspective is incorrect, which is practiced in massage classes. Therefore, massage contributes for this development stage.

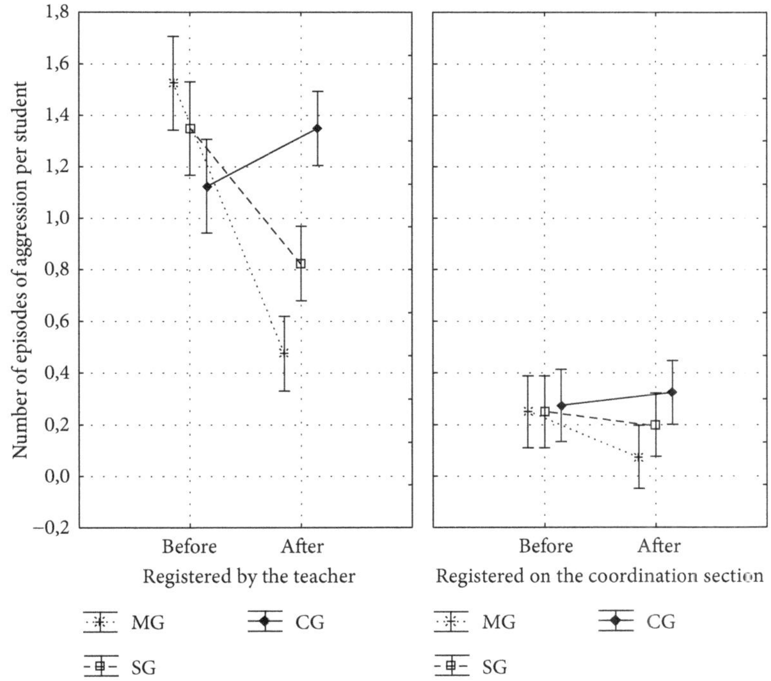

FIGURE 2: Records of teachers and coordination register books, in which aggression episodes involving students and students and parents complaints are registered. Before the intervention: observations from April/May were analyzed. After the intervention: observations from September/October were analyzed.

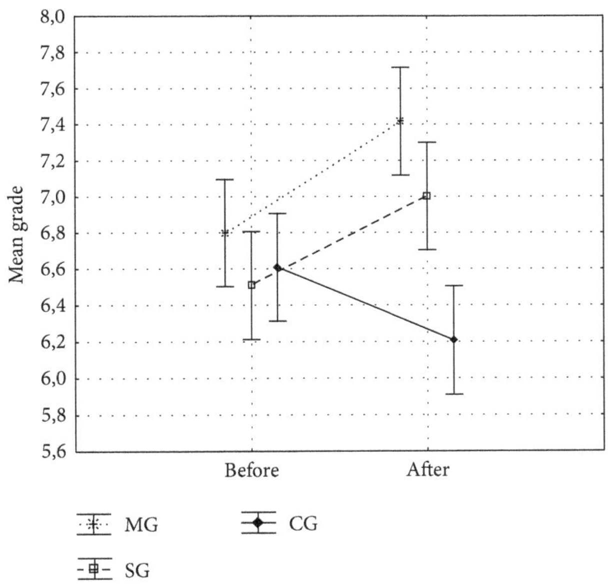

FIGURE 3: Mean grade obtained by each group before and after the intervention. Before the intervention: the exams of the last week of April were considered. After the intervention: the exams of the last week of September were considered.

4.2. The Beneficial Effects of Storytelling. Storytelling reduced the number of aggressive behaviors and improved academic performance in 6–8-year-old students attending elementary school. Children of SG showed improvement in social behavior. Our findings are in agreement with the ones reported in the literature, showing that storytelling decreases anxiety and provides joy, confidence, and relaxation [10, 20]. Storytelling stimulates creativity, language, and memory, promoting the healthy development and coping processes in situations of social disorganization or illness [21].

Children aged 6–8 years are in the transition to the concrete operational stage, according to Piaget's theory of cognitive development [22]. This stage is characterized by the appropriate use of logic, with thoughts more mature and "adult like," which can be extensively practiced in storytelling. Telling and retelling stories provide children projection and introspection, inspired by the struggles of the characters, fighting their battles and enjoying the pleasure of defeating giants and monsters. These projections can improve empathic and cooperative behaviors and reduce aggression.

To sum up, both massage and storytelling seemed to facilitate interpersonal connection. Both approaches seemed to improve not only self-caring and self-regulation, but also affection, empathy, and respect. Such changes impacted positively in social behavior and academic performance at school.

4.3. Other Impacts on the Community. We found teachers who were motivated and available to continue with the massage and storytelling classes. The activities were offered to all students aged 5–9 years as extra classes, after the postintervention observation period.

Teachers of Physical Education and Portuguese became engaged in organizing massage and storytelling activities, respectively. We believe that this action is the result of the interest of teachers in children's mental health, which contributes to the humanization of educational processes. Massage and storytelling can act in line with educational goals, as a way of approaching collaborative and motivating new educational projects.

Children who exhibit high rates of conduct problems at school often experience chronic difficulties in both academic and social domains. Many of these students come from a background of early adversity (poverty, family instability, parenting difficulties, and violence exposure) [1, 6, 23]. The high rate of school failure and dropout experienced by students with conduct problems, compared with other students with disabilities, underscores the difficulties schools face in serving these children effectively [6]. For this reason, strategies with positive effects on aggressive behaviors are important to assure better social and academic development of elementary school children and teachers.

4.4. Limitations. Although teachers were not informed about the hypothesis and aims of the present study, they may have made some inferences correlating massage, storytelling, and aggressive behaviors. We had to keep the same teachers giving the extra class and assessing aggressive behaviors of each group (one teacher for MG, another for SG, and another for CG), due to professional/time unavailability. Another limitation is that we could not randomly assign the students to the groups. Also, evaluating only one (public) school is a limitation, because children living in different social contexts were not compared.

4.5. Future Studies. Future studies should assess larger samples and interview parents about possible beneficial effects of massage and storytelling outside school environment.

5. Conclusion

Interventions with massage and storytelling seemed to affect behavior and academic performance positively in 6–8-year-old children from an elementary public school of São Paulo, Brazil. These strategies should be explored as children's education and health promotion approaches.

Additional Points

Relevance to Clinical Practice. Massage and storytelling positively seemed to affect the behavior and academic performance of elementary school children. *Limitations.* Although we followed 105 children, only one public school participated in the study. *Recommendations for Future Research.* To investigate the impacts of massage and/or storytelling in longer follow-ups and other age ranges.

Competing Interests

All authors state that they have no conflict of interests.

References

[1] Y.-G. Yoo, D.-J. Lee, I.-S. Lee et al., "The effects of mind subtraction meditation on depression, social anxiety, aggression, and salivary cortisol levels of elementary school children in South Korea," *Journal of Pediatric Nursing*, vol. 31, no. 3, pp. e185–e197, 2016.

[2] P. Reebye, "Aggression during early years: infancy and preschool," *The Canadian Child and Adolescent Psychiatry Review*, vol. 5, no. 14, pp. 16–20, 2005.

[3] D. Murray-Close and J. M. Ostrov, "A longitudinal study of forms and functions of aggressive behavior in early childhood," *Child Development*, vol. 80, no. 3, pp. 828–842, 2009.

[4] J. Bae, H. Park, and M. Yang, "Effects of a self-discovery program for ego resilience, self-esteem, stress and depression in elementary school students," *Journal of Korean Academy of Psychiatric and Mental Health Nursing*, vol. 21, no. 3, p. 210, 2012.

[5] H. S. Ez-Elarab, S. M. Sabbour, M. A. Gadallah, and T. A. Asaad, "Prevalence and risk factors of violence among elementary school children in Cairo," *Journal of the Egyptian Public Health Association*, vol. 82, no. 1-2, pp. 127–146, 2007.

[6] S. De Laet, H. Colpin, E. Vervoort et al., "Developmental trajectories of children's behavioral engagement in late elementary school: both teachers and peers matter," *Developmental Psychology*, vol. 51, no. 9, pp. 1292–1306, 2015.

[7] S. Fossum, B. H. Handegård, M. Martinussen, and W. T. Mørch, "Psychosocial interventions for disruptive and aggressive behaviour in children and adolescents: a meta-analysis," *European Child and Adolescent Psychiatry*, vol. 17, no. 7, pp. 438–451, 2008.

[8] American Academy of Child and Adolescent Psychiatry, *Facts for Families: Conduct Disorders*, 2004, http://aacap.org/aacap/families_and_youth/facts_for_families/fff-guide/Conduct-Disorder-033.aspx.

[9] World Health Organization, March 2016, http://www.who.int/school_youth_health/en/.

[10] K. A. Schonert-Reichl, E. Oberle, M. S. Lawlor et al., "Enhancing cognitive and social-emotional development through a simple-to-administer mindfulness-based school program for elementary school children: a randomized controlled trial," *Developmental Psychology*, vol. 51, no. 1, pp. 52–66, 2015.

[11] S. Woods and D. Wolke, "Direct and relational bullying among primary school children and academic achievement," *Journal of School Psychology*, vol. 42, no. 2, pp. 135–155, 2004.

[12] M.-T. Wang and J. S. Eccles, "Social support matters: longitudinal effects of social support on three dimensions of school engagement from middle to high school," *Child Development*, vol. 83, no. 3, pp. 877–895, 2012.

[13] B. Wonglorsaichon, S. Wongwanich, and N. Wiratchai, "The influence of students school engagement on learning achievement: a structural equation modeling analysis," *Procedia—Social and Behavioral Sciences*, vol. 116, pp. 1748–1755, 2014.

[14] Y. Li and R. M. Lerner, "Trajectories of school engagement during adolescence: implications for grades, depression, delinquency, and substance use," *Developmental Psychology*, vol. 47, no. 1, pp. 233–247, 2011.

[15] D. Nesdale, E. Milliner, A. Duffy, and J. A. Griffiths, "Group membership, group norms, empathy, and young children's intentions to aggress," *Aggressive Behavior*, vol. 35, no. 3, pp. 244–258, 2009.

[16] L. Powell and L. Potter, "Report on an intervention involving massage and yoga for male adolescents attending a school

for disadvantaged male adolescents in the UK," *International Journal of Special Education*, vol. 25, no. 2, pp. 47–54, 2010.

[17] S. Beider, N. E. Mahrer, and J. I. Gold, "Pediatric massage therapy: an overview for clinicians," *Pediatric Clinics of North America*, vol. 54, no. 6, pp. 1025–1041, 2007.

[18] A. Slominski and J. Wortsman, "Neuroendocrinology of the skin," *Endocrine Reviews*, vol. 21, no. 5, pp. 457–487, 2000.

[19] A.-L. Von Knorring, A. Söderberg, L. Austin, and K. Uvnäs-Moberg, "Massage decreases aggression in preschool children: a long-term study," *Acta Paediatrica*, vol. 97, no. 9, pp. 1265–1269, 2008.

[20] T. A. Amabile, *Growing Up Creative*, The Creative Education Foundation Press, Buffalo, NY, USA, 1989.

[21] R. Isbell, J. Sobol, L. Lindauer, and A. Lowrance, "The effects of storytelling and story reading on the oral language complexity and story comprehension of young children," *Early Childhood Education Journal*, vol. 32, no. 3, pp. 157–163, 2004.

[22] J. Piaget, "The role of action in the development of thinking," in *Knowledge and Development*, pp. 17–42, Springer, New York, NY, USA, 1977.

[23] C. J. Powers, K. L. Bierman, and D. L. Coffman, "Restrictive educational placements increase adolescent risks for students with early-starting conduct problems," *The Journal of Child Psychology and Psychiatry*, vol. 57, no. 8, pp. 899–908, 2016.

9

Everyday Activities for Children with Mitochondrial Disorder

Marieke Lindenschot[1,2,3,4] **Imelda J. M. de Groot**[4] **Saskia Koene,**[5] **Ton Satink,**[2,3,6] **Esther M. J. Steultjens,**[2,3] **and Maria W. G. Nijhuis-van der Sanden**[1,4]

[1]*Department IQ Healthcare, Research Institute for Health Sciences, Radboud University Medical Center Nijmegen, Postbus 9101, 6500 HB Nijmegen, Netherlands*
[2]*Department of Occupational Therapy, HAN University of Applied Sciences, Postbus 6960, 6503 GL Nijmegen, Netherlands*
[3]*Research Group Neurorehabilitation, HAN University of Applied Sciences, Nijmegen, Netherlands*
[4]*Department of Rehabilitation, Donders Center for Neuroscience, Radboud University Medical Center Nijmegen, Postbus 9101, 6500 HB Nijmegen, Netherlands*
[5]*Department of Pediatrics, Radboud Center for Mitochondrial Medicine, Radboud University Medical Center Nijmegen, Geert Grooteplein Zuid 10, 6525 GA Nijmegen, Netherlands*
[6]*European Masters of Science in Occupational Therapy, Amsterdam University of Applied Sciences, Amsterdam, Netherlands*

Correspondence should be addressed to Marieke Lindenschot; marieke.lindenschot@radboudumc.nl

Academic Editor: Jodie A. Copley

Background. Engagement in everyday activities is important for the health and wellbeing of children. Children with mitochondrial disorders have impaired energy production leading to limitations in activity. It is unknown which activities these children perform and if the nature of activities of low-functioning children differs from average-functioning children. Therefore, this pilot study explored the activities reported in patient records of a heterogeneous group of children with genetically confirmed mitochondrial disorders. *Methods.* A retrospective qualitative directed content analysis by health care professionals reported activities (as part of their professional reasoning obligations) in hospital patient records of children with mitochondrial disorder. *Results.* Seventeen patient records, presenting notes on capacities and performed activities, showed an overview of everyday activities that covered the categories: self-care, house chores, therapy, school, computing, hobby, play, sports, and mobility/ transport. The activity categories of low-functioning children did not differ from average-functioning children, although descriptions of specific activities differed between groups. *Conclusion.* This pilot exploration indicates that the types of activities that children with mitochondrial disorders perform are not necessarily linked to the child's impairments. However, differences in levels of independence, assistive device usage, and energy costs seem to exist. Future research should address the child's perspective on, and meaning of, activity performances.

1. Introduction

Performing everyday activities is viewed as an important factor for the wellbeing of an individual and is an important determinant of health [1–3]. If children are unable to be engaged in everyday activities, they do not have the opportunity to explore their environment and are less able to grow up as unique individuals [4]. Although children with disabilities might enjoy the same activities and have similar desires as their healthy developing peers [5, 6], they can experience limitations in activities, leading to restrictions in their participation in daily life.

Mitochondrial disorders, with an estimated prevalence of 23 in 100,000, are one of the most common inherited errors of metabolism [7]. Mitochondrial disorders can be caused by mutation of genes encoded by either nuclear DNA (nDNA) or mitochondrial DNA (mtDNA) [8]. Mutations have been identified in more than 230 different genes [8, 9], and the number of identified genes associated with mitochondrial disorder is continuously increasing [10]. This genetic heterogeneity is also reflected in the clinical phenotypes associated with mitochondrial disorder, with a large range of symptoms and impairments [11–13]. It was previously found that children (when we talk about children in this article, we mean children and adolescents in the age of 0–18 years) with mitochondrial disorders are less physically active and engage less in vigorous activities compared to healthy peers [14]. Children with a mitochondrial disorder experience these limitations in performing everyday activities due to motor and cognitive impairments including muscle weakness, balance problems, concentration problems, and intellectual disability [13]. These impairments have consequences for daily living activities and participation. The extent of perceived limitations in activities and participation of children with mitochondrial disorders varies from none to extremely high [13]. While some children remain in a mainstream school and achieve normal milestones, others barely interact with their environment [15].

Although literature states that children with mitochondrial disorder experience limitations in activities, a clear overview of their everyday activities is lacking. It is commonly expected that the nature of activities differs based on the global functioning of the child. Knowledge of these possible differences and similarities is important to choose or develop assessments for this population, to evaluate the outcome of treatment on participation, and to be able to tailor the assessments and treatment to the child's and parent's specific wishes. As healthcare professionals make clinical decisions based on information about the child's capacities and activities, we expect that information concerning the activities of the child is reported in patient records. Therefore, this pilot study is aimed at exploring which everyday activities of children with genetically confirmed mitochondrial disorders are reported in patient records by health care professionals and understanding the profile of activities these children participate in.

2. Methods

A retrospective chart review [16, 17] was performed. A directed content analysis [18] was used to explore which everyday activities were reported in patient records and to explore if they differed among the functional profiles of the children.

2.1. Participants. The participants of this study were children (0–18 years) with a genetically confirmed mitochondrial disorder who were periodically evaluated in the so-called "MitoRoute," a multidisciplinary, medical, and allied health care screening program at Radboud Center for Mitochondrial Medicine (RCMM), Radboud University Medical Center (Radboudumc), Nijmegen. During MitoRoute, the children were evaluated by a team consisting of several physicians of different disciplines and allied health professionals, including a physical therapist, occupational therapist, speech therapist, dietitian, social worker, and psychologist. The goal of this screening program was to establish a detailed overview of the consequences of the disorder for the child on different dimensions of the International Classification of Functioning, Disability and Health for Children and Youth (ICF-CY) [19], to prevent and detect possible complications and formulate treatment advice. The patient records of all children with a genetically proven mitochondrial disorder who were screened from May 2015 to May 2016 in the Radboudumc were included in this study.

2.2. Data Collection. Qualitative data concerning activities of children with mitochondrial disorders were extracted from clinical notes of (allied) health care professionals (MitoRoute) in the electronic patient records. The patient records contained unprompted written information relevant to the assessment and conversations performed by (allied) health care professionals, as they were not asked to collect data specific to this study.

2.3. Stratification. As motor function, cognitive abilities, and communication influence participation in activities [20, 21], these characteristics were used to construct functional capacity profiles of the children. To ensure the quality of the stratification into the profiles, a log was kept documenting thought processes and tracked decision-making. Member checking with health care professionals was used to verify the profiles. Functional capacities were stratified as the following: *Cognitive development* (based on the age-related norm-referenced test used for each child): 1 = extremely low cognitive functioning, 2 = low cognitive functioning, 3 = average cognitive functioning, and 4 = good cognitive functioning; *Ambulation* (Hoffer scale [22], with the normal ambulation level added by Schoenmakers et al. [23]): 1 = nonambulation, 2 = nonfunctional ambulation, 3 = household ambulation, 4 = community ambulation, and 5 = normal ambulation; and *Speech abilities* (Radboud dysarthria assessment [24]): 1 = no oral communication possible, 2 = communication with a known person, 3 = frequent repetitions (frequently repeating themselves to guarantee that they will be understood), 4 = incidental repetitions, 5 = effective despite small problems, and 6 = effective communication.

Other patient characteristics collected included gender, age, gross motor development (based on norm-referenced tests), performance in daily activities (based on Pediatric Evaluation of Disabilities Inventory (PEDI) [25]), and fatigue (measured with Pediatric Quality of Life Inventory Multidimensional Fatigue Scale (PedsQL-MFS) [26]). These characteristics were not used in defining the profiles but were used as descriptive outcomes linked to each profile.

2.4. Profiles Based on Functional Capacities. Three profiles could be defined based on the functional capacities of the children:

Global low functioning: children with an extremely low or low cognitive developmental level and limited motor functioning which lead to nonfunctional outdoor ambulation and nonfunctional communication.

Low cognitive functioning with a moderate to normal ambulation: children with extremely low or low cognitive developmental level and some limitations in motor functioning but able to have functional ambulation. Speech abilities in this profile differ among the children.

Global moderate functioning: children with average cognitive developmental level and some limitations in motor functioning but able to have functional ambulation. Speech abilities are sufficient to make themselves understandable.

2.5. Data Analysis. In this exploratory study, the method of directed content analysis [18] was used on the text fragments extracted from the patient records [27–29]. The text fragments were focused on information reported by the health care professionals regarding the experiences of children and parents in their daily life situations. Before starting the analysis of the patient records, two preliminary steps were conducted:

(1) Identify the key concept "activity" as initial coding category

(2) Operationalize the concept "activity" using theory

In step 2 of the data analysis, the term "activity" was defined based on the ICF-CY [19] and occupational therapy literature [30–32] as an activity that is the meaningful targeted performance of tasks and/or actions by an individual, like playing guitar, dressing yourself, eating, and cycling.

For the analysis of the patient records, the following steps were conducted by one of the researchers:

(1) Read text and highlight all text that appears to represent activity

(2) Code the highlighted text with codes fitting the concept activity

(3) Categorize the codes into groups of activities

(4) Organize the categories (the different groups of activities) into three occupational performance areas of Reed and Sanderson [33]: personal maintenance, productivity, and leisure

The procedure of the analysis and the result of steps 4 and 6 were peer reviewed by the fourth author (TS).

2.6. Ethical Considerations. The data used in this research were obtained during the medical care for which the child and parents gave approval to use anonymously for research (ethical board approval number 2013-287). Data were deidentified before analysis. The research was conducted conforming to the ethical principles of the Declaration of Helsinki [34].

3. Results

Patient records of seventeen children (five girls and twelve boys) were included. The age of the children varied from 4 to 18 years old. Eight children had a mutation on their nuclear DNA and nine children on mitochondrial DNA. Five children demonstrated a global low-functioning profile, five children demonstrated a low cognitive-functioning profile with a moderate to normal ambulation, and seven children demonstrated a global moderate-functioning profile. The clinical and genetic characteristics of the children are presented in Table 1. More clinically relevant priorities hindered scheduling of the fatigue assessment in two cases. Therefore, they were not available in the chart.

As mentioned before, the activities were organized in three occupational performance areas of Reed and Sanderson: personal maintenance, productivity, and leisure [33]. Personal maintenance activities permit a person to maintain individual life support needs, for example, getting dressed or taking a shower. Productivity activities assist society to facilitate each person to meet individual needs by the use of collective resources, for example, going to work or doing homework. Leisure activities permit the individual to express needs for creative outlet, for example, drawing or swimming [33]. The outcome of step 5 of the analysis was the activity categories: self-care, house chores, therapy, school, computing, hobby, play, sports, and mobility/transport. Some activity categories could be placed under two occupational performance areas as the meaning or value of the activity was not noted. For instance, mobility/transport activities could be performed as personal maintenance but also as leisure. The results, including any double placement, are presented in Figure 1.

3.1. Personal Maintenance. The area under personal maintenance included all the activities that children do to take care of themselves and organize their lives. It comprises the following categories: self-care, house chores, and mobility/transport. Across the three profiles, the (allied) health care professionals reported on all three different categories in personal maintenance. The patient records showed similarities across the profiles in self-care activities like showering, eating, taking rest, and getting dressed. In the category mobility/transport activities, cycling and taking the bus were commonly reported activities. Although in this category and the category house chores, the activities showed more differences among the profiles. The activities varied from doing the dishes to mowing the lawn.

The notes in the patient records indicate that there was a difference in the support or assistance that the children received when they performed the activity. For instance, the activity eating was mentioned as "*she can eat independently*," "*with spreading butter and cutting he gets help*," and "*he uses an eating device which makes him able to move the cutlery independently to his mouth*." In several activities, receiving assistance or using assistive devices or adaptations were mentioned. For instance, getting dressed and showering were mentioned as "with help" or as "independent." Occasionally, no notes about the support or assistance were written.

3.2. Productivity. The area under productivity featured all the activities that children do to learn and work. It included the following categories: school activities and therapy activities. However, therapy activities can also be seen as personal maintenance. Across the three profiles the (allied) health care professionals documented notes that fit within both categories in productivity. Children within the global low-functioning profile all attended to special education, some

Table 1: Clinical and genetic characteristics of the children.

Gender (A)	Age (years)	Level of cognitive development (B)	Level of motor development (C)	Score on Hoffer scale (D)	Level of speech ability (E)	Level of functional abilities of daily activities (F)	Fatigue score (G)	Gene (H)	Mutation
Profile: global low functioning ($N = 5$)									
F	5	1	2	1	4	2	71	*OPA1*	c.910C>T
M	6	1	3	1	1	1	40	*FBXL*	c.1361A>C
M	12	1	2	2	3	2	49	*SDHA*	c.64-2A>G
M	18	1	2	1	3	3	?	*RARS2*	c.442A>G; c.1519G>A
M	18	1	2	3	3	2	49	*ATP6*	m.09176T>C
Profile: low cognitive functioning and moderate to normal ambulation ($N = 5$)									
M	13	2	4	4	6	4	58	*MT-TL1*	m.3243A>G
F	13	1	2	5	5	3	?	*RARS2*	c.442A>G; c.1519G>A
M	14	1	3	5	3	2	49	*MTFMT*	c.626C>T; c.766C>T
M	16	1	3	4	2	3	32	*ATP6*	m.8993T>G
F	17	1	3	5	6	4	54	*MT-TL1*	m.3243A>G
Profile: global moderate functioning ($N = 7$)									
M	4	3	3	4	5	3	65	*TAZ*	c.788_794del
M	4	3	4	4	3	3	72	*ATP6*	m.8993T>G
F	5	3	3	4	6	3	72	*NDUFS7*	c.364G>A
F	5	3	4	4	6	3	39	*MT-TL1*	m.3243A>G
M	7	3	2	4	6	3	66	*ATP6*	m.09185T>C
M	7	3	4	4	6	3	38	*mt-tRNASer*	m.7507A>G
M	13	3	3	4	5	4	58	*MT-TL1*	m.3243A>G
Total									
F: $N = 5$ M: $N = 12$	Range: 4–18	1: $N = 9$ 2: $N = 1$ 3: $N = 7$ 4: $N = 0$	1: $N = 0$ 2: $N = 6$ 3: $N = 7$ 4: $N = 4$ 5: $N = 0$	1: $N = 3$ 2: $N = 1$ 3: $N = 1$ 4: $N = 9$ 5: $N = 3$	1: $N = 1$ 2: $N = 1$ 3: $N = 5$ 4: $N = 1$ 5: $N = 3$ 6: $N = 6$	1: $N = 1$ 2: $N = 2$ 3: $N = 11$ 4: $N = 3$	Range: 32–72 2 unknown		

A: M = male, F = female; B: 1 = extremely low, 2 = low, 3 = average, 4 = good; C: 1 = spasticity, 2 = ataxia, 3 = extremely delayed, 4 = delayed, 5 = normal development; D: 1 = nonambulation, 2 = nonfunctional ambulation, 3 = household ambulation, 4 = community ambulation, 5 = normal ambulation; E: 1 = no oral communication possible, 2 = communication with a known person, 3 = frequent repetitions, 4 = incidental repetitions, 5 = effective despite small problems, 6 = effective communication; F: 1 = not self-independent, 2 = minimal self-independent, 3 = sufficient self-independent, 4 = fully self-independent; G: the higher the score, the better the (by fatigue impacted) health-related quality of life, unknown = missing data; H: OPA1 = optic atrophy 1; FBXL = F-box and leucine-rich repeat proteins; SDHA = succinate dehydrogenase complex, subunit A; RARS2 = arginyl-tRNA synthetase 2; ATP6 = ATP synthase 6; MT-TL1 = mitochondrial tRNA leucine; MTFMT = mitochondrial methionyl-tRNA formyltransferase; TAZ = taffazin; NDUFS7 = NADH-ubiquinone oxidoreductase Fe-S protein 7; mt-tRNASer = mitochondrial tRNA serine.

with training for future work positions: "*He goes to secondary special education, while doing two days of workplace training in an employment center for people with intellectual disabilities.*" Three children from the low cognitive level with a moderate to normal ambulation profile attended to special education, while two children attended to regular education. Two of the children with the global moderate-functioning profile attended to special education, while five attended to regular education. Sometimes, small adaptations were made: "*She goes to regular education, but when she is too tired she stays at home for the afternoon.*" This quote also illustrate that the energy level is used as a deciding factor in performing or avoiding the activity. Notes about the energy level as the deciding factor were present in all occupational performance areas. Although the type of education varied from special to regular education, the range of activities did not differ among the three profiles. Most children attended classes that included writing, spelling, and calculating, as well as physical and/or occupational therapy.

3.3. Leisure. The area under leisure featured all the activities that children do to play or occupy their free time. It included the following categories: computing, hobbies, play, and sports. In each of the three profiles, the (allied) health care

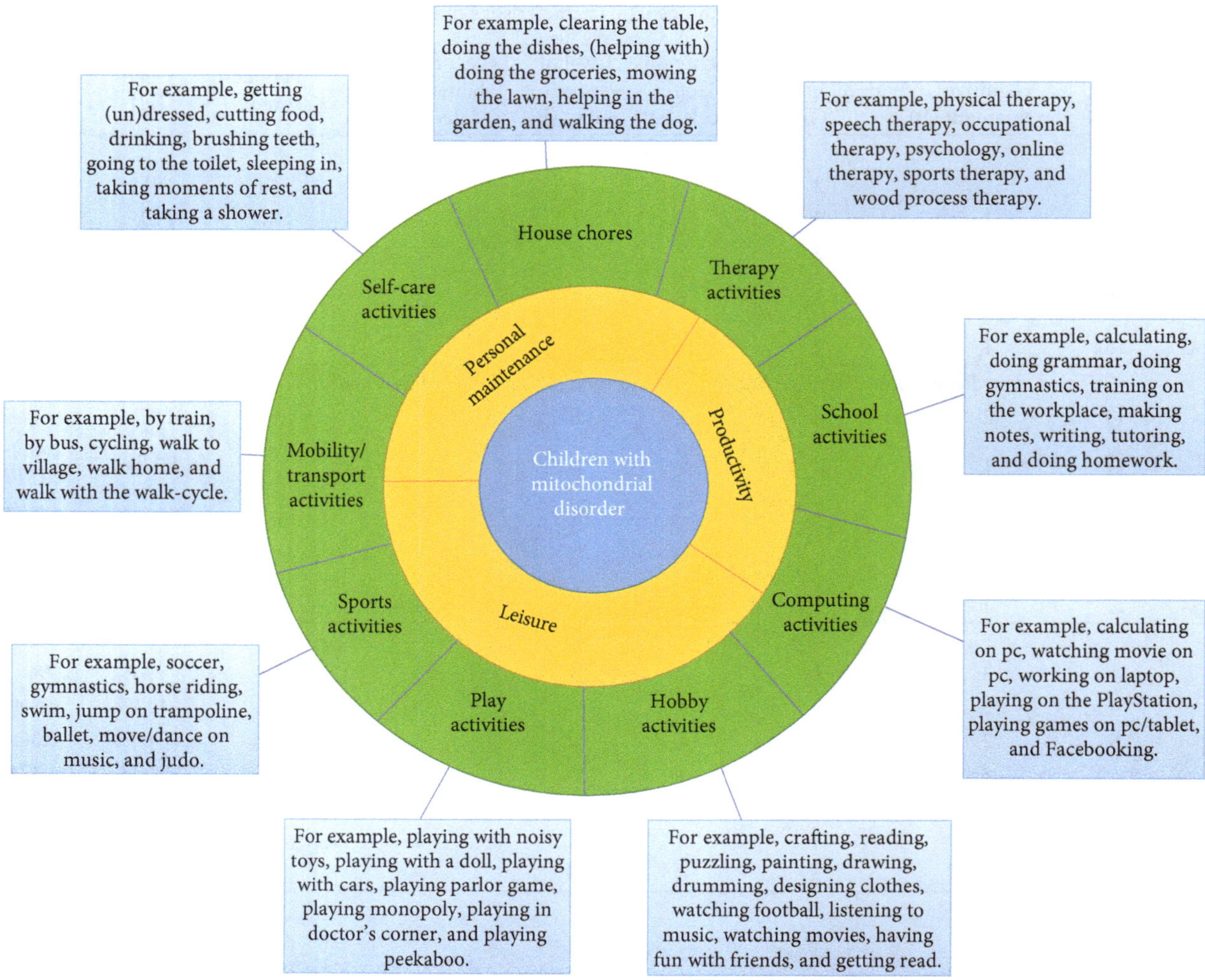

Figure 1: Activities, activity categories, and occupational performance areas of children with mitochondrial disorder.

professionals noted all four different categories in leisure. The physically passive activities were reported more in the global low-functioning profile than the other two profiles. For instance, it was mentioned that: "*After school he is tired and uses his laptop or tablet to play games, uses Facebook or watches movies.*" In the profiles of children with a better ambulation, there were more regular physically active activities, for instance, "*After finishing his homework he usually goes outside and jumps on the trampoline or plays soccer.*" The analysis showed that the children performed individual leisure activities, for example, horse riding, jumping on the trampoline, watching football, or going to Bible study. Some activities were more popular, including swimming, gymnastics, watching television, or a movie.

4. Discussion

This study provides a first overview of the activity categories of children with a mitochondrial disorder. Three occupational performance areas: personal maintenance, productivity, and leisure [33] comprised, as reported by allied health professionals in patient records, nine activity categories: self-care, house chores, therapy, school, computing, hobby, play, sports, and mobility/transport. Contrary to our expectations, we found that all activity categories were present in each global-functioning profile. This is congruent with the guiding principles for children's rehabilitation in the Netherlands, which stipulate that children with disabilities are full participants in everyday life [35].

The activities performed by children with mitochondrial disorders, as identified in this study, resemble the activities of typically developing children identified in the PACS Pediatric Activity Card Sort: the PACS [36], with one exception: "therapy activities". The PACS was developed based on typical activities of childhood that are relevant for all, not only for typically developing children. This means that this instrument has potential for use as an outcome measure for children with mitochondrial disorders. Although the current study did not compare the activities of children with mitochondrial disorders to healthy peers, the results appear to echo the findings of Shields et al. [6] and King et al. [37] who found that there were more similarities than differences in the participation of children with intellectual disabilities and their typically developing peers. The current findings and existing literature emphasize the fact that the type of activities a child engages in is not necessarily linked to the child's disabilities, but the nature of the performance differs.

Within and between the activities, we found diversity in the amount of support or assistance provided and the equipment used among the children to facilitate successful participation. For example, cycling was reported as performed differently, for example, on a regular bike, a walk-cycle or duo bicycle and with guidance or independently. Also, eating was an activity that was reported as performed independently, with help or with an eating device. It can be reasoned that the regular use of the PEDI [25] could have influenced the notes in the patient files as assistive devices or support is measured with this assessment. However, only the occupational therapist used the PEDI, the other (allied) health professionals did not, yet they also reported the amount of assistance or assistive devices. In addition to the notes on independence, there were also notes about energy levels as a deciding factor in performing or avoiding activities. This is not surprising, given that in the professional literature describing the care of children with mitochondrial disorder, fatigue is a frequently mentioned burden [13]. Although the study design did not allow for a comparison between the amount of assistance or adaptations to energy levels in performing activities, there are indications that differences exist in levels of independence, assistive devices, and energy costs across the children. When children have limited abilities or are more dependent, a higher burden is placed on parents to facilitate participation and autonomy [38, 39]. This suggests that future research should focus on the differences in levels of independence and assistive devices in relation to energy costs and caregiver burden.

We found clear activity categories that represent the different activities and could be organized into frequently used occupational performance areas [33] as described in the literature. The activity categories are also consistent with the (sub)domains of the ICF-CY [19]. We organized the activities in categories based on the typical purpose of the activities for children, which best fit the three occupational performance areas of Reed and Sanderson [33]. It was noticed that some activity categories could be linked to more occupational performance areas than others. For instance, computing activities are used to learn or work (productivity) but also for leisure. This supports the idea that the meaning of the activity can be viewed from different perspectives, can differ for each child and that activity categories are not solely linked to a certain occupational performance area [40]. To confirm to which activity categories an activity belongs, we need to gain insight in the perspectives of the children on the individual meaning each activity has for them. The categorization of activities by the children themselves is therefore suitable for use in future research.

Using patient records resulted in some limitations in interpreting the findings. As the written information was unprompted, not every (allied) health professional reported the same information. Another consequence of using patient records is that it was not always clear if the activities that were performed during therapy had a relationship to the activities that the children performed and experienced as meaningful in the daily life situation. For example, "*The child found the pencils and immediately started coloring.*" This note about a test situation in one of the patient records can imply that the child likes to color, but this is disputable. Outcomes of test situations cannot be seen as representative of the child's daily life [41]. In this research, we focused on activity performance, which describes what a person actually does in daily life, expressing the individual's involvement in a life situation [42]. Interviewing the children themselves would provide knowledge about their self-reported activity performance and experience in daily life.

Another limitation of the study is the small sample size and stratification of the sample into three global-functioning profiles. However, the sample size overall is suitable for an exploratory study taking into account the low prevalence of the disease. In each profile, there were even smaller numbers of participants; however, this was necessary to address the difference in functioning levels of the children. Prediction of the activity profile based on the level of impairments in this population is difficult given the unpredictable nature of the condition. Nonetheless, our study showed a large diversity of functional capacities, which indicates that we covered the broad spectrum of impairments and limitations seen in this population [43]. Stratification into the functional capacity profiles enhanced the insight into activity categories of the total study population and each profile separately. Conversely, a selection bias might have occurred because solely reports of children within the specific MitoRoute were included. Pediatricians refer all children with mitochondrial disorder to be screened at the MitoRoute for different reasons (e.g., new diagnosis, two-yearly screening, or a deterioration in the clinical condition). Although not all parents and/or children with mitochondrial disorder agree to participate in the MitoRoute, it is not sure whether and how this will lead to selection bias. Despite this, we think that the findings may provide an overview of activity categories for possibly all children with mitochondrial disorders. Future research should include a representative sample, on all characteristics, of children with mitochondrial disorders.

The clinical implications of the large variation of reported activities found in this study could be that health care professionals need to consider all nine activity categories in their assessment and therapy. In addition, clinicians should consult children on the meaning they attach to an activity to decide on activity category to which it belongs. Furthermore, assessments and interventions should be tailored enough to encompass the diversity in activities performed as seen in the global functional capacity profiles of the children and the individual preferences in performance of activities.

5. Conclusions

This exploratory pilot retrospective chart review gives insight into the everyday activities performed by children with mitochondrial disorders as reported by professionals. Nine activity categories were identified that represent regular childhood activities. We found that, although the children varied in capacities and limitations, all activity categories were present in each global-functioning profile. There are indications that children perform activities differently in terms of the level of independence, assistive device usage, and energy costs. This study provides a foundation for a qualitative study on the activities of children with a mitochondrial disorder and whether allied health care professionals support their practice. Furthermore, it supports the need for personalized and strength-based care, which puts emphasis on involving the children's perspective in care.

Conflicts of Interest

The authors report no conflicts of interest.

Acknowledgments

The authors thank the professionals in the MitoRoute at the Radboudumc, Nijmegen, Netherlands, namely, (i) Kim van de Loo, MSc, and Dr. José Clusters, psychologists; (ii) Marjo van Gerven, speech therapist; (iii) Dr. Anjo Janssen, pediatric physical therapist; and (iv) Yvonne Veenhuizen, MSc, and Anita van der Molen, occupational therapists. The authors used their data to categorize the children into three profiles: global low functioning, low cognitive functioning with a moderate to normal ambulation, and global moderate functioning. For the ability to study all patient records, the authors would like to thank Professor Dr. J. A. M. Smeitink, head of the Radboud Centre for Mitochondrial Medicine. The authors also thank him for his critical review of the manuscript and the suggested improvements.

References

[1] M. Asbjørnslett and H. Hemmingsson, "Participation at school as experienced by teenagers with physical disabilities," *Scandinavian Journal of Occupational Therapy*, vol. 15, no. 3, pp. 153–161, 2008.

[2] R. M. Bendixen and C. M. Kreider, "Review of occupational therapy research in the practice area of children and youth," *The American Journal of Occupational Therapy*, vol. 65, no. 3, pp. 351–359, 2011.

[3] M. Law, C. Missiuna, N. Pollock, and D. Stewart, "Foundations for occupational therapy practice with children," in *Occupational Therapy for Children*, J. Case-Smith, Ed., pp. 53–87, Elsevier Mosby, St. Louis, MO, USA, 2005.

[4] G. King, M. Lawm, S. King, P. Rosenbaum, M. K. Kertoy, and N. L. Young, "A conceptual model of the factors affecting the recreation and leisure participation of children with disabilities," *Physical & Occupational Therapy In Pediatrics*, vol. 23, no. 1, pp. 63–90, 2003.

[5] T. Heah, T. Case, B. McGuire, and M. Law, "Successful participation: the lived experience among children with disabilities," *Canadian Journal of Occupational Therapy*, vol. 74, no. 1, pp. 38–47, 2007.

[6] N. Shields, M. King, M. Corbett, and C. Imms, "Is participation among children with intellectual disabilities in outside school activities similar to their typically developing peers? A systematic review," *Developmental Neurorehabilitation*, vol. 17, no. 1, pp. 64–71, 2014.

[7] G. S. Gorman, A. M. Schaefer, Y. Ng et al., "Prevalence of nuclear and mitochondrial DNA mutations related to adult mitochondrial disease," *Annals of Neurology*, vol. 77, no. 5, pp. 753–759, 2015.

[8] W. J. Koopman, P. H. Willems, and J. A. Smeitink, "Monogenic mitochondrial disorders," *The New England Journal of Medicine*, vol. 366, no. 12, pp. 1132–1141, 2012.

[9] A. Rötig, "Genetics of mitochondrial respiratory chain deficiencies," *Revue Neurologique*, vol. 170, no. 5, pp. 309–322, 2014.

[10] J. B. WJ Koopman, C. W. Fung, S. Koene, R. J. Rodenburg, P. H. Willems, and J. A. Smeitink, "Mitochondrial disorders in children: toward development of small-molecule treatment strategies," *EMBO Molecular Medicine*, vol. 8, no. 4, pp. 311–327, 2016.

[11] A. Dassler and P. J. Allen, "Mitochondrial disease in children and adolescents," *Pediatric Nursing*, vol. 40, p. 150, 2014.

[12] J. E. Kisler, R. G. Whittaker, and R. McFarland, "Mitochondrial diseases in childhood: a clinical approach to investigation and management," *Developmental Medicine & Child Neurology*, vol. 52, no. 5, pp. 422–433, 2010.

[13] S. Koene, S. B. Wortmann, M. C. de Vries et al., "Developing outcome measures for pediatric mitochondrial disorders: which complaints and limitations are most burdensome to patients and their parents?," *Mitochondrion*, vol. 13, no. 1, pp. 15–24, 2013.

[14] A. M. Martens, H. Gorter, R. G. Wassink, and H. Rietman, "Physical activity of children with a mitochondrial disease compared to children who are healthy," *Pediatric Physical Therapy*, vol. 26, no. 1, pp. 19–26, 2014.

[15] S. Koene, M. Jansen, C. M. Verhaak, R. L. A. De Vrueh, I. J. M. De Groot, and J. A. M. Smeitink, "Towards the harmonization of outcome measures in children with mitochondrial disorders," *Developmental Medicine & Child Neurology*, vol. 55, no. 8, pp. 698–706, 2013.

[16] D. R. Hess, "Retrospective studies and chart reviews," *Respiratory Care*, vol. 49, no. 10, pp. 1171–1174, 2004.

[17] M. Vassar and M. Holzmann, "The retrospective chart review: important methodological considerations," *Journal of Educational Evaluation for Health Professions*, vol. 10, p. 12, 2013.

[18] H. F. Hsieh and S. E. Shannon, "Three approaches to qualitative content analysis," *Qualitative Health Research*, vol. 15, no. 9, pp. 1277–1288, 2005.

[19] World Health Organization, *International Classification of Functioning, Disability, and Health: Children & Youth Version: ICF-CY.*, World Health Organization, 2007.

[20] M. KVN Braun and D. L. Yeargin-Allsopp, "Activity limitations among young adults with developmental disabilities: a population-based follow-up study," *Research in Developmental Disabilities*, vol. 30, no. 1, pp. 179–191, 2009.

[21] O. V. MK Bult, M. J. Jongmans, E. Lindeman, and M. Ketelaar, "What influences participation in leisure activities of children and youth with physical disabilities? A systematic review," *Research in Developmental Disabilities*, vol. 32, no. 5, pp. 1521–1529, 2011.

[22] E. MM Hoffer, R. Feiwell, J. Perry, and C. B. Perry, "Functional ambulation in patients with myelomeningocele," *The Journal of Bone & Joint Surgery*, vol. 55, no. 1, pp. 137–148, 1973.

[23] M. A. Schoenmakers, V. A. Gulmans, R. H. Gooskens, and P. J. Helders, "Spina bifida at the sacral level: more than minor gait disturbances," *Clinical Rehabilitation*, vol. 18, no. 2, pp. 178–185, 2004.

[24] S. Knuijt, J. G. Kalf, B. M. G. Van Engelen, B. J. M. De Swart, and A. C. H. Geurts, "The Radboud dysarthria assessment: development and clinimetric evaluation," *Folia Phoniatrica et Logopaedica*, vol. 69, no. 4, pp. 143–153, 2017.

[25] J. Wassenberg-Severijnen and J. Custers, *Handleiding PEDI-NL*, Pearson, 2005.

[26] J. W. Varni, *Scaling and Scoring of the Pediatric Quality of Life Inventory™ (PedsQL™)*, Mapi Research Trust, Lyon, 14 edition, 2014.

[27] H. Priest, P. Roberts, and L. Woods, "An overview of three different approaches to the interpretation of qualitative data. Part 1: theoretical issues," *Nurse Researcher*, vol. 10, no. 1, pp. 30–42, 2002.

[28] S. Elo and H. Kyngäs, "The qualitative content analysis process," *Journal of Advanced Nursing*, vol. 62, no. 1, pp. 107–115, 2008.

[29] M. Stanley, "Qualitative descriptive," in *Qualitative Research Methodologies for Occupational Science and Therapy*, S. Nayar and M. Stanley, Eds., Routledge, 2015.

[30] R. Hagedorn, *Foundations for Practice in Occupational Therapy*, Elsevier Health Sciences, 2001.

[31] M. le Granse and M. J. Hartingsveldt, *Grondslagen van de Ergotherapie*, Reed Business, 2012.

[32] A. A. Wilcock, *An Occupational Perspective of Health*, Slack Incorporated, 2006.

[33] K. L. Reed and S. N. Sanderson, *Concepts of Occupational Therapy*, Lippincott Williams & Wilkins, 1999.

[34] World Medical Association, "World Medical Association Declaration of Helsinki. Ethical principles for medical research involving human subjects," *Bulletin World Health Organization*, vol. 79, pp. 373-374, 2001.

[35] A. H. M. Mulders, M. J. Meihuizen-de Regt, and J. M. H. de Moor, "Kinderrevalidatie: een plaatsbepaling," in *Kinderrevalidatie*, M. J. Meihuizen-de Regt, J. M. H. Moor, and A. H. M. Mulders, Eds., pp. 1–48, Koninklijke Van Gorcum BV, Assen, 2009.

[36] A. Mandich, H. Polatajko, L. Miller, and C. Baum, *The Pediatric Activity Card Sort (PACS)*, Canadian Occupational Therapy Association, Ottawa, 2004.

[37] M. King, N. Shields, C. Imms, M. Black, and C. Ardern, "Participation of children with intellectual disability compared with typically developing children," *Research in Developmental Disabilities*, vol. 34, no. 5, pp. 1854–1862, 2013.

[38] B. Piškur, A. J. Beurskens, M. J. Jongmans et al., "Parents' actions, challenges, and needs while enabling participation of children with a physical disability: a scoping review," *BMC pediatrics*, vol. 12, no. 1, p. 177, 2012.

[39] B. Piškur, M. K. AJ Beurskens, M. J. Jongmans, B. M. Casparie, and R. J. Smeets, "Daily actions, challenges, and needs among Dutch parents while supporting the participation of their child with a physical disability at home, at school, and in the community: a qualitative diary study," *BMC Pediatrics*, vol. 17, no. 1, p. 12, 2017.

[40] D. Persson, L. Erlandsson, M. Eklund, and S. Iwarsson, "Value dimensions, meaning, and complexity in human occupation—a tentative structure for analysis," *Scandinavian Journal of Occupational Therapy*, vol. 8, no. 1, pp. 7–18, 2001.

[41] C. Morris, "Measuring participation in childhood disability: how does the capability approach improve our understanding?," *Developmental Medicine & Child Neurology*, vol. 51, no. 2, pp. 92–94, 2009.

[42] M. E. Michielsen, M. de Niet, G. M. Ribbers, H. J. Stam, and J. B. Bussmann, "Evidence of a logarithmic relationship between motor capacity and actual performance in daily life of the paretic arm following stroke," *Journal of Rehabilitation Medicine*, vol. 41, no. 5, pp. 327–331, 2009.

[43] S. Koene and J. Smeitink, "Mitochondrial medicine: entering the era of treatment," *Journal of Internal Medicine*, vol. 265, no. 2, pp. 193–209, 2009.

10

Facilitators and Barriers of Assistive Technology and Learning Environment for Children with Special Needs

Suchitporn Lersilp,[1] **Supawadee Putthinoi**,[1] **and Theeratorn Lersilp**[2]

[1]*Department of Occupational Therapy, Faculty of Associated Medical Sciences, Chiang Mai University, Thailand*
[2]*Department of Special Education, Faculty of Education, Chiang Mai Rajabhat University, Thailand*

Correspondence should be addressed to Suchitporn Lersilp; suchitporn.l@cmu.ac.th

Academic Editor: Lynette Mackenzie

The purpose of this research was to study the facilitators and barriers of assistive technology (AT) and the learning environment for children with special needs in special education schools in Chiang Mai, Thailand. The informants were one hundred and sixteen children with special needs, who studied in nursery to Grade 12, or with their caregivers. The instrument was a questionnaire applied by the International Classification of Functioning, Disability and Health (ICF) and examined for content validity by five specialists. The results in terms of AT showed that a majority of children with physical disability needed it for mobility and use of school buildings and those with hearing disability for communication. However, most of the children did not need to use AT for culture, recreation, or sports, while many considered it as a facilitator for education. In terms of the learning environment, most characteristics of the physical environment were facilitators for children with special needs, as were those of the social environment for all groups of such children. The results of this study were useful in providing information for AT and design of a learning environment relating to the varied characteristics of children with special needs in special education schools.

1. Introduction

Education is an occupation performance area that is meaningful for children, in that the school system can provide direct impact on their occupation [1]. Children with special needs require a specific education program and related services that encourage them to learn with peers in schools and participate in social activities as children do in general. Children with special needs include those with visual, hearing, physical, and intellectual disability, autism, and language and communication disorders as well as multiple disabilities. They have various needs depending on severity and context. Some children with disabilities are encouraged to study in mainstreaming schools, where they meet their needs successfully, but others do not. A number of children need more specific help and services in order to be suitable for study in special education schools.

Assistive Technology (AT) is any product, instrument, strategy, service, or practice used by people with disabilities and also the elderly. It is produced specially or availed generally to prevent, compensate, relieve, or neutralize impairment, disability, or handicap and improve the individual's autonomy and quality of life (QOL) [2]. AT users vary from children to elderly people. The purpose of AT use depends on age relating to requirement, lifestyle, and the environment in which it is used [2]. Children with special needs can use AT as a way of improving functions and encouraging learning, especially when participating in a school environment. In the school year 2015–2016, survey data of the US Department of Education indicated that a higher percentage of students aged between 3 and 21 years received special education services [3]. This high percentage showed that most of these students had learning disabilities and studied in general schools. The trend for mainstreaming and inclusive education schools is increasing in order to encourage and enable students with special needs to have the same learning environment as that of their peers without disabilities [4]. However, due to policy and socio-cultural factors, most children with special needs in Thailand enroll in special education schools, including those for the blind and with hearing, physical, and intellectual disability. Students in special education schools are provided AT from the Ministry of Education. AT items are found in schools that are related to the disabilities of their students, for example, magnifiers, Braillers, slates, and styluses in schools for the blind; hearing aids, cochlear implants, and sign language interpreters in schools for students with hearing disability; walkers, crutches, canes, wheelchairs, and Augmentative and Alternative Communication (AAC) in schools for students with physical disability; and Computer-Assisted Instruction (CAI) and educational board games in schools for students with intellectual disability [5]. Some studies reported that all types of AT items were provided to students with disabilities in special education schools. Students with visual disability were given and used more AT items than other students with disabilities, in both special education schools and universities [5, 6]. Moreover, students with visual disabilities needed AT the most, while those with hearing and physical disabilities did not need it so much [6]. Previous studies surveyed AT provision, problems, and needs, but they did not study or explore the facilitators and barriers of AT for students in the context of their learning environment. Although matching equipment with the needs and characteristics of disabled students is not always difficult, understanding the nature of their tasks or functions and environment and preferences is necessary [2]. Thus, the perspectives of students with special needs on AT as facilitators and barriers are useful for service providers when choosing, planning, and encouraging these people to reach their potential.

A learning environment refers to the diverse physical locations, contexts, and cultures in which students learn [7]. Thus, the learning environment is not only the typical classroom but also a collaboration area that can be characterized as a place for active interactions between learner and instructor or between learner and other learners [8]. Some studies found that the learning environment, especially the classroom, had a positive impact on the academic performances of the students [9, 10], and it is very important for those with special needs. A positive learning environment can facilitate the performance areas in daily life, education, play, leisure, and social participation for the students. On the other hand, a negative learning environment can obstruct their performances and skills.

International Classification of Functioning, Disability and Health (ICF) was adopted in 2001 by the World Health Organization (WHO) [11]. The ICF provides a common language to describe human functioning in people with and without disabilities. In fact, it can be a model that guides selection measures, treatment goals, and outcomes [12]. The definition of "environmental factors" in the ICF is a component that makes up the physical, social, and attitudinal environment in which people live and conduct their lives [11]. These factors include products and technology, natural environment and human-made changes to the environment, support and relationships, attitudes and services, and systems and policies. These environmental factors may act as facilitators and also barriers in meaningful activities, in which persons are able to participate [12].

The context in this study was placed on special education schools for students with disabilities, including schools for the blind, deaf and hard of hearing, and those for students having physical and intellectual disability. These schools are placed in urban areas, except for those for physical disability, which are located in suburban areas. The students are selected for admission to a school by type of disability. In addition, the schools have an evaluating team that generally comprises special education teachers, occupational therapists, and school administrators who consider minimum performances that students are expected to have, particularly regarding communication and self-care performance. Most of the students are provided AT by the rights of children with disabilities, as indicated in the Acts of the Ministry of Health. However, in some cases, students still do not receive AT; therefore, the Individual Education Plan (IEP) team plays a role in considering suitable AT for students through the rights in the Acts of the Ministry of Education. School buildings for students in need are designed in the same way as general schools and each one has three to four floors. Not all of them have elevators. However, the buildings of the school for students with physical disability do have slopes between each floor and wide walkways to facilitate wheelchairs and walking aids for the students.

In fact, AT and the learning environment are able to improve the study and participation of students with disabilities to the level of their peers. However, different types of students have varied needs. As AT and the learning environment are considered as both facilitators and barriers in schools where disabled students can participate in learning and social activities, this study is aimed at exploring these factors for providing appropriate AT and setting a suitable learning environment for these people.

2. Methods

This research studied the facilitators and barriers of AT and the learning environment for students with disabilities in special education schools, in Chiang Mai, Thailand. The participants were selected by stratified random sampling from all four special education schools in Chiang Mai such as those for students with physical, intellectual, hearing, and visual disability. They comprised 115 students with disabilities, including 10 kindergarten, primary, and secondary students from each school, except for only 6 kindergarten students from the school for the blind. Most of the students were boarders, but some attended day school. Students who had multiple disabilities were not included in this study.

The instrument used was a questionnaire that applied to the ICF and consisted of two parts: AT and the learning environment (Table 1). The questionnaire also was examined for content validity by five related specialists. The AT part (IOC = 0.91) included 63 items and comprised five types of AT such as that for mobility (IOC = 0.93), communication (IOC = 0.93), education (IOC = 0.94), culture, recreation, and sports (IOC = 1.00), and school buildings (IOC = 0.88). The learning environment part (IOC = 0.95) consisted of two types: physical (IOC = 0.94) and social environment (IOC = 1.00).

TABLE 1: Applying ICF to the questionnaire on facilitators and barriers of assistive technology and the learning environment.

ICF domains in environmental factors	The questionnaire
Chapter 1: products and technology	*Part 1 assistive technology*
Products or substance for personal consumption (e110)	Not included
Products and technology for personal use in daily living (e115)	Applied in (i) Assistive technology for mobility (ii) Assistive technology for communication
Products and technology for personal indoor and outdoor mobility and transportation (e120)	Applied in assistive technology for mobility
Products and technology for communication (e125)	Applied in assistive technology for communication
Products and technology for education (e130)	Applied in assistive technology for education
Products and technology for employment (e135)	Not included
Products and technology for culture, recreation, and sport (e140)	Applied in assistive technology for culture, recreation, and sports
Products and technology for the practice of religion and spirituality (e145)	Not included
Design, construction and building products, and technology of buildings for public use (e150)	Applied in assistive technology for buildings
Design, construction and building products, and technology of buildings for private use (e155)	Applied in assistive technology for buildings
Products and technology for land development (e160)	Not included
Assets (e165)	Not included
Chapter 2: natural environment and human-made changes to the environment	*Part 2 the learning environment*
Physical geography (e210)	Not included
Population (e215)	Applied in the physical environment
Flora and fauna (e220)	Not included
Climate (e225)	Applied in the physical environment
Natural events (e230)	Not included
Human-caused events (e235)	Not included
Light (e240)	Applied in the physical environment
Time-related changes (e245)	Not included
Sound (e250)	Not included
Vibration (e255)	Not included
Air quality (e260)	Not included
Chapter 3: support and relationships	
Immediate family	Not included
Extended family	Not included
Friends	Applied in the social environment
Acquaintances, peers, colleagues, neighbors, and community members	Applied in the social environment
People in positions of authority	Applied in the social environment
People in subordinate positions	Not included
Personal care providers and personal assistants	Applied in the social environment
Strangers	Not included
Domesticated animals	Not included
Health professionals	Not included
Health-related professionals	Not included
Chapter 4: attitudes	Not included
Chapter 5: services, systems, and policies	Not included

There were four qualifier scales in the questionnaire (F = Facilitator, B = Barrier, NO = No Opportunity, and NA = Not Applicable). An AT facilitator was defined as a convenience with positive effect on accessibility to learning and socializing activities in the school context. An AT barrier was defined as an inconvenience with negative effect on accessibility to learning and socializing activities in the school context. No Opportunity was defined as students who were aware that AT was useful for them, or they needed to use it, but did not have the opportunity to do so. Not Applicable was defined as students who did not consider AT as being necessary. The definitions of these four qualifier scales were explained to the participants individually.

An individual interview was carried out directly in the data collection process by using the questionnaire with students who had good communication skills in the Thai language. However, if the students were too young or had communication problems, the caregivers or teachers gave the interview instead. All of the kindergarten students and the adults responded to the questions in this study. Most of the primary school students (70.00%) and all of the secondary ones responded to the questions by themselves. Twenty-four adults responded to the questions on behalf of the kindergarten and 30% of the primary school students, including 8 special education teachers, 4 occupational therapists, and 12 guardians. The special education teachers and occupational therapists responded on behalf of more than one student. The conditions under which data were collected consisted of an individual interview in a quiet room. The time-span for completing the questionnaire was about 30–45 minutes. If the students or informants did not know about any type of AT, the researchers and two research assistants could give more explanation and present pictures. Then, data were analyzed by descriptive statistics for examining and summarizing the facilitators and barriers of AT and the learning environment for students with disabilities in special education schools.

Table 2: Characteristics of children with disabilities ($n = 116$).

Characteristics	Numbers (percentage)				Total
	PD	ID	HD	VD	
Gender					
Male	9	20	13	8	50
Female	21	10	17	18	66
Age (years old)					
6 and below	2	10	8	4	24
7–9	12	4	6	2	24
10–12	5	5	4	6	20
13–18	11	11	12	14	48
Class level					
Nursery	10	10	10	6	36
G1–G6	10	10	10	10	40
G7–G12	10	10	10	10	40
Medical condition					
No	30	30	28	26	114
Yes	0	0	2	0	2
(i) Hepatitis B	0	0	1	0	1
(ii) Seizures	0	0	1	0	1

VD = visual disability; HD = hearing disability; PD = physical disability; ID = intellectual disability.

3. Results

The students with disabilities comprised 30 with physical (25.86%), 30 with intellectual (25.86%), 30 with hearing (25.86%), and 26 with visual disability (22.42%). Most of them were female (56.90%) and 13–18 years old (41.38%). The oldest students were 18 years old and the youngest 5. In addition, two students with hearing disability had medical conditions such as hepatitis B (0.86%) and seizures (0.86%), as presented in Table 2.

The results in terms of AT showed that most of the students did not need to use it for communication, mobility, or use of school buildings, except for those with hearing and physical disability. Most of them did not need to use it for culture, recreation, or sports, and most considered AT for education as a facilitator. In terms of AT for mobility (as shown in Table 3), most of the students with physical disability perceived it as a facilitator, especially the standard wheelchair. On the other hand, many of them had no opportunity to use highly functional mobility aids such as an electric wheelchair, a scooter, or hand bicycle. In addition, many students with visual disability perceived a white cane and reflective tape as facilitators. These AT items were necessary mobility devices for students with visual disability, but it was interesting that some of them had no opportunity to use them, which were nonetheless low-tech devices that were not difficult to provide.

In terms of AT for communication (as shown in Table 4), most of the students with disabilities realized the importance of this AT as a facilitator, particularly those with hearing disability, as they probably needed it to help them. It was interesting that many students with visual disability considered AT for communication as a facilitator, even though they had no obvious communication barriers. When considering detail, this study found that most students with visual disability perceived AT for communication as a facilitator for written communication.

In terms of AT for education (as shown in Table 5), most of the students perceived this AT as not necessary for this purpose. However, most of those with intellectual disability indicated that concentration training software was a facilitator for them in education, while students with physical disability needed AT items for participating in classroom educational activities such as pen and notebook, concave table, and touch screen computer.

In terms of AT for recreation (as shown in Table 6), many of the students perceived the importance of AT for recreation as a facilitator. At the same time, many of them had no opportunity to use it, except for those with visual disability. This finding showed that although this AT was in the educational context, the students perceived it as necessary.

In terms of AT for school buildings (as shown in Table 7), most of the students with physical disability reported that this AT was a facilitator, particularly the guide post for all types of these students. However, even though a low number of students with visual disability reported on AT for school buildings, they indicated that the permanent and movable slope was a barrier for them. This information is useful, as it shows that not all AT is a facilitator for all students with disabilities. It depends on what their disabilities are. That is

TABLE 3: Facilitators and barriers of AT for mobility.

Items	PD ($n = 30$)				ID ($n = 30$)				HD ($n = 30$)				VD ($n = 26$)			
	B	F	NO	NA	B	F	NO	NA	B	F	NO	NA	B	F	NO	NA
White cane	/	/	/	30	/	/	/	30	/	/	/	30	/	13	3	10
Reflective tape	/	/	/	30	/	1	/	29	/	/	/	30	/	11	6	9
Walker	/	5	/	25	/	/	/	30	/	/	/	30	/	/	/	26
Crutch	/	2	/	28	/	/	/	30	/	/	/	30	/	/	/	26
Cane	/	2	/	28	/	/	/	30	/	/	/	30	/	/	/	26
Standard wheelchair	/	23	/	7	/	/	/	30	/	/	/	30	/	/	/	26
Electric wheelchair	/	1	18	11	/	/	/	30	/	/	/	30	/	/	/	26
Hand bicycle	/	2	12	16	/	/	/	30	/	/	/	30	/	/	/	26
Scooter	/	/	15	15	/	/	/	30	/	/	/	30	/	/	/	26

TABLE 4: Facilitators and barriers of AT for communication.

Items	PD				ID				HD				VD			
	B	F	NO	NA	B	F	NO	NA	B	F	NO	NA	B	F	NO	NA
Hearing aids (behind ears)	/	/	/	30	/	/	/	30	/	27	1	2	/	/	/	26
Hearing aids (in-ears)	/	/	/	30	/	/	/	30	/	25	3	2	/	/	/	26
Cochlea implant	/	/	/	30	/	/	/	30	/	18	12	/	/	/	/	26
FM system	/	/	/	30	/	/	/	30	/	16	14	/	/	/	/	26
Mobile phone	/	6	6	18	/	7	7	16	/	12	5	13	/	12	/	14
Binoculars	/	/	3	27	/	1	/	29	/	2	1	27	/	6	3	17
Slate and stylus	/	/	/	30	/	1	/	29	/	2	/	28	/	22	3	1
CCTV	/	/	/	30	/	2	/	28	/	4	/	26	/	/	/	26
Brailler	/	/	/	30	/	/	/	30	/	1	/	29	/	23	1	2
Thermoform Brailon duplicator	/	/	/	30	/	1	/	29	/	/	/	30	/	12	7	7
Braille notebook computer	/	/	/	30	/	/	/	30	/	/	/	30	/	20	/	6
Optical character recognition	/	/	/	30	/	1	/	29	/	/	/	30	/	3	6	17
Book reader software	/	2	/	28	/	1	/	29	/	/	/	30	/	16	1	9
Tone bar	/	/	/	30	/	1	/	29	/	1	3	26	/	/	1	25
Listen and speech training device	/	2	/	28	/	4	1	25	/	17	12	1	/	/	/	26
Sign language interpreter	/	/	/	30	/	/	/	30	/	30	/	/	/	/	/	26
Remote control	/	4	7	19	/	1	/	29	/	11	3	16	/	/	/	26

to say, some AT is able to be a facilitator for some types of students with disabilities but not for others.

There are two parts in terms of the learning environment, including the physical and social environment. Results for the physical environment showed that it was mostly a facilitator for students with physical disability, except for the colored bands on school building stairs, braille keypads, and elevators, which were not applicable. The physical environment for students with intellectual disability was mostly a facilitator, except for obstacles in school buildings, such as the barriers of slopes and steep stairs. In addition, the students had no opportunity to use the colored bands on stairs or elevators in school buildings. The physical environment for students with hearing disability was mostly a facilitator, except for the barriers of slopes and colored bands on school building stairs. In addition, results indicated that stairs, slopes, colored bands on stairs, classroom doors, steps in front of classroom doors and position of handles in a classroom, use of the doorknob in the classroom, weight of a chair, and use of an elevator in a school building were not applicable. The physical environment for students with visual disability was mostly a facilitator, except for the elevator, which the students had no opportunity to use (as shown in Table 8).

In terms of the social environment, all four groups of students with special needs perceived it as a facilitator (as shown in Table 9). However, except for those with physical disability, the students perceived this AT as a barrier in relation to the school context. Furthermore, some students with intellectual and hearing disability reported that help from assistant teachers was not necessary for them.

4. Discussion and Conclusion

This study is aimed at exploring the facilitators and barriers of AT and the learning environment for students with special

TABLE 5: Facilitators and barriers of AT for education.

Items	PD				ID				HD				VD			
	B	F	NO	NA	B	F	NO	NA	B	F	NO	NA	B	F	NO	NA
Adjustable chair	/	2	9	19	/	/	/	30	/	1	1	28	/	/	/	26
Electric desk	/	/	16	14	/	/	/	30	/	1	1	28	/	/	/	26
Concave table	/	19	4	7	/	1	/	29	/	/	1	29	/	/	/	26
Adapted keyboard	/	/	18	12	/	/	/	30	/	/	1	29	/	/	/	26
Keyboard controller	/	/	8	22	/	/	/	30	/	/	/	30	/	/	/	26
Prism glasses	/	/	/	30	/	1	/	29	/	2	/	28	/	/	/	26
Book holder	/	4	14	12	/	5	/	25	/	2	1	27	/	/	/	26
Writing and typewriting device	/	/	6	24	/	/	/	30	/	2	/	28	/	/	/	26
Book opening device	/	/	6	24	/	/	/	30	/	/	/	30	/	/	/	26
Word recognition software	/	/	2	28	/	1	/	29	/	2	1	27	/	/	/	26
Touch screen	/	19	2	9	/	13	2	15	/	5	1	24	/	/	/	26
Word prediction software	/	2	4	24	/	4	1	25	/	5	2	23	/	/	/	26
Concentration training software	/	10	4	16	/	25	/	5	/	8	1	21	/	/	/	26
Pen and notebook	/	27	/	3	/	19	10	1	/	16	/	14	/	/	/	26

TABLE 6: Facilitators and barriers of AT for recreation.

Items	PD				ID				HD				VD			
	B	F	NO	NA	B	F	NO	NA	B	F	NO	NA	B	F	NO	NA
Sport wheelchair	/	16	/	14	/	/	/	30	/	/	2	28	/	/	/	26
Adapted sport devices	/	14	4	12	/	2	/	28	/	/	1	29	/	/	/	26
Adapted musical instruments	/	5	13	12	/	9	2	19	/	2	4	24	/	6	/	20
Adapted educational games	/	18	4	8	/	27	/	3	/	14	11	5	/	16	/	10
Web camera	/	1	3	26	/	6	4	20	/	13	1	16	/	1	/	25

TABLE 7: Facilitators and barriers of AT for school buildings.

Items	PD				ID				HD				VD			
	B	F	NO	NA	B	F	NO	NA	B	F	NO	NA	B	F	NO	NA
Permanent slope	/	28	/	2	/	4	/	26	/	1	/	29	1	/	/	25
Movable slope	/	18	8	4	/	3	/	27	/	/	/	30	1	/	/	25
Automatic door	/	18	10	2	/	3	/	27	/	1	9	20	/	/	/	26
Adapted handle	/	22	6	2	/	/	1	29	/	3	/	27	/	/	/	26
Guide post	/	29	/	1	/	29	/	1	/	22	/	8	/	26	/	/

needs in special education schools in Chiang Mai, Thailand, by using a questionnaire that applied to the ICF. The results of this study found not all students indicating AT for mobility as a barrier. Most of these AT items were perceived as facilitators by the students with physical disability, while no students with hearing disability saw them as such. On the other hand, most AT items for communication were perceived as a facilitator for students with hearing disability. These findings indicated that not all AT is necessary for all students with disabilities, but necessity depends on their type of disability [12]. Students with physical disability have the problem of general mobility, while those with visual disability frequently need AT to help them move and gain access to where they need to communicate and participate in social activities [13, 14]. In fact, students with communication difficulty, such as those with hearing and intellectual disability as well as cerebral palsy, also need AT for accessing and participating in their daily activities [15]. However, some AT items might be a facilitator and barrier simultaneously. For instance, while AT for school buildings might be a facilitator to enable access for students with physical disability, it might be a barrier in the case of those with visual disability. Therefore, awareness of the students' perspectives should be considered, and they should be able to participate in the process of AT design and provision if possible [16]. These findings relate to previous studies [5, 6], which also indicated that most AT items were perceived as facilitators by students with disabilities, but their necessity depends on the students' disability. For example, the slopes in school buildings are a facilitator for students with physical disability, while being a

Table 8: Facilitators and barriers of the physical environment.

Items	PD				ID				HD				VD			
	B	F	NO	NA	B	F	NO	NA	B	F	NO	NA	B	F	NO	NA
Buildings																
Floor texture around the building	3	27	/	/	10	20	/	/	10	13	/	7	/	26	/	/
Steps around the building	/	30	/	/	12	16	/	2	/	11	/	19	2	24	/	/
Barriers around the building	3	20	7	/	12	9	/	9	12	5	2	11	7	19	/	/
Rail around the building	/	30	/	/	/	20	3	7	1	23	/	6	/	13	11	2
Slope into the building	/	30	/	/	/	13	5	12	12	1	2	15	/	26	/	/
Rail of slope	/	30	/	/	/	15	3	12	1	21	/	8	/	26	/	/
Barriers on the slope	/	21	/	9	15	3	2	10	12	5	3	10	1	19	6	/
Rail along the steps	/	18	2	10	/	28	/	2	2	21	/	7	/	26	/	/
Floor texture of steps	/	22	2	6	10	20	/	/	11	12	2	5	/	26	/	/
Height of each step	3	13	2	12	16	14	/	/	10	13	/	7	1	25	/	/
Width of each step	3	19	2	6	14	16	/	/	/	21	/	9	/	26	/	/
Colored tape on each step	/	6	1	23	/	6	21	3	10	9	1	10	/	16	/	10
Classroom																
Door sill	/	29	/	1	13	15	/	2	/	10	4	16	6	20	/	/
Door step	/	30	/	/	16	12	/	2	/	9	3	18	6	20	/	/
Floor texture at the entrance	/	30	/	/	/	17	/	13	1	22	/	7	/	26	/	/
Position of door handle	3	25	2	/	2	26	/	2	2	11	/	17	/	26	/	/
Width of door	/	30	/	/	/	30	/	/	1	21	/	8	/	26	/	/
Floor texture	/	30	/	/	/	30	/	/	1	23	/	6	/	26	/	/
Object arrangement	/	30	/	/	/	30	/	/	1	25	/	4	/	26	/	/
Number of students	/	30	/	/	12	16	2	/	13	15	/	2	/	26	/	/
Temperature	/	30	/	/	/	30	/	/	1	27	/	2	/	26	/	/
Lights	/	30	/	/	/	30	/	/	/	30	/	/	1	24	/	1
Position of switches	4	16	10	/	/	30	/	/	/	27	/	3	1	18	7	/
Elevator																
Width of door	/	28	2	/	/	1	26	3	1	8	3	18	/	/	26	/
Height of bottoms	1	27	2	/	/	1	26	3	1	6	2	21	/	/	26	/
Braille bottoms	/	13	2	15	/	1	26	3	2	4	3	21	/	/	26	/
Rail in elevator	/	28	2	/	/	1	26	3	/	11	2	17	/	/	26	/
Floor texture	/	28	2	/	/	1	26	3	/	11	2	17	/	/	26	/
Voice notification	/	27	3	/	/	1	26	3	/	1	26	3	/	/	26	/
Desk and chair																
Height of desk	/	30	/	/	13	17	/	/	/	16	/	14	/	26	/	/
Width of desk	/	30	/	/	13	17	/	/	/	25	/	5	1	25	/	/
Texture of desk	/	30	/	/	10	17	/	3	1	15	/	14	/	26	/	/
Weight of desk	/	28	/	2	13	14	/	2	1	16	/	13	6	20	/	/
Height of chair	/	30	/	/	13	17	/	/	1	16	/	13	/	26	/	/
Width of chair	/	30	/	/	10	20	/	/	1	15	/	14	/	26	/	/
Texture of chair	/	30	/	/	10	17	/	3	1	15	/	14	/	26	/	/
Weight of chair	/	28	/	2	13	17	/	/	2	13	/	15	6	20	/	/

barrier for students with visual disability, although slopes are designed universally for all people. When considering the design of slopes in school buildings for blind students, this study found that most slopes had no rail on either side. For this reason, some blind students might fall down when walking along the edge of a slope. In other words, whether AT items are facilitators or not depends on how they are able to compensate for disability, and this is why awareness of the students' perspectives should be considered in the process of AT design and provision. Besides AT being provided for all students with disabilities, there must be awareness of quality and design. Moreover, the findings showed that students

TABLE 9: Facilitators and barriers of the social environment.

Items	PD				ID				HD				VD			
	B	F	NO	NA	B	F	NO	NA	B	F	NO	NA	B	F	NO	NA
Relationship with teachers																
Help from classroom teachers	/	30	/	/	/	30	/	/	/	30	/	/	/	26	/	/
Help from other teachers in the school	/	30	/	/	/	30	/	/	/	30	/	/	/	26	/	/
Help from assistant teachers	/	30	/	/	/	21	/	9	1	26	/	3	/	26	/	/
Relationship with peers																
Interpersonal activities	/	30	/	/	1	29	/	/	1	29	/	/	1	25	/	/
Help each other	/	30	/	/	/	30	/	/	/	30	/	/	1	25	/	/
Relationship with other students in school																
Interpersonal activities	/	30	/	/	/	30	/	/	/	30	/	/	1	25	/	/
Help each other	/	30	/	/	/	30	/	/	/	30	/	/	1	25	/	/
Relationship with other school staff members																
Help from other school staff members	/	30	/	/	/	30	/	/	/	29	/	1	/	26	/	/

reported NO for most AT items or they did not have the opportunity to use high-tech AT. Students with physical disability did not have the opportunity to use high-tech AT related to mobility and education such as an electric wheelchair or adapted keyboard. Students with intellectual disability did not have the opportunity to use high-tech AT such as a mobile phone, which related to communication. Students with hearing disability did not have the opportunity to use high-tech AT such as an FM system, which also related to communication. Lastly, students with visual disability did not have the opportunity to use high-tech AT such as a Thermoform Brailon Duplicator, which related to communication as well. This information reflected that some needs for high-tech AT items were not reached by children with disabilities, although they were addressed in the rights of students with disabilities under ministerial regulations. This was due to a problem with management policy and national socio-economic status. Most high-tech AT items are expensive and so many steps have to be taken before receiving them. In addition, the AT items addressed in ministerial regulations are provided only for students who studied in mainstreaming schools and are in the Individual Education Plan (IEP). On the other hand, most students with disabilities are placed in special education schools in Thailand and some have no IEP. These problems are barriers against AT provision and interesting points for further study.

This study found that the physical environment, in terms of the learning environment, is a facilitator for all types of students with disabilities. This is because this study researched in special education schools that were designed for specific disabilities and suitable for limiting each type of disability. These schools are based on a universal design concept in order to encourage, particularly students with physical disability, to be able to access classrooms, because the way buildings are constructed has direct impact on student participation [17]. In addition, these findings indicated that the physical environment is as important as the social one. In fact, besides the physical environment, the lack of understanding and positive perspectives in society leads to barriers against improving the occupational performance of students with special needs [18]. When these students have a good relationship with their teachers, peers, other students, and other school staff, they will be motivated to improve their learning and increase their opportunity to participate in school activities [19, 20]. The findings in terms of the learning environment indicated that students and adults perceived both the physical and social environment as facilitators in special education schools by responding to the questionnaire. It is of interest that as some of the students in the physical environment need facilitators, others see them as barriers, and special education schools do not need the same building construction plans. Instead, they should construct with a barrier-free design for each type of disability. Furthermore, the social environment, including relationships with teachers, peers, other students, and other school staff, is important for all of the students. In providing information to build understanding and a positive attitude in school societies, facilitators encourage children with disabilities to participate in school and social activities in the same way as people do in general.

Previous researches surveyed the AT items that students with disabilities needed, used, and had problems using. This study provides more findings in terms of student perspectives on AT and the learning environment as facilitators or barriers. Moreover, this study reflected findings on the opportunities for students with disabilities to receive high-tech AT in provincial areas of a developing country. In addition, this study is useful for related service providers such as educators, school therapists, and administrators in that it examines the individual needs of each student and presents the AT that will meet them. These people have to be aware of a safe design for AT together with environmental evaluation and encouragement in understanding students with disabilities, in order to relate with people and build relationships in the school context. The limitation of this study was the specific area of Chiang Mai province. Further research should expand to wider areas and study mainstreaming schools that include various types of students with disabilities in the same school. Furthermore, the roles of school-based occupational therapists should cover devices and environmental adaptation, and studies on their effectiveness would be interesting for students with disabilities. In addition, further studies might research other aspects and their correlation with, for example, physical environment and mobility, social environment and communication, or learning environment and education.

Conflicts of Interest

The authors declare no conflict of interest.

Acknowledgments

This research was supplied with tools and equipment by the Department of Occupational Therapy, Faculty of Associated Medical Sciences, Chiang Mai University, Thailand.

References

[1] J. W. Solomon and J. C. O'Brien, *Pediatric Skills for Occupational Therapy Assistants*, Mosby, 3rd edition, 2011.

[2] H. Pain, L. McLellan, and S. Gore, *Choosing Assistive Devices: A Guide for Users and Professionals*, Library of Congress Cataloging in Publication Data, PA, USA, 2003.

[3] National Center for Education Statistics, "Children and youth with disabilities," October 2018, https://nces.ed.gov/programs/coe/indicator_cgg.asp#.

[4] T. Minou, "New trends in education of children with disabilities," *Procedia - Social and Behavioral Sciences*, vol. 15, pp. 1955–1959, 2011.

[5] S. Lersilp, S. Putthinoi, and N. Chakpitak, "Model of providing assistive technologies in special education schools," *Global Journal of Health Science*, vol. 8, no. 1, pp. 36–44, 2016.

[6] T. Lersilp, "Access to information for learning by using assistive technology for undergraduate students with disabilities in Northern Thailand," *Information*, vol. 7, no. 4, p. 54, 2016.

[7] S. Abbott, Ed., "Hidden curriculum," *The glossary of Education reform*, August 2014, http://edglossary.org/hidden-curriculum.

[8] H.-J. So and T. A. Brush, "Student perceptions of collaborative learning, social presence and satisfaction in a blended learning environment: relationships and critical factors," *Computers & Education*, vol. 51, no. 1, pp. 318–336, 2008.

[9] P. Barrett, Y. Zhang, J. Moffat, and K. Kobbacy, "A holistic, multi-level analysis identifying the impact of classroom design on pupils' learning," *Building and Environment*, vol. 59, pp. 678–689, 2013.

[10] P. Barrett, F. Davies, Y. Zhang, and L. Barrett, "The impact of classroom design on pupils' learning: final results of a holistic, multi-level analysis," *Building and Environment*, vol. 89, pp. 118–133, 2015.

[11] World Health Organization, *International Classification of Functioning, Disability and Health (ICF)*, World Health Organization, Geneva, 2001.

[12] A. Majnemer, *Measures for Children with Developmental Disabilities: An ICF-CY Approach*, Mac Keith Press, London, 2012.

[13] D. M. Cowan and Y. Khan, "Assistive technology for children with complex disabilities," *Current Paediatrics*, vol. 15, no. 3, pp. 207–212, 2005.

[14] H. Hemmingsson, H. Lidstrom, and L. Nygard, "Use of assistive technology devices in mainstream schools: students' perspective," *American Journal of Occupational Therapy*, vol. 63, no. 4, pp. 463–472, 2009.

[15] F. Stasolla, A. O. Caffo, L. Picucci, and A. Bosco, "Assistive technology for promoting choice behaviors in three children with cerebral palsy and severe communication impairments," *Research in Developmental Disabilities*, vol. 34, no. 9, pp. 2694–2700, 2013.

[16] L. Benton and H. Johnson, "Widening participation in technology design: a review of the involvement of children with special educational needs and disabilities," *International Journal of Child-Computer Interaction*, vol. 3-4, pp. 23–40, 2015.

[17] S. I. Mihaylov, S. N. Jarvis, A. F. Colver, and B. Beresford, "Identification and description of environmental factors that influence participation of children with cerebral palsy," *Developmental Medicine and Child Neurology*, vol. 46, no. 5, pp. 299–304, 2004.

[18] M. Law, M. Haight, B. Milroy, D. Willms, D. Stewart, and P. Rosenbaum, "Environmental factors affecting the occupations of children with physical disabilities," *Journal of Occupational Science*, vol. 6, no. 3, pp. 102–110, 1999.

[19] A. E. Brophy, A. D. Smith, J. Olds, E. Fitzpatrick, C. Duquette, and J. Whittingham, "Facilitators and barriers to the integration of orally educated children and youth with hearing loss into their families and communities," *Volta Review*, vol. 107, no. 1, pp. 5–36, 2007.

[20] Y.-T. Chen, "A study to explore the effects of self-regulated learning environment for hearing- impaired students," *Journal of Computer Assisted Learning*, vol. 30, no. 2, pp. 97–109, 2014.

11

A Cognitive Occupation-Based Programme for People with Multiple Sclerosis: A Study to Test Feasibility and Clinical Outcomes

Sean Reilly and Sinéad M. Hynes

Discipline of Occupational Therapy, National University of Ireland Galway, Galway, Ireland

Correspondence should be addressed to Sinéad M. Hynes; sinead.hynes@nuigalway.ie

Academic Editor: Jodie A. Copley

Cognitive impairments are common in MS and affect personal, social, and occupational functioning. There is a developing body of evidence highlighting the role of cognitive rehabilitation, but there is still no evidence for a validated holistic approach. The aim of this study was to assess the effectiveness of Cognitive Occupation-Based Programme for People with Multiple Sclerosis (COB-MS) for improving daily life and cognitive impairment. This study used an experimental pretest/posttest design with eight-week follow-up. Participants were recruited from MS networks using convenience sampling. The primary outcome measure was the GAS. Secondary outcomes included the OSA-DLS, CVLT-II, BVMT-R, SDMT, TMT, BRIEF-A, and EMQ-R. Twelve participants were recruited, aged 39–73 years (mean: 55.08; SD: 9.61). There were statistically significant improvements in the GAS ($p < .002$), CVLT-II: total free recall ($p < .000$), short delay free recall ($p < .018$), long delay free recall ($p < .008$), BVMT-R total recall ($p < .000$), TMT part B ($p < .044$), and EMQ-R ($p < .006$). Except for the BRIEF-A, clinically significant improvements were observed in secondary outcome measures at posttest and follow-up. Limitations include selection bias and subtle practice effects in cognitive measures. Results suggest that a larger scale study is justified considering improvements seen in daily life and cognitive measures.

1. Background

Multiple Sclerosis (MS) is a demyelinating disease of the central nervous system, characterised by the development of lesions in the brain and spinal cord [1]. According to Amato et al. [2], the prevalence of cognitive difficulties in MS ranges from 43% to 70%. The most commonly affected cognitive domains in people with MS are memory, attention, processing speed, and executive functions [3]. Cognitive difficulties affect the daily lives of people with MS in several ways. Cognitive impairment resulting from MS has been found to be associated with impaired social functioning [4], reduced employability [5], and decreased quality of life [6].

Cognitive rehabilitation (CR) is an intervention that aims to improve cognitive impairment through using compensatory and restorative approaches [7]. There are many unique factors to be considered when developing interventions for people with MS such as the disease's fluctuating nature, associated fatigue, and the emotional well-being of the person [8]. To date, most studies examining CR in MS have mainly involved computer-based interventions [9–12], although others have investigated non-computer-based (face to face) interventions that use educational methods [13, 14]. Research has found that computer-based interventions, specifically targeting the domain of attention (e.g., [9, 10]), are effective at improving outcomes on cognitive measures for people with MS. Computer-based interventions that target several cognitive domains [15] also found significant improvements in objective and subjective cognitive outcome measures. In contrast, many computerised interventions that specifically target memory did not lead to improvements (e.g., [16, 17]). It is apparent that non-computer-based interventions are more beneficial for improving memory [18] and several cognitive domains [19, 20] than computerised interventions. Group interventions and frequent professional contact appear to be important components in the effectiveness of CR for people with MS.

Despite the findings from individual studies being generally positive, the pooled results of a meta-analysis in a Cochrane review [21] suggest that the effectiveness of cognitive rehabilitation for people with MS is far from being conclusive. In two recent reviews [22, 23], the authors found low-level evidence that CR reduces cognitive difficulties in MS. Both reviews concluded that CR in MS is in its relative infancy. There is a clear need for more randomised control trials of sound methodological quality before conclusions can be drawn on the possibility of improving function through CR. In addition, both reviews recommended that future studies should examine interventions that aim to increase occupational participation and use outcomes that measure impact on daily life—cognitive interventions adopting a specific approach may not necessarily generalise to functional domains. Findings and recommendations provided the rationale for the current study.

From the current evidence and recommendations provided in the literature, there was a clear need for a holistic cognitive intervention targeting several domains using a functional approach that is measured by and focuses on occupational participation. A Cognitive Occupation-Based Programme for People with Multiple Sclerosis (COB-MS) was developed in response to this noted clinical treatment gap, and it focuses on facilitating people with MS to engage more effectively in everyday occupations that they find difficult as a result of their cognition [24].

Thus, the purpose of this current study was to establish clinical outcomes of COB-MS in relation to daily life and cognition. This study will contribute towards COB-MS' proof of principle and add to the paucity of research in the field of MS and CR.

Specifically, the following research questions were addressed:

(i) Will people who receive COB-MS have improved daily life scores?

(ii) Will people who receive COB-MS see improvements in their cognition?

We were interested if any gains seen were also maintained at follow-up of 8 weeks.

2. Method

2.1. Recruitment. Information regarding the study was available to participants through MS networks such as the monthly MS Ireland newsletter, biannual MS Ireland eZine, and research section of MS Ireland website and Facebook page. Recruitment posters were also hung, with permission, in the outpatient department of University Hospital Galway. Study details and the second author's contact information were available on all recruitment material.

2.2. Participants. Participants were self-selected by contacting the second author via phone or email if they were interested in taking part. To be part of the convenience sample, participants had to meet the following inclusion criteria: (i) be aged 18 years of age or older, (ii) be fluent in written and spoken English, (iii) have a diagnosis of MS, (iv) have mild cognitive difficulties as shown by a score of >22 on the MSNQ, (v) be clinically stable, (vi) can provide informed consent, (vii) do not have neurologic history other than MS, including evidence of current dementia, (viii) do not have history of major depressive disorder, schizophrenia, or bipolar disorder I or II, (ix) do not have history of diagnosed substance use or dependence disorder, and (x) live in the community. Exclusion criteria were the following: (i) cognitive impairment that would affect reliable participation or capacity to give informed consent and (ii) being incarcerated or institutionalised.

Eligibility was determined by the second author during the initial contact. If deemed ineligible, the participant was thanked for their time and the reasons were explained. For eligible participants who were satisfied with the study requirements, verbal consent was sought and their availability was noted to allow for scheduling of COB-MS sessions. Once individual and group sessions were confirmed by the second author, the first author then contacted the participants via phone to schedule the baseline assessment. The first author posted an information sheet to participants for the study. The first author also went through the information sheet with participants at the beginning of the baseline assessment and answered any questions the participants had before signing the written consent form.

2.3. COB-MS Programme. The COB-MS programme consists of eight sessions: two being individual and six being group-based. The focus of the COB-MS is on managing the demands of employment and daily life by using compensatory strategies and routines and learning new techniques that can be integrated into daily occupations and contexts in order to make it meaningful to the participant. The programme was facilitated by the second author. The programme consisted of eight sessions over 9 weeks, beginning one week after baseline assessments and finishing one week before posttest assessments. The COB-MS programme takes a three-pronged approach to cognitive rehabilitation using education, remediation, and adaption to help people meet their goals while managing their cognitive challenges. The programme is informed by the Person-Environment-Occupational Performance model [25].

Table 1 summarises the content of each of the 60-minute sessions.

2.4. Outcome Measures. Participants completed a total of eight assessments. The Goal Attainment Scaling (GAS) [26] was the primary outcome measure of this current study and allowed participants to set meaningful goals related to daily life, which could be measured in a systematic way. Given the emphasis placed on goal-setting in COB-MS and the importance of personal goals as a source of motivation for participants, goal achievement reflected the practical benefit of COB-MS.

Table 1

Session	Brief content
Session 1 (individual)	*Focus on you* (i) Initial meeting with the OT: briefing on what will be involved in COB-MS (ii) Goal setting with the person on occupations that they wish to target
Session 2 (group)	*You and your cognition* (i) Education about the brain and cognition (ii) Discussion on how MS can impact cognitive function (iii) Discussion on the impact of cognitive difficulties on day-to-day occupations
Session 3 (group)	*You, the centerpiece* (i) How the cognitive difficulties affect you? (ii) What changes can be made by you? (iii) Discussion and application of strategies
Session 4 (group)	*You, the person* (i) Further concepts on what changes can be made by you (ii) Internal strategies to practice and apply (iii) Discussion around sleep and sleep diaries
Session 5 (group)	*Your environment* (i) How does the environment impact cognition? (ii) What can we change that might help? (iii) Application of external memory strategies (iv) Managing distraction and the impact of other factors
Session 6 (group)	*Focus on doing* (i) How are our occupations and daily life affected? (ii) What can we do to help integrate strategies into daily life? (iii) Examples of how to adapt or remediate occupations
Session 7 (group)	*Seeking new challenges* (i) Seek new challenges with strategies that support success (ii) Set goals for yourself (iii) Stay motivated, maintain progress and on-going adaptation (iv) Group conclusion and debrief
Session 8 (individual)	*Testing the application* (i) Review goals and strategies used (ii) Plan for future (iii) Discussion around useful groups and services (iv) Debrief and summary

Secondary outcomes included measures of occupational competence [Occupational Self-Assessment-Daily Living Scales (OSA-DLS) [27]], verbal memory [California Verbal Learning Test-II (CVLT-II) [28]], visual memory [Brief Visuospatial Memory Test-Revised (BVMT-R) [29]], processing speed [Symbol Digit Modality Test (SDMT) [30]], divided attention [Trail Making Test (TMT) [31]], perceived executive functioning [Behaviour Rating Inventory of Executive Function-Adult Version (BRIEF-A) [32]], and self-reported memory difficulties [Everyday Memory Questionnaire-Revised (EMQ-R) [33]].

Data was collected by the researcher at three time points: one week before the first COB-MS session (baseline), one week after the final COB-MS session (posttest), and eight weeks after the final COB-MS session (follow-up). Except for the GAS, all assessments were administered at three time points, with alternate forms used where possible.

2.5. Statistical Analysis. SPSS Version 23 was utilised to analyse the data. Descriptive statistics were used to describe the characteristics of the sample regarding gender, age, education, work status, MS type, disease duration, and MSNQ score. To answer the research questions, inferential statistics were utilised. The Friedman test measured changes in mean daily life and cognitive scores over three time points, whereas the Wilcoxon signed-rank test measured changes over two time points.

3. Results

In total, 1 male and 11 female participants received COB-MS. The types of MS varied between participants and included relapsing remitting ($n = 5$) or primary progressive ($n = 3$) types. Four participants were unsure of their MS type. Participants' work status also varied and included long term disability ($n = 5$), staying at home parent ($n = 3$), or being retired ($n = 4$).

A full data set was obtained, as the twelve participants completed outcome measures at each of the three time points. Descriptive statistics were expressed as a mean, standard

TABLE 2: Demographic data of the sample.

	Mean	SD	Minimum	Maximum
Age (years)	55.08	9.61	39	73
Duration (years)	14.25	7.61	3	31
Education (years)	16.42	2.31	13	20
MSNQ	26.58	2.27	23	30

TABLE 3: Wilcoxon signed-rank test results for the GAS.

	Time 1			Time 3			z-value	p value
	Mean	SD	Median	Mean	SD	Median		
GAS	37.02	0.88	37.5	56.23	10.60	52.7	−3.061	.002*

*p value is statistically significant at $p < .05$.

TABLE 4: Friedman test results for the OSA-DLS.

	Time 1			Time 2			Time 3			p value
	Mean	SD	Median	Mean	SD	Median	Mean	SD	Median	
Competence	30.58	7.50	31.00	31.67	6.77	33.00	31.33	7.55	34.00	.822
Importance	31.42	6.54	31.00	31.92	8.59	35.00	31.67	8.19	31.00	1.000

deviation (SD), minimum, and maximum. Table 2 illustrates the demographic data of the sample in relation to age, disease duration, education, and MSNQ score.

3.1. Daily Life. After receiving COB-MS, participants' goal achievement improvement in scores on the GAS (Table 3) was statistically significant ($z = -3.061$; $p = .02$). This shows that the meaningful goals set in relation to daily life were achieved by follow-up. Table 4 shows that occupational competence scores on the OSA-DLS were clinically significant as posttest and follow-up scores were greater than baseline.

3.2. Cognition. Findings from cognitive outcome measures are shown in Table 5. Statistically significant improvements were observed in verbal memory on the CVLT-II: in total free recall ($p = .000$), short delay free recall ($p = .018$), and long delay free recall ($p = .008$). In visual memory, a statistically significant difference was obtained on the BVMT-R in total recall ($p = .000$). In part B of the TMT, improvements in divided attention were statistically significant ($p = .044$). Although results for part A of the TMT and the SDMT were not statistically significant, results show that processing speed improved across the three time points. Participants reported significantly fewer memory difficulties in daily life on the EMQ-R ($p = .006$). In contrast to the trend of results, perceived executive functioning scores on the BRIEF-A at follow-up did not improve when compared to baseline.

3.3. Post Hoc Tests. After establishing that there were statistically significant differences somewhere among the three time points in Friedman test results for the CVLT-II, BVMT-R, TMT, and EMQ-R, post hoc tests were used to identify changes between individual time points (Table 6). Wilcoxon signed-rank tests were used to compare Time 1 with Time 2, Time 2 with Time 3, and Time 1 with Time 3.

To control for Type 1 errors, a Bonferroni adjustment was applied to the alpha values. This involved dividing the original alpha level of .05 by the total number of tests used (.05/3 = .01666). Thus, the adjusted alpha level for determining statistical significance was .0167.

4. Discussion

Results suggest that people who receive COB-MS have significantly higher mean daily life scores at posttest and eight-week follow-up. The GAS, which was the primary outcome measure of the study, showed a statistically significant increase in goal achievement with a large effect size. This adds to the findings of Mantynen et al. who observed similar changes in the GAS and showed that personal goals for their computer-based and non-computer-based interventions were well achieved [34]. However, it is important to note that the goals set by participants in this study related to leisure, self-care, and productivity occupations in their daily lives and not just the intervention as seen in Mantynen et al.'s work [34]. Therefore, the improvements observed in the GAS in this study reflect the practical benefit of COB-MS and acknowledge the real-world implications of COB-MS in daily life.

Although there was no statistically significant increase in the OSA-DLS, scores at posttest and follow-up were greater than baseline and are indicative of clinical significance. With regard to the trend of competence scores in the OSA-DLS, it appears that people who receive COB-MS feel that they improve their ability to sustain a pattern of occupational behaviour, which is both satisfying and productive. Therefore, the perceived ability to perform activities of daily living (ADLs) and instrumental activities of daily living (IADLs) increased after receiving COB-MS. Similarly, the importance placed on daily life occupations was also greater at posttest and follow-up. Unfortunately, no comparisons with other

TABLE 5: Friedman test results for cognitive outcome measures.

	Time 1			Time 2			Time 3			p value
	Mean	SD	Median	Mean	SD	Median	Mean	SD	Median	
CVLT-II										
Total free recall	45.92	6.83	45.00	58.00	7.10	56.00	54.50	9.85	52.00	.000*
Short delay free recall	9.00	2.09	9.00	12.17	2.41	13.00	11.25	3.22	13.00	.018*
Long delay free recall	9.67	2.81	10.00	12.33	2.06	13.00	11.58	2.84	12.00	.008*
BVMT-R										
Total recall	45.67	9.87	44.00	51.33	12.61	52.00	57.33	10.22	60.00	.000*
Delayed recall	48.83	12.77	49.00	52.42	14.87	56.00	57.58	8.22	61.00	.103
SDMT	38.42	8.08	38.00	39.83	10.20	37.00	41.75	9.28	37.00	.127
TMT										
Part A	35.92	12.07	31.00	34.33	11.51	33.00	33.75	15.39	33.00	.368
Part B	95.92	47.96	79.00	69.17	31.57	56.00	67.33	27.58	62.00	.044*
BRIEF-A										
Behavioural regulation index	58.83	9.71	58.00	57.58	8.55	60.00	59.33	7.98	61.00	.376
Metacognition index	61.58	11.31	61.00	61.08	7.83	63.00	63.00	7.94	63.00	.862
Global executive composite	61.17	10.05	63.00	60.25	8.01	62.00	61.25	8.21	61.00	.320
EMQ-R	19.83	10.85	18.00	15.67	12.46	14.00	16.00	11.07	14.00	.006*

* p value is statistically significant at $p < .05$.

TABLE 6: Wilcoxon signed-rank test results for post hoc tests.

	Time 1	Time 2	Time 3
CVLT-II: total free recall	.002*	.181	.003*
CVLT-II: short delay free recall	.008*	.058	.052
CVLT-II: long delay free recall	.012*	.311	.044
BVMT-R: total recall	.028	.012*	.022
TMT: part B	.077	.610	.016*
EMQ-R	.040	.563	.022

* p value is statistically significant at $p < .0167$.

studies can be made as the OSA-DLS was not used as an outcome measure in previously reviewed literature. However, there is an abundance of literature pertaining to the Model of Human Occupation which illustrates the meaning of the OSA-DLS results [35]. It has been stated by Lee et al. that a person's motivation for occupation, often referred to as volition, is influenced by personal causation, values, and interests [36]. Volition is also recognised as a fundamental factor in the achievement of goals. Thus, this is in line with findings in the current study as higher competence scores (personal causation) and importance scores (values and interests) appear to have contributed towards people achieving their daily life goals after receiving COB-MS.

With regard to cognition, results suggest that people who receive COB-MS have statistically significant improvements in verbal memory scores at posttest and follow-up, as shown on the CVLT-II. This finding is similar to verbal memory improvements seen in computer-based interventions [11, 37], non-computer-based interventions [38, 39], and studies that investigated computer-based and non-computer-based interventions [40, 41]. While one may think that an intervention that specifically trained memory would result in better verbal memory outcomes than a nonspecific intervention, this is not the case. For example, two computer-based interventions specifically targeting memory failed to find statistically significant improvements in verbal memory [12, 17], whereas the nonspecific intervention in this current study did. This observation supports the argument that interventions for people with MS are more effective in the presence of a healthcare professional [20].

Findings from this current study also suggest that people who receive COB-MS improve statistically in visual memory, as shown in the BVMT-R. These findings are reminiscent of those by computer-based interventions [15, 40] and interventions using a combination of computer-based and non-computer-based training [37, 41, 42]. Once again, there is evidence supporting the argument by Jonsson et al., as interventions that involved frequent input from a healthcare professional appear to be more effective for improving visual memory [39]. It appears that regular contact with a professional is required as people may not comply with the intervention if they are not monitored weekly [14]. In addition, qualitative research suggests that people enjoy the social element of group interventions [13], which is absent in individual and computer-based interventions. In COB-MS, each session involves discussion around cognitive difficulties, whereby the facilitator explains various strategies and techniques that can be applied to improve occupational performance in daily life. A group-based design is a feasible and cost-efficient method to deliver interventions in a healthcare setting, making the COB-MS meaningful to frontline health professionals. The format of the COB-MS, importantly, allows for individualisation through the two individual sessions coupled with goal setting.

Although results pertaining to processing speed and working memory on the SDMT did not improve statistically, they were nonetheless clinically significant. From the literature reviewed which utilised the SDMT as an outcome measure, no study identified a statistically significant improvement [9, 10, 14, 16, 38]. However, it is interesting to note that people who received COB-MS improved in the SDMT at each time point (follow-up > posttest > baseline). Considering that there are minimal practice effects in the SDMT [43], it would appear that the 8-week gap between posttest and follow-up allowed people to integrate and generalise strategies learned in COB-MS into their daily lives. This finding validates the purpose of a follow-up assessment in the current study.

There was also a clinically significant improvement for processing speed in part A of the TMT. Similar to the SDMT, participants performed better at each time point. It must be noted that, at one-month intervals, part A is susceptible to practice effects after the first trial [44]. However, according to the same research by Craddick and Stern [44], there were no practice effects for part B in the current study as it was only utilised at three time points. Thus, it was positive to discover statistically significant improvements for divided attention in part B after receiving COB-MS. While clinical improvements in the TMT were frequently observed in the literature [10, 34, 41], few studies identified statistically significant changes. Although Amato et al. identified statistically significant improvements in both parts of the TMT, their computer-based intervention specifically targeted attention, which means that the results were unsurprising [9].

Results suggest that people who receive COB-MS perceive fewer difficulties with memory in daily life. Although a statistically significant improvement was observed after the Friedman test, the improvement was not statistically significant when using a Bonferroni adjustment. This is similar to Carr et al. who also identified a clinically but not statistically significant improvement [13]. It is possible that the small sample size in both studies may have led to the lack of a statistically significant difference. Furthermore, the use of a Bonferroni adjustment to reduce the chance of Type 1 error made the significance level more conservative. However, it is correct practice to use a Bonferroni adjustment when making multiple comparisons.

Although participants perceived fewer difficulties with executive functioning at posttest, scores at follow-up show that there was a greater frequency of difficulties reported in comparison with baseline. However, similar to the OSA-DLS, it is difficult to draw comparisons as the BRIEF-A was not used as an outcome measure in previously reviewed literature. While some studies have identified statistically significant improvements in objective executive functioning [41, 42], it has been argued by Sullivan et al. that subjective cognitive functioning often correlates poorly with the objective equivalent [45]. It may have been that, given the period of reflection that comes with follow-up assessment, participants became more aware of the metacognitive domains (e.g., planning and monitoring) and their difficulties in these areas. The subjective scores they provided may not necessarily reflect objective measurement but an increased insight and awareness of difficulties.

The results from this study suggest that people who receive COB-MS improve significantly (statistically or clinically), in all daily life outcome measures and most cognitive outcome measures, at posttest and follow-up. These findings are encouraging given the fact that this was a pilot study with a small number of participants. Considering that a nonspecific intervention was used in this study, it is not surprising that there were only two statistically significant improvements in cognitive outcome measures. As MS is a degenerative disease, cognitive difficulties are likely to worsen [1]. Therefore, it could be argued that a nonspecific intervention that addresses daily life, by targeting difficulties with cognition, will produce longer lasting benefits for people with MS rather than attempting to improve a specific cognitive domain. Thus, the validity of COB-MS is supported by statistically significant improvements in the primary outcome measure, the GAS, and clinically significant improvements in the OSA-DLS. However, there are some factors that limit the generalisability of findings.

Firstly, there is a high risk of self-selecting bias in this study. Therefore, the participants may have been highly motivated to learn and apply strategies from COB-MS in their daily lives. However, treatment contamination is incredibly difficult to control when recruiting community-dwelling participants. Although the prevalence of MS is reported to be three times more common in females [46], there was only one male participant and this limits generalisability to males. The lack of disease course data on the entire sample as well as the substantial variation in disease duration is also noted as a limitation. Another significant limitation that relates to participant selection is the use of the MSNQ. This measurement device was used as a self-report screening tool for cognitive impairment as part of the inclusion criteria, whereby participants required a score of at least 22 or more. However, the observation of ceiling effects in the results suggests that this cut-off score may have been too low, and previous studies have shown weak correlations between subjective and objective cognitive impairments [47, 48]. Nonetheless, it was decided to include people who had self-reported cognitive impairment (as shown in the MSNQ) without objective evidence because (i) this was a pilot study, which aimed to ensure that COB-MS was feasible in the largest possible sample of people with MS, (ii) some people may have experienced cognitive difficulties in daily life but would not be classified as impaired on an objective measure, and (iii) it was felt that the people would be more motivated to learn if they felt they had cognitive difficulties.

Secondly, despite using alternative assessment forms (CVLT-II and BVMT-R) and research stating minimal practice effects (SDMT and TMT part B), subtle practice effects cannot be completely ruled out in cognitive outcome measures. There are two types of practice effects: "test-specific," which refers to people knowing the assessment format, and "item-specific," which refers to people learning the actual content of the assessment (e.g., word lists or geometric figures [49, 50]). Although item-specific practice effects were mitigated by using alternative forms, test-specific practice effects were unavoidable. For example, at baseline assessments, participants were unaware that there was a delayed recall in the CVLT-II. However, at posttest and follow-up, it is likely that participants knew that they would have to recall the words and may have been internally listing them. In addition, the use of nonparametric tests to analyse outcomes is a limitation. The Friedman test and Wilcoxon signed-rank test are less sensitive than the equivalent parametric techniques, one-way repeated-measures ANOVA and paired-samples t-test, respectively. Thus, it is possible that statistically significant differences may have been missed [51].

5. Conclusion

Future research should use outcome measures related to daily life. It was highlighted in the literature review that it is unclear whether improvements in cognitive outcome measures are indicative of improvements in daily life [52]. The use of daily life assessments would also facilitate comparisons between studies, an issue that was observed in the current study. In addition, subjective cognitive assessments should continue to be used. Although Sullivan et al. argue that subjective and objective cognitive assessments correlate poorly with each other [45], findings from this current study suggest that they trend in the same direction. It appears that different concepts are being measured, with objective tools measuring how a person performs in a structured test, whereas subjective devices measure how a person feels they perform in daily life. Furthermore, outcome assessors should be blinded, and a follow-up period of approximately 6–12 months should be used to determine if improvements are maintained over the long term.

Occupational therapists and people with MS reported that COB-MS may be more beneficial for people who are newly diagnosed [24]. Thus, future studies of COB-MS could consider comparing its effectiveness for people who are newly diagnosed versus people who have been diagnosed for some time. Considering that Chiaravalloti et al. [18] found that people with moderate cognitive impairment benefitted more than those with mild cognitive impairment, it may be worth comparing the effectiveness of COB-MS for a group of moderately versus mildly impaired participants. These recommendations could also be integrated into occupational therapy practice, whereby COB-MS is provided to people with MS who are newly diagnosed and/or have similar levels of cognitive impairment. Previous studies found that older participants were more adherent in completing CR at home than younger participants [15, 41]. Therefore, future COB-MS studies should monitor completion of homework activities to determine adherence to the programme. In addition, the paucity of qualitative research indicates that participants of future COB-MS studies should be interviewed to determine benefits of the programme that cannot be detected in quantitative measures, as shown in Carr et al. [13].

The primary implication for occupational therapy practice is that this study provides an occupation-based intervention that is specific to the cognitive difficulties faced by people with MS. COB-MS is a step-by-step evidence-based intervention that can be facilitated by occupational therapists and enable people to identify, understand, and implement strategies to simultaneously manage cognitive impairment and improve function in daily life.

To conclude, this pilot study established the clinical outcomes of COB-MS in relation to daily life and cognition. This study provides foundational evidence to support COB-MS as the most suitable intervention for people with MS who experience cognitive difficulties in daily life and adds to the paucity of research in the field of MS and CR.

Conflicts of Interest

The authors declare that there are no conflicts of interest regarding the publication of this article.

Acknowledgments

This research was supported by funding from the National University of Ireland Galway Millennium Fund 2016/2017.

References

[1] B. K. Tsang and R. McDonnell, "Multiple sclerosis: diagnosis, management and prognosis," *Australian family physician*, vol. 40, no. 12, pp. 948–959, 2011.

[2] M. P. Amato, V. Zipoli, and E. Portaccio, "Multiple sclerosis-related cognitive changes: a review of cross-sectional and longitudinal studies," *Journal of the Neurological Sciences*, vol. 245, no. 1-2, pp. 41–46, 2006.

[3] D. W. Langdon, "Cognition in multiple sclerosis," *Current Opinion in Neurology*, vol. 24, no. 3, pp. 244–249, 2011.

[4] M. Filippi, G. Riccitelli, F. Mattioli et al., "Multiple sclerosis: effects of cognitive rehabilitation on structural and functional MR imaging measures—an explorative study," *Radiology*, vol. 262, no. 3, pp. 932–940, 2012.

[5] N. D. Chiaravalloti and J. DeLuca, "Cognitive impairment in multiple sclerosis," *The Lancet Neurology*, vol. 7, no. 12, pp. 1139–1151, 2008.

[6] A. Brenk, K. Laun, and C. G. Haase, "Short-term cognitive training improves mental efficiency and mood in patients with multiple sclerosis," *European Neurology*, vol. 60, no. 6, pp. 304–309, 2008.

[7] S. H. Pierson and N. Griffith, "Treatment of cognitive impairment in multiple sclerosis," *Behavioural Neurology*, vol. 17, no. 1, pp. 53–67, 2006.

[8] T. A. M. Siepman, A. C. J. W. Janssens, I. De Koning, C. H. Polman, J. B. Boringa, and R. Q. Hintzen, "The role of disability and depression in cognitive functioning within 2 years after multiple sclerosis diagnosis," *Journal of Neurology*, vol. 255, no. 6, pp. 910–916, 2008.

[9] M. P. Amato, B. Goretti, R. G. Viterbo et al., "Computer-assisted rehabilitation of attention in patients with multiple sclerosis: Results of a randomized, double-blind trial," *Multiple Sclerosis Journal*, vol. 20, no. 1, pp. 91–98, 2014.

[10] A. Cerasa, M. C. Gioia, P. Valentino et al., "Computer-assisted cognitive rehabilitation of attention deficits for multiple sclerosis: a randomized trial with fMRI correlates," *Neurorehabilitation and Neural Repair*, vol. 27, no. 4, pp. 284–295, 2013.

[11] M. Lanz, J. Kraus, H. Hahn, B. Schwarze, G. Schwendemann, and H. Hildebrandt, "Cognitive training in MS: effects and relation to brain atrophy," *Aktuelle Neurologie*, vol. 32, no. S 4, 2005.

[12] L. Mendozzi, L. Pugnetti, A. Motta et al., "Computer-assisted memory retraining of patients with multiple sclerosis," *Italian Journal of Neurological Sciences*, vol. 19, no. 6, pp. S431–S438, 1998.

[13] S. E. Carr, R. Das Nair, A. F. Schwartz, and N. B. Lincoln, "Group memory rehabilitation for people with multiple sclerosis: A feasibility randomized controlled trial," *Clinical Rehabilitation*, vol. 28, no. 6, pp. 552–561, 2014.

[14] N. B. Lincoln, A. Dent, J. Harding et al., "Evaluation of cognitive assessment and cognitive intervention for people with multiple sclerosis," *Journal of Neurology, Neurosurgery & Psychiatry*, vol. 72, no. 1, pp. 93–98, 2002.

[15] E. Shatil, A. Metzer, O. Horvitz, and A. Miller, "Home-based personalized cognitive training in MS patients: A study of adherence and cognitive performance," *NeuroRehabilitation*, vol. 26, no. 2, pp. 143–153, 2010.

[16] L. M. Hancock, J. M. Bruce, A. S. Bruce, and S. G. Lynch, "Processing speed and working memory training in multiple sclerosis: A double-blind randomized controlled pilot study," *Journal of Clinical and Experimental Neuropsychology*, vol. 37, no. 2, pp. 113–127, 2015.

[17] A. Solari, A. Motta, L. Mendozzi et al., "Computer-aided retraining of memory and attention in people with multiple sclerosis: a randomized, double-blind controlled trial," *Journal of the Neurological Sciences*, vol. 222, no. 1-2, pp. 99–104, 2004.

[18] N. D. Chiaravalloti, J. DeLuca, N. B. Moore, and J. H. Ricker, "Treating learning impairments improves memory performance in multiple sclerosis: A randomized clinical trial," *Multiple Sclerosis Journal*, vol. 11, no. 1, pp. 58–68, 2005.

[19] F. Fink, E. Rischkau, M. Butt, J. Klein, P. Eling, and H. Hildebrandt, "Efficacy of an executive function intervention programme in MS: A placebo-controlled and pseudo-randomized trial," *Multiple Sclerosis Journal*, vol. 16, no. 9, pp. 1148–1151, 2010.

[20] E. Shevil and M. Finlayson, "Pilot study of a cognitive intervention program for persons with multiple sclerosis," *Health Education Research*, vol. 25, no. 1, pp. 41–53, 2010.

[21] E. M. Rosti-Otajärvi and P. I. Hämäläinen, "Neuropsychological rehabilitation for multiple sclerosis.," *Cochrane Database of Systematic Reviews*, vol. 2, p. CD009131, 2014.

[22] R. das Nair, K. J. Martin, and N. B. Lincoln, "Memory rehabilitation for people with multiple sclerosis," *The Cochrane Library*, 2016.

[23] A. R. O'Brien, N. Chiaravalloti, Y. Goverover, and J. DeLuca, "Evidenced-Based Cognitive Rehabilitation for Persons With Multiple Sclerosis: A Review of the Literature," *Archives of Physical Medicine and Rehabilitation*, vol. 89, no. 4, pp. 761–769, 2008.

[24] S. M. Hynes and S. J. Forwell, "A Cognitive Occupation-Based Programme for People with Multiple Sclerosis (COB-MS): the development of a new occupational therapy intervention," in Press.

[25] C. Christiansen, C. M. Baum, and J. Bass, "The Person-Environment-Occupational-Performance Model," in *Foundations for Practice in Occupational Therapy*, S. E. A. Duncan, Ed., pp. 93–104, Elsevier, London, UK, 5th edition, 2011.

[26] T. J. Kiresuk and R. E. Sherman, "Goal attainment scaling: A general method for evaluating comprehensive community mental health programs," *Community Mental Health Journal*, vol. 4, no. 6, pp. 443–453, 1968.

[27] P. Scott, *Occupational Self Assessment - Daily Living Scales*, Model of Human Occupation, Clearinghouse, 2016.

[28] J. Baños, "California Verbal Learning Test-Second Edition D. Delis, J. Kramer, E. Kaplan, B. Ober. San Antonio, TX. The Psychological Corporation, 2000," *Archives of Clinical Neuropsychology*, vol. 17, no. 5, pp. 509–512.

[29] R. H. Benedict, *Brief visuospatial memory test–revised: professional manual*, PAR, 1997.

[30] A. Smith, *Symbol digit modality test (SDMT): manual (revised)*, Psychological Services, Los Angeles, Cakif, USA, 1982.

[31] R. M. Reitan and D. Wolfson, "The Trail Making Test as an initial screening procedure for neuropsychological impairment in older children," *Archives of Clinical Neuropsychology*, vol. 19, no. 2, pp. 281–288, 2004.

[32] R. M. Roth, P. K. Isquith, and G. A. Gioia, *Behavior Rating Inventory of Executive Function - Adult Version, Professional Manual*, Psychological Assessment Resources, 2005.

[33] J. Royle and N. B. Lincoln, "The Everyday Memory Questionnaire - Revised: Development of a 13-item scale," *Disability and Rehabilitation*, vol. 30, no. 2, pp. 114–121, 2008.

[34] A. Mantynen, E. Rosti-Otajärvi, K. Koivisto, A. Lilja, H. Huhtala, and P. Hämäläinen, "Neuropsychological rehabilitation does not improve cognitive performance but reduces perceived cognitive deficits in patients with multiple sclerosis: A randomised, controlled, multi-centre trial," *Multiple Sclerosis Journal*, vol. 20, no. 1, pp. 99–107, 2014.

[35] G. Kielhofner, *A model of human occupation: Theory and application*, Williams and Wilkins, Baltimore, MD, USA, 4th edition, 2008.

[36] S. W. Lee, R. Taylor, G. Kielhofner, and G. Fisher, "Theory use in practice: a national survey of therapists who use the model of human occupation," *The American Journal of Occupational Therapy*, vol. 62, no. 1, pp. 106–117, 2008.

[37] H. Brissart, M. Leroy, E. Morele, C. Baumann, E. Spitz, and M. Debouverie, "Cognitive rehabilitation in Multiple sclerosis," *Neurocase*, vol. 19, no. 6, pp. 553–565, 2013.

[38] A. K. Stuifbergen, H. Becker, F. Perez, J. Morison, V. Kullberg, and A. Todd, "A randomized controlled trial of a cognitive rehabilitation intervention for persons with multiple sclerosis," *Clinical Rehabilitation*, vol. 26, no. 10, pp. 882–893, 2012.

[39] A. Jonsson, E. M. Korfitzen, A. Heltberg, M. H. Ravnborg, and E. Byskov-Ottosen, "Effects of neuropsychological treatment in patients with multiple sclerosis," *Acta Neurologica Scandinavica*, vol. 88, no. 6, pp. 394–400, 1993.

[40] A. Vogt, L. Kappos, P. Calabrese et al., "Working memory training in patients with multiple sclerosis - Comparison of two different training schedules," *Restorative Neurology and Neuroscience*, vol. 27, no. 3, pp. 225–235, 2009.

[41] J. Gich, J. Freixanet, R. García et al., "A randomized, controlled, single-blind, 6-month pilot study to evaluate the efficacy of MS-Line!: A cognitive rehabilitation programme for patients with multiple sclerosis," *Multiple Sclerosis Journal*, vol. 21, no. 10, pp. 1332–1343, 2015.

[42] N. Tesar, K. Bandion, and U. Baumhackl, "Efficacy of a neuropsychological training programme for patients with multiple sclerosis - A randomised controlled trial," *Wiener Klinische Wochenschrift*, vol. 117, no. 21-22, pp. 747–754, 2005.

[43] R. H. B. Benedict, J. A. Duquin, S. Jurgensen et al., "Repeated assessment of neuropsychological deficits in multiple sclerosis using the symbol digit modalities test and the MS neuropsychological screening questionnaire," *Multiple Sclerosis Journal*, vol. 14, no. 7, pp. 940–946, 2008.

[44] R. A. Craddick and M. R. Stern, "Practice effects on the trail making test," *Perceptual and Motor Skills*, vol. 17, no. 3, pp. 651–653, 1963.

[45] M. J. L. Sullivan, K. Edgley, and E. Dehoux, "A survey of multiple sclerosis. Part 1: Perceived cognitive problems and compensatory strategy use," *Canadian Journal of Rehabilitation*, vol. 4, no. 2, pp. 99–105, 1990.

[46] A. D. Sadovnick, "European Charcot Foundation Lecture: The natural history of multiple sclerosis and gender," *Journal of the Neurological Sciences*, vol. 286, no. 1-2, pp. 1–5, 2009.

[47] J. M. Bruce, A. S. Bruce, L. Hancock, and S. Lynch, "Self-reported memory problems in multiple sclerosis: influence of psychiatric status and normative dissociative experiences," *Archives of Clinical Neuropsychology*, vol. 25, no. 1, pp. 39–48, 2010.

[48] S. W. Kinsinger, E. Lattie, and D. C. Mohr, "Relationship between depression, fatigue, subjective cognitive impairment, and objective neuropsychological functioning in patients with multiple sclerosis," *Neuropsychology*, vol. 24, no. 5, pp. 573–580, 2010.

[49] R. H. B. Benedict and D. J. Zgaljardic, "Practice effects during repeated administrations of memory tests with and without alternate forms," *Journal of Clinical and Experimental Neuropsychology*, vol. 20, no. 3, pp. 339–352, 1998.

[50] D. J. Zgaljardic and R. H. B. Benedict, "Evaluation of practice effects in language and spatial processing test performance," *Applied Neuropsychology*, vol. 8, no. 4, pp. 218–223, 2001.

[51] J. Pallant, *SPSS survival manual: A step by step guide to data analysis using IBM SPSS*, McGraw-Hill Education, Berkshire, UK, 5th edition, 2013.

[52] B. A. Wilson, "Neuropsychological rehabilitation," *Annual Review of Clinical Psychology*, vol. 4, pp. 141–162, 2008.

12

Enhancing a Client-Centred Practice with the Canadian Occupational Performance Measure

A. Enemark Larsen,[1] B. Rasmussen,[1] and J. R. Christensen[2,3]

[1]*Department of Occupational Therapy, Institute of Medwifery and Therapy, University College Copenhagen, Sigurdsgade 26, DK-2200 N Copenhagen, Denmark*
[2]*Department of Public Health, University of Southern Denmark, JB Winsløwsvej 9A, 5000 Odense, Denmark*
[3]*Department of Sports Science and Clinical Biomechanics, University of Southern Denmark, Campusvej 55, 5230 Odense, Denmark*

Correspondence should be addressed to A. Enemark Larsen; anel@phmetropol.dk

Academic Editor: Mélanie Levasseur

Background. The active participation of clients is an important aspect of rehabilitation quality as conceptualized in client-centred practice (CCP). A recommended outcome measure for enhancing CCP is the Canadian Occupational Performance Measure (COPM). However, the relationship between COPM use and CCP enhancement has not been documented. *Aim.* The aim of this study was to examine whether the use of the COPM enhanced CCP. *Methods.* We performed a scoping review in five steps: (1) *identifying* a search strategy with inclusion and exclusion criteria; (2) *screening* relevant databases for published and unpublished studies by using selected keywords and by manually scrutinizing reference lists; (3) agreeing on *eligible* papers between authors in terms of inclusion and exclusion criteria; (4) charting *included* data; and (5) *analysing* data using qualitative content analysis. *Results.* Twelve studies were included in the review. The results indicated enhanced CCP in two themes when using the COPM. These themes appeared to influence each other; therefore, the first theme, *Conditions for enhancing CCP when using the COPM*, represented the circumstances needed for the second theme, *Enhancing CCP when using the COPM*, to be fulfilled. *Conclusion.* The use of the COPM seems to enhance CCP if certain conditions are present.

1. Introduction

The active participation of clients is an important aspect of the quality of rehabilitation processes and the aim in healthcare institutions around the world [1, 2]. Similar in Denmark, since 2013, the hospital staff have endeavoured the active involvement of clients through a systematic collection of information from clients about their experiences during rehabilitation [3]. The information has been collected within the Danish Model of Quality in the Healthcare System (DDKM) and used to improve the quality of hospital services [3]. Thus, active participation of clients is included as a key component in the 2020 visions of healthcare systems in many countries [4]. The 2020 visions aim to create a healthcare system that is suited to each individual and more responsive to each client's preferences, needs, and values [4]. However, fulfilling this aim is difficult [5, 6]. A recent study showed that although the aim is the active participation of clients in the rehabilitation process, the process often does not truly reference the client's wishes and goals and is not collaborative [7]. Another study showed that clients experienced inadequate rehabilitation that did not emphasize their individual and emotional needs [8]. Furthermore, clients who require help to manage uncertainties have experienced unaddressed problems [8, 9]. All this evidence illustrates the need to optimize efforts to enhance client participation in the rehabilitation process [10].

One conceptual framework that includes the active participation of clients is "client-centred practice" (CCP), described by Carl Rogers as practice that is nondirective and focuses on the concerns expressed by the client [6, 11]. In occupational therapy (OT), CCP has always been an integrated value and a fundamental element [12]. Research on CCP has increased over the last few decades [6, 13–15]. A systematic review revealed five thematic conceptual elements that should be addressed when working with CCP, namely, power, listening and communicating, partnership, choice, and hope [6].

A recommended method believed to enhance CCP in the rehabilitation process is the use of the Canadian Occupational Performance Measure (COPM) [16]. The COPM is designed to identify changes in the client's personal perceptions of occupational performance over time, and studies show that the identification of self-perceived occupational performance problems (OPPs) seems to enhance client motivation and the relevance of the individualized goals in rehabilitation [16–20]. The COPM consists of the following five steps and three scores: (1) the clients identify their OPPs within the areas of self-care, productivity, and leisure and score their *importance* on a scale ranging from 1, not important, to 10, extremely important. (2) The clients prioritize up to five OPPs on which to focus during the intervention. (3) The clients rate their *performance* and (4) their *satisfaction with performance* of the identified OPPs. Both scales range from 1 to 10, with higher values indicating better performance and greater satisfaction. (5) Performance and satisfaction with performance are reassessed after an appropriate interval of time, normally between three to six months, and changes in the clients' perceptions of their occupational performance can be calculated [16].

Generally, studies on concurrent and content validity that included a variety of clients and OT practitioners show that the COPM is a valid measure of occupational performance [20]. Studies have also documented the COPM's utility in providing an individualized perspective of the client's values, judgements, and preferences regarding occupational performance and thus its ability to facilitate clinical decision-making and monitor functional progress [19, 20].

Given that the aim of the COPM interview is not only to identify, prioritize, and score the OPPs but also to enhance CCP, it seems important to evaluate whether the latter aim is actually fulfilled. Studies of the COPM have also reported the ability of the COPM interview to enhance CCP [17–20]. Additionally, in the systematic review by Parker and Sykes, the COPM interview enabled clients to name and frame their problems, allowed them to be experts on their own circumstances, and empowered them to be more critical of their own performance, that is, the use of the COPM seemed to support CCP [21]. However, a review from 2011 that examined the COPM and other measurements identified a paucity of literature concerning the client's experiences with the COPM, leaving the question of whether the use of the COPM can enhance CCP [22]. Thus, the aim of the current study was to examine the literature and determine whether the use of the COPM can enhance CCP.

2. Materials and Method

2.1. Design. The current scoping review followed the recommendations from the commentary of Colquhoun et al. [23], which advised the use of the following methodological steps outlined in the Arksey and O'Malley framework [24] and further enhanced by Levac et al. [25]: (1) identification: identify the research questions. (2) Screening: find the relevant studies. (3) Eligibility: select the studies relevant to the question. (4) Inclusion: chart the data. (5) Analysis: collate, summarize, and report the results. Because our aim was to examine the *literature* on the COPM, the optional 6th step of the scoping review procedure, consultation with stakeholders as a required knowledge translation component, was not applied in this review [23–25].

2.2. Procedure

2.2.1. Identification. We developed a search strategy with inclusion and exclusion criteria and used the PICO (population, intervention, comparison, outcome) model to identify keywords relevant to our research question [26] as we wanted to examine whether the COPM (the 'I') would enhance CCP (the 'O'). Thus, in our search strategy, we included all kinds of populations from all kinds of settings (the 'P's), but we did not include any comparisons (the 'C').

2.2.2. Screening. The literature search was performed in two steps between September and December 2016 (last search: 18.12.2016). First, an initial literature search in PubMed and CINAHL was performed to identify relevant keywords, synonyms, word modifications, and thesaurus terms to use to adjust the O criteria—the clarification of the term "client-centred" [26]. Several searches using different word combinations were performed until we found a search strategy that seemed to identify studies on the COPM and CCP. Keywords were narrowed to the framework of "client-centred" as this is the term used in the COPM and the OT profession, for which the COPM was developed. Other concepts such as "patient-centred" or "patient-focused care" were not included, because although similar, they define an organizational process rather than a conceptual approach to ensure the participation and engagement of clients. Thus, we used the following keywords: ((COPM) OR "Canadian Occupational Performance Measure") AND ((client-center*) OR client-centre*)).

Second, database-specific searches using PubMed, CINAHL, OTseeker, PEDro, Web of Science, and SCOPUS were conducted using the thesaurus terminology for each database. Truncations were used when relevant. The above-mentioned keywords were also used to search for unpublished items on interventions of interest in SwePub and NORA. Google Scholar was also examined using the terms "COPM" and "CCP".

2.2.3. Eligibility. The selection of papers eligible for inclusion was guided by inclusion and exclusion criteria based on the research question. The papers were selected by agreement among the authors. The *inclusion criteria* were the following: (I) studies of all kinds of interventions in all settings, addressing all adult clients ≥ 18 years to whom the COPM had been administered. (II) Studies that revealed the OTs' or their clients' experiences with the use of the COPM to enhance CCP. (III) Published and unpublished qualitative and quantitative studies. (IV) Studies published from January 2005 to August 2016 as the research on the COPM and CCP has increased over the past decade. The *exclusion criteria* included the following: (I) studies in which the COPM only was used as an outcome measure, without data on the participants perception of the use of the COPM. (II) Studies focussing on children. (III) Studies written in languages other than English, Danish, Swedish, or Norwegian. (IV) Editorials, commentaries, interviews, lectures, periodicals, and abstracts.

The two first authors conducted the study selection. Agreement was reached by discussion between the authors, and the third author was consulted if unresolved disagreements occurred. All studies were entered into an Excel sheet to identify and exclude duplicates. The titles and abstracts of the remaining studies were assessed for the inclusion and exclusion criteria, thus facilitating the exclusion of studies that did not fit the research question. The remaining studies were read in full, and studies that were unfit to answer the research question were excluded. Finally, the reference lists of the studies that were read were examined to identify additional studies eligible for inclusion in the scoping review.

2.2.4. Inclusion. As recommend by Levac et al. [25], the authors collectively conducted first assessment of the included studies to determine which descriptive variables to extract to answer the research question. Because the included studies were mostly qualitative, we followed the recommendations of Levac et al. and used a qualitative content analysis approach [25, 27].

2.2.5. Analysis. The qualitative content analysis was based on the recommendations of Graneheim and Lundman, focussing on latent context analysis centred on an in-depth interpretation of the underlying meaning of the text [27]. The two first authors performed the analysis. The included studies were read independently to obtain a general sense of the entire pool of included studies. Then, each author performed a systematic identification of textual information, located the important structures and information from each study, and entered these textual units into a table to identify how these "constellation of words" related to the central meaning. The two tables were compared, and the differences were discussed to subsequently form a common table of significant "meaning units" that had been identified and agreed upon. To ensure that all relevant content was identified, the authors reread all studies while searching for text in accordance with the identified "meaning units" and entered new findings into the table. The content of the meaning units was condensed and abstracted to identify adequate labels, or codes, to represent each condensed meaning unit. The authors compared the codes to identify differences and similarities and sorted the codes into themes and subthemes related to the research question. Finally, all studies were reread to ensure that all the information had been extracted into the themes and subthemes, and dialogues with the third author ensured that nothing in the studies contradicted the themes [27].

3. Results

As presented in Figure 1, we identified 174 studies, and 90 studies remained after duplicates were removed. After the titles and abstracts were screened, 22 studies remained for full-text readings. The authors independently read the 22 studies and discussed their inclusion and exclusion, which left eight studies. After a careful examination of the reference lists of the eight studies, four studies were added.

The twelve studies included one systematic review [28], one opinion paper [29], one quantitative study [30], four qualitative studies [1, 31–33], and five mixed-method studies [19, 34–36], including one unpublished PhD dissertation [11]. The contents of each study, including their aims, methods, samples, and settings, are summarized in Table 1.

The analysis of the literature on the ability of the COPM to enhance CCP revealed two main themes, with five subthemes in the first theme and four subthemes in the second. The two main themes seemed to influence and affect each other; thus, the first theme represented the circumstances required for the second theme to be fulfilled. The first theme considered the prerequisite conditions for CCP when conducting a COPM interview. Some of these conditions related to the OTs' skills and attitudes, specifically in relation to *communication* and *willingness to listen to the clients' points of view*. Others related to how *the environment* seemed to affect the ability of the COPM interview to enhance CCP, particularly in terms of the institutional *commitment to CCP* and the willingness to *share the power with the client.*

The second theme concerned the aspects of CCP that a COPM interview seemed to enhance. These aspects included how the interview could lead to an increase in the OT's awareness of the client's preferences, needs, and values, such as that the OT *got to know the client* and was able to *enhance the client's self-awareness*. Additionally, the use of the COPM interview seemed to enable the processes of *forming a partnership* and *develop collaborative goals*. When these aspects of CCP occurred, they seemed to positively strengthen and increase the OT's behaviours and the environmental conditions under which the COPM was administered. The themes are narratively presented, and an example of the analysis and translation from meaning units to themes is shown in Table 2.

3.1. Conditions for Enhancing CCP When Using the COPM. Our analysis of the included studies indicated that certain conditions should be met if CCP is to be enhanced by the use of the COPM. The OTs' skills and their willingness to *communicate with* and *listen to* the clients' points of view are necessary for the COPM to enhance CCP [11, 19, 30, 31, 33, 36]. A statement by one of the OTs in one of the studies supported the importance of these factors: "It takes very expert communication skills to use [the COPM] in the way it is designed and for it to actually have a therapeutic benefit" [33]. Tuntland et al. reported that personnel without bachelors-level qualification felt a need for additional training in the COPM interview and CCP, indicating that they regarded their expertise as insufficient [30]. Stevens et al. focused on the OTs' communication skills: "It's about the skillful interview in the initial stages and communication to establish what the client is having difficulties with and negotiate with them the areas they want to work on... being honest with them ... [and] provide and renegotiate ... goals..." [28].

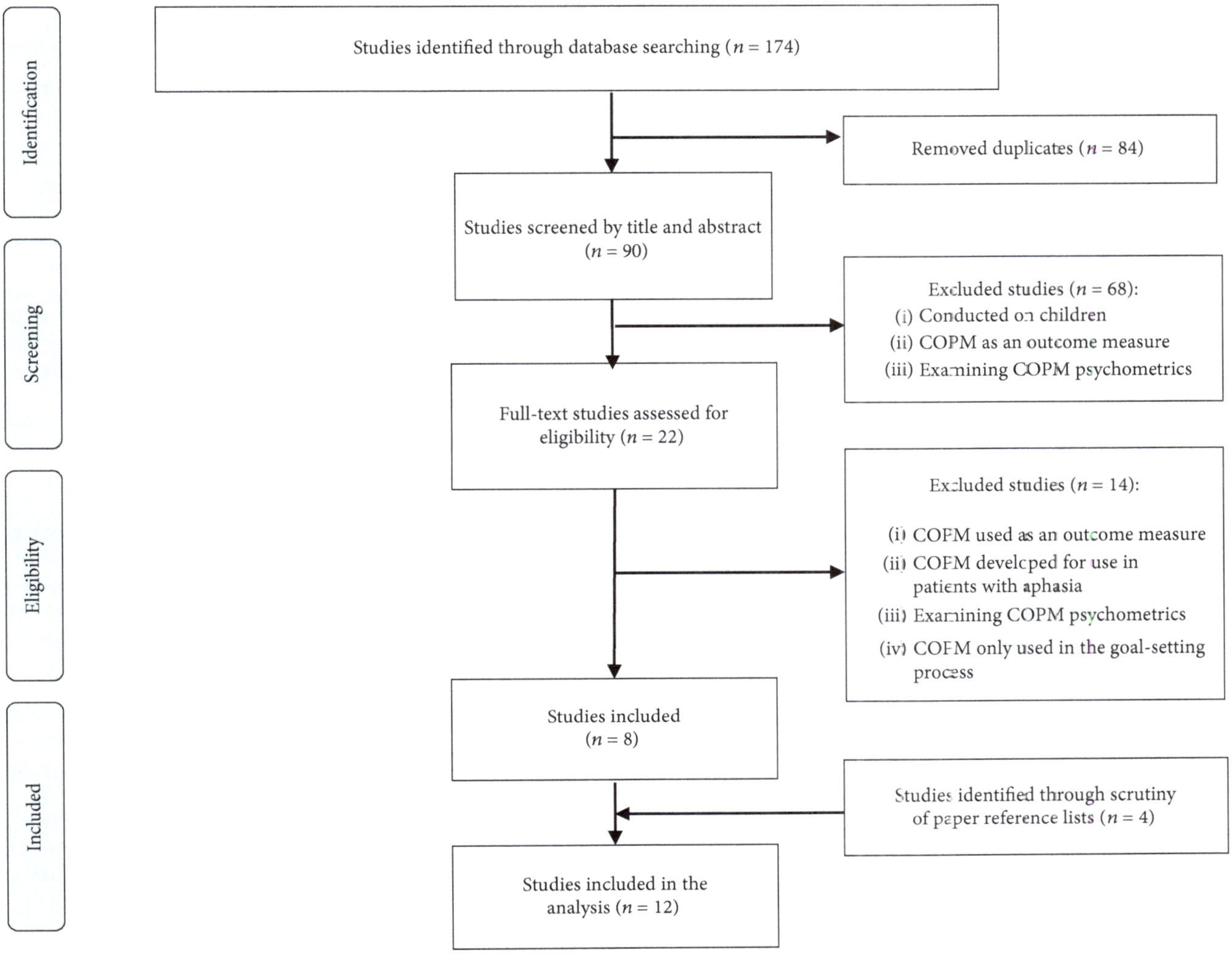

FIGURE 1: Study flow.

Other studies indicated that for the COPM interview to facilitate CCP, a *commitment to CCP* that included an acceptance of the client's opinion, that is, *sharing the power*, was important [1, 11, 19, 28, 29, 33, 36]. Further, the OT's reluctance to use the COPM and his or her commitment to CCP could be interpreted as depending on *the environment* in which the rehabilitation occurred. For instance, if the OT focused on restoring physical function while working in a hospital, contradictory paradigms such as the traditional biomedical model would be inconsistent with the use of the COPM, which is based on a holistic approach [1, 19]. It seemed that therapy was influenced by the environmental conditions of the respective institutions and that this could lead to differences in expectations between clients and OTs [1, 19, 28, 36]. The OTs felt uncomfortable having to listen to and go along with their clients and expressed ambivalence when dealing with the clients' wishes if these wishes differed from the OTs' own [1, 19, 28]. This process was difficult if the OTs found the clients' goals unrealistic as the OTs felt they had the expertise to know what was best for the client [1, 28]. Stevens et al. found that "Some [OTs] indicated that involving patients even undermined the therapy and reduced the patient's motivation, reporting that they [the patients] set unrealistic goals or had unrealistic expectations" [28]. Thus, in some settings, an OT's reluctance to use the COPM to determine the client's point of view and to power were identified as impediments [1, 28], and discrepancies between client aspirations and OT expectations were observed [1, 19, 32, 36]. In a survey on CCP, Parker found that although only 6% of participating OTs agreed with the statement that "the therapist should set the treatment goals," 27% of the OTs agreed that "the therapist has different goals than those of the client" [11]. In the studies by Richard and Knis-Matthews [1] and Engelbrecht et al. [36], differences in the goals of the therapy were observed. The clients identified goals outside the context of the residence programme, such as returning to work or school, whereas the OTs focused on achieving goals within the residence programme [1]. In these studies, the OTs' ideas of feasibility seemed to limit collaborative goal setting [1, 36]. These limitations were related to the clients' constitutions, for example, if the clients had just become ill or did not have the cognitive ability to conduct a COPM

TABLE 1: An overview of the included papers ($n = 12$).

Reference name/ number	Goal/aim	Study design	Method	Materials (sample and context)
Bjørkedal et al. [31]	To qualitatively evaluate the feasibility of client-centred OT intervention focused on enabling meaningful occupations and supporting the recovery process for individuals with schizophrenia in the early phases of recovery.	Qualitative study.	A qualitative study comprising an eight-week client-centred OT intervention and semistructured interviews with five of the six clients out of 10 who completed the intervention. The COPM was used to initiate and guide the intervention, and the Canadian Model of Client-Centred Enablement was used for the client-therapist relationship.	Ten participants with schizophrenic disorders, five of whom (three women and two men) participated in postintervention semistructured interviews. They were recruited from the community and lived in their own apartments.
Colquhoun et al. [34]	To survey OTs currently using the COPM to gather their perceptions about the use of the COPM on a routine basis. A secondary objective was to propose a meaningful template for summarizing routine COPM data.	Mixed method study.	The OTs were given a short-answer written questionnaire that focused on the key areas, derived from the literature, in the routine outcome measures used. These questions related to the feasibility of the COPM and the value of the data. In addition, the resulting five months of COPM data were summarized into a proposed template based on what the OTs found meaningful.	Three female OTs, with six, eight, and 31 years of practice. They had been working in the geriatric unit for one year, five years, and one year, respectively.
Colquhoun et al. [35]	To determine whether COPM administration was associated with changes in eight dimensions of OT practice.	Mixed-method study.	A before-and-after study with repeated tests. The eight practice dimensions were assessed after three months of usual care (no COPM use) and after three months of intervention (COPM use) using chart-stimulated recall (CSR) interviews and chart audit.	24 OTs working in eight inpatient geriatric rehabilitation facilities across two large urban centres. Potential sites were identified by geographic area and the presence of inpatient geriatric rehabilitation units.
Donovan et al. [32]	To describe the occupational concerns and goals of mothers who care for children with disabilities.	Qualitative study.	A qualitative design analysing retrospective data collected using the COPM.	38 mothers of children with disabilities.
Enemark Larsen and Carlsson [19]	To evaluate the utility of the COPM in an interdisciplinary geriatric rehabilitation context (RCC) in Copenhagen in terms of (a) its utility to both OTs and physiotherapists, (b) its utility to document change, and (c) the therapists' experiences with the administration and usability of the COPM.	Mixed-method study.	Data were collected from a pre- and postassessment with the COPM and a questionnaire answered by all participating therapists.	18 therapists (11 physiotherapists and seven OTs) participated in the project group. 185 elderly clients referred to the RCC by home care personnel or general practitioners participated in the study through consecutive sampling over a period of eight months.
Engelbrecht et al. [36]	To determine whether healthcare workers could successfully identify the occupational performance priorities of adult people with disabilities (PWD) living in a Kwaguqa community in the Mpumalanga province of South Africa.	Mixed-method study.	A nonexperimental descriptive design using descriptive survey questionnaires, for example, the COPM, which captured quantitative and qualitative data.	25 adults (17 men and 8 women) from the Thembelihle Self Help Centre and the Kwaguqa Association for the Disabled Workshop with mobility or dexterity problems, aged 18 to above 60 years of age, plus seven female healthcare workers responsible for the service in the Kwaguqua area.

Table 1: Continued.

Reference name/ number	Goal/aim	Study design	Method	Materials (sample and context)
Gustafsson et al. [33]	To investigate the goal-setting process and clinical utility of the COPM from the perspective of OTs within a spinal cord injury unit (SIU).	Qualitative study.	A focus group interview was conducted with seven OTs working in an SIU to explore their experiences and use of goalsetting and the COPM. Inductive thematic analysis identified key themes from their comments.	Seven female OTs, with a mean age of 29.7 (SD 8.38) years. Their clinical experience working in the hospital SIU ranged from less than 6 months to more than 20 years.
Hannah [29]	To summarize the psychological impact of severe hand injuries, to discuss coping strategies for the social impacts of severe hand injuries, and to outline assessments and strategies that can be used by hand therapists to treat the whole person, develop patient-centred goals, and improve therapy outcomes.	An opinion study based on a literature review.	Opinion based on a literature review.	No material included as due to the study format.
Parker [11]	To determine clients' and OTs' perceptions of the CCP in OT in the UK	PhD dissertation. Different studies—a review, a survey, and a qualitative design.	A mixed-method study examining the views of clients and therapists was undertaken using a systematic review to examine global evidence of client-centred outcome measures, a survey of the experiences of a sample of therapists and individual client and OT interviews.	Study (1): 25 OTs opted to attend the focus group. The gender profile of the group was 3 males and 22 females. Study (2): 230 questionnaires were sent to OTs, and 25% were returned. Study (3): four OTs with 4–30 years of education and four clients aged 35–81 years.
Richard and Knis-Matthews [1]	To compare the intervention goals identified by clients and an OT using the COPM.	Qualitative study.	In-depth interviews were conducted with an OT and her clients in conjunction with the use of the COPM.	Seven clients living in a long-term residential programme and diagnosed with schizophrenia and one OT who had worked at the programme for three years at the time of the study.
Stevens et al. [28]	To identify the currently available patient-specific measurement instruments used in the process of goalsetting and to assess their feasibility.	A qualitative systematic review.	After a systematic search in PubMed, EMBASE, CINAHL, PsychINFO, and REHABDATA, patient-specific instruments were included, structured within a goal-setting practice framework and subjected to a qualitative thematic analysis of feasibility.	25 patient-specific instruments were identified, and 11, one of which was the COPM, were included.
Tuntland et al. [30]	To investigate the validity, responsiveness, interpretability, and feasibility of the COPM when used by various health professions in home-dwelling older adults receiving assistance.	A quantitative study on psycometrics.	A quantitative study following the COSMIN guidelines and recommendations for evaluating methodological quality.	The sample included 225 participants, mean age 80.8 years, in need of rehabilitation for various health conditions. Data collection was conducted at baseline and at a 10-week follow-up. The assessments were conducted by 12 nurses, 33 OTs, 27 physiotherapists, five auxiliary nurses, and one social educator.

interview, or the environmental conditions, for example, what the OTs were expected to address or the available facilities [19, 28, 30, 35, 36]. However, if the environmental values aligned with CCP, the OTs seemed to translate the client requirements into goals based on the COPM interview [19].

Table 2: Meaning units, condensed meaning units, subthemes, and themes from the content analysis.

Examples of meaning units	Condensed meaning unit/interpretation of the underlying meaning	Subthemes	Theme
The participants found that the COPM made the challenges and barriers that they experienced in their everyday lives tangible, helping them set suitable personal goals and initiate the intervention ([31], p. 102).	The COPM helped the clients to comprehend their everyday lives and set suitable goals for intervention.		
The COPM proved to be a suitable measure for determining occupational performance priorities from the perspectives of both the PWD and the healthcare workers (HCWs), although this initially resulted in diverse lists of priorities ([36], p. 13).	The COPM helped the clients and the OTs identify OPPs. The identified OPPs differed between clients and OTs.		
The OTs felt that the COPM facilitated discussions with clients about functional independence and the formulation of OT-related goals. They felt that until they actually performed the COPM with a person, they did not really have a sense of the person's needs. The COPM was also thought to aid in increasing client motivation and the client's sense of control over their rehabilitation; it made the rehabilitation process meaningful for the client and provided OTs with client-centred directions and priorities for therapy. An OT stated, "[The COPM] also assists in your assessment of knowing the person's insight and adjustment to their disability" ([33], p. 340).	The COPM helped the OTs get to know their clients. The COPM also helped the clients and facilitated insights for both the OTs and the clients.	*Getting to know the client* and *Enhancing clients' self-awareness*	*Enhancing CCP with the COPM.*
The participants felt that the COPM interview led to greater awareness of their daily lives and to a feeling of being seen and listened to. They also reported that the interview enhanced their motivation to focus on improving occupational performance and that the information brought forward during the interview and scoring process was useful as a basis for developing rehabilitation goals ([30], p. 419).	The COPM led the clients to a greater awareness of their daily lives and enhanced motivation and development of goals.		

3.2. Enhancing CCP When Using the COPM. In all the studies, there was agreement regarding the benefits of using the COPM, most frequently expressed as the ability that the COPM provided for the OTs *to get to know the client.* This awareness was two sided; the OTs familiarized themselves with the clients and their aspirations, and *the clients gained better insight* and awareness of what they wanted and what to expect from the intervention. This often *facilitated partnerships* in the CCP through *collaborative goals.*

It seemed that the use of the COPM provided a positive starting point for CCP because it improved the OT's knowledge of the client's everyday life and aspirations and encouraged the collaborative formation of goals based on the identified OPPs [19, 28, 30–33]. Apparently, using the COPM could emphasize the importance of clinical judgement for guidance [31, 33]. In the study by Donovan et al., the use of the COPM increased equality in the therapeutic relationship by enhancing the understanding of individual clients' perspectives and shifting perceptions, attitudes, and behaviours towards occupations that are meaningful in the clients' lives [32]. In the study by Tuntland et al., the OTs considered the COPM to be very useful in planning and evaluating the intervention [30]. The majority (82%) of the clients stated that they felt the COPM interview and scoring were useful [30].

In addition to the OT's positive experiences with the COPM, the COPM also seemed to improve interdisciplinary teamwork around the client, providing broader information regarding the client, increased information on occupational performance, and a greater emphasis on team goal setting [11, 19, 28, 30].

Colquhoun et al. found evidence that OT knowledge of what matters to the client shows statistically significant improvements when using the COPM [34]. In hand therapy, the use of the COPM was thought to help the therapists focus on issues and goals that would assist the client in fulfilling important life roles [29].

Tuntland et al. found that the COPM was useful for determining goals, and clients felt that the COPM contributed information about "what is important to me" [30]. The COPM interview encouraged the clients to increase their attentiveness to their problems and enhanced their motivation, cooperation, and responsibility for their own therapy [28, 31], thus facilitating a process of self-awareness [19, 32]. The COPM interview seemed to improve the clients' understanding of their own issues, making difficult experiences in everyday life tangible, and thereby facilitated the client-centred partnership [31, 33]. As the COPM interview increased awareness of daily life and acknowledged the clients [30], it helped improve the degree to which the rehabilitation was client centred [33]. The importance of being acknowledged was also supported by Parker, in whose study clients expressed the overwhelming importance of how they were treated [11]. The clients expressed a fundamental need to be valued as individuals, indicating that the attitudes of the OTs in these relationships are more important than their actions [11].

4. Discussion

The assumption that the use of the COPM facilitates CCP led to the objective of this study to examine the literature to determine whether CCP is enhanced when the COPM is used. The scoping review found that the use of the COPM seemed to enhance CCP and that certain conditions were necessary for the COPM interview to have this desired effect.

4.1. The Use of the COPM Seemed to Enhance an Awareness That Goes beyond Assessments. The process of identifying OPPs seemed to change the clients' awareness of their self-perceived needs, which further appeared to affect the client's motivation, cooperation, and responsibility through the subsequent rehabilitation. The COPM interview seemed to influence the clients' attentiveness to and understanding of their problems, which seemed to facilitate a process of self-awareness, making difficult experiences in everyday life more tangible. Thus, starting a rehabilitation process with a COPM interview might help the client begin to come to terms with life. In this way, the COPM interview appeared to initiate a process similar to what Antonovsky called a "sense of coherence" (SOC) [37]. Studies have shown that a SOC contributes to a client's quality of life, health, and satisfaction with daily occupations [37, 38]. Provided that the COPM interview has this positive influence on the client's self-awareness, the COPM interview might facilitate CCP beyond the assessment by influencing the rehabilitation outcome itself.

4.2. The Use of the COPM Helped with Forming a Partnership and Making Collaborative Goals. The COPM interview led to an increased awareness of the client's preferences, needs, and values and helped the OT and the client form a partnership with meaningful and collaborative goals [11, 19, 28, 29, 31–33]. An important aspect of CCP is the establishment of a client-centred partnership in which the client plays an active role in defining goals [6]. Forming a partnership with clients and collaborating in goal setting have always been valued processes in OT [5, 6, 11, 12, 39, 40] that are described as ethical values in both national and international OT associations [41, 42]. Because partnerships and collaborative goalsetting have a positive effect on the outcomes of rehabilitation [15, 43], these aspects are important parts of healthcare politics and have formed the basis for many government policies in recent years [4, 44].

This scoping review revealed that using the COPM to examine client perceptions might help to minimize the OTs' misinterpretation of client needs, goals, and wishes [1, 32]. The included studies showed a discrepancy between goals of the OTs and those of their clients. Similar discrepancies between therapists and clients have been seen in other studies, for example, in stroke rehabilitation [15, 43]. Here, the OTs prioritized goals characterized by short timeframes, conservative estimates of outcomes, and physical function, that is, focused on impairments, independent self-care, and locomotion [15, 43], whereas the clients focused on resuming their predisease status and participating in social activities [15, 43].

4.3. Environmental and Therapeutic Factors Seemed to Affect If a COPM Interview Enhanced CCP. This review showed that the OTs' commitments to CCP, their willingness and ability to share power with the client, and the environment in which the rehabilitation occurred were important factors determining whether the COPM interview would positively affect CCP. Environmental factors affected the possibility of conducting a COPM interview as the OTs were reluctant to perform a COPM interview if the focus was on physical functions, that is, in settings where a medical paradigm was dominant [15, 19–21]. Some of the reluctance seemed to be an attempt to avoid the dilemma of different goals. This was also seen in the study of Mortenson and Dyck in which the OTs avoided the use of the COPM because they feared it would reveal differences between what the clients wanted to achieve and what the OTs were expected to deliver [45]. Other reasons for not using the COPM were that the clients had suddenly became ill or been hospitalized or that they did not have the cognitive ability to undergo a COPM interview [21]. When clients experience an acute disease, a preoccupation with the body's condition, symptoms, and prognosis may follow [46, 47], in addition to feelings of loss, decreased self-esteem, frustration, and anger [48]. Accordingly, in the early stages of a rehabilitation process, clients may ignore or be unaware of OPPs, which explains why it might be difficult to use the COPM under such circumstances [19, 21, 47]. However, the OTs' disinclination to use the COPM in the early stages of their clients' illnesses may reflect CCP in which the OTs acknowledged their clients' fragility and use of counselling for client-centred care [49]. Thus, although the COPM interview seems to enhance CCP, it can be argued that sometimes CCP is better provided without the COPM.

However, some OTs' reluctance to implement CCP could be due to the notion that the OTs considered themselves the experts and thus believed that they knew what was best for the clients. This illustrated a contradiction of paradigms, for example, the traditional biomedical model, with the therapist as the expert, versus the occupational model of the COPM, the Canadian Model of Occupational Performance (the CMOP), in which the client is considered the expert [12, 16]. It seems that the more therapists align with the medical paradigm for example, in hospitals, the lower their use of the COPM interview [15, 19]. This was also the case in a study of implementing the COPM in Taiwan. In that study, practice was driven by the biomedical model; thus, the concepts of COPM and CCP seemed unfamiliar and required adjustments from both therapists and their clients [49].

4.4. The COPM Interview Requires Advanced Communication Skills. Effective communication skills appeared to be vital to the successful use of the COPM and the enhancement of CCP. Corresponding findings have been reported in other studies on CCP, which describe a focus on interviewing skills, for example, the ability to listen actively, communicate in an appropriate language, and share information that aligns with the clients' needs [4–7, 20, 21, 38, 39]. Studies on how to support the successful implementation of the COPM have shown that introductory courses, ongoing support, and follow-up supervision during the implementation process are beneficial [19, 33–35]. Regular reviews might also be beneficial since Colquhoun et al. found that despite support, sustained use of the COPM was not observed [35].

4.4.1. Methodological Considerations. Despite rigorous measures, such as using two reviewers for all sources, this study has limitations that are inherent to scoping reviews in general, such as the synthesis of both published and unpublished studies and qualitative and quantitative research to balance broadness and depth. Since a scoping review is not meant to be exhaustive but rather to provide a good sense of the literature in a particular area, it is likely that some relevant publications were not included in this study. Moreover, given the global nature of the COPM, the exclusion of studies published in languages other than English or Scandinavian makes it unlikely that all relevant studies are included. The number of studies may also have been limited because we narrowed our keywords to the framework of "client-centred," the term used by the COPM and the OT profession. However, by screening the references of the included articles, we attempted to limit the number of missed articles.

5. Conclusion

This scoping review examined whether the use of the COPM could enhance CCP. Twelve studies were identified that used different designs and a range of clients in various settings. The review found that the use of the COPM seems to enhance CCP, specifically by improving awareness of client perspectives, wishes and hopes for the future, thereby reinforcing a partnership with collaborative goalsetting. However, to use the COPM interview to enhance CCP, professional communication skills, power sharing, and an institutional commitment are required.

Conflicts of Interest

The authors declare that there are no conflicts of interest regarding the publication of this paper.

References

[1] L. F. Richard and L. Knis-Matthews, "Are we really client-centered? Using the Canadian Occupational Performance Measure to see how the client's goals connect with the goals of the occupational therapist," *Occupational Therapy in Mental Health*, vol. 26, no. 1, pp. 51–66, 2010.

[2] D. T. Wade, "Editorial," *Clinical Rehabilitation*, vol. 21, no. 12, pp. 1059–1062, 2007.

[3] Institut for Kvalitet og Akkreditering i Sundhedsvæsenet (IKAS), *Den Danske Kvalitets Model. Akkrediteringsstandarder for Sygehuse, 2012*, Department of Quality and Accreditation in the health service. The Danish Quality Model. Accreditation Standards for Hospitals, 2012, Danish. http://www.ikas.dk/FTP/PDF/D12-6522.pdf.

[4] I. Kickbusch, T. Behrendt, and Organisation mondiale de la santé. Bureau régional de l'Europe, *Implementing a Health 2020 Vision: Governance for Health in the 21st Century: Making it Happen*, World Health Organization, Regional Office for Europe, 2013.

[5] G. Palmadottir, "Client-therapist relationships: experiences of occupational therapy clients in rehabilitation," *British Journal of Occupational Therapy*, vol. 69, no. 9, pp. 394–401, 2006.

[6] T. Sumsion and M. Law, "A review of evidence on the conceptual elements informing client-centred practice," *Canadian Journal of Occupational Therapy*, vol. 73, no. 3, pp. 153–162, 2006.

[7] M. Freil, A. Wandel, L. Pedersen, A. B. R. Jönsson, and M. NyborgLæger og sygeplejerskers forståelse af patientinddragelse, "En spørgeskemaundersøgelse blandt ansatte på hospitaler," in *Doctors and Nurses' Understanding of Patient Involvement. A Questionnaire Survey among Employees in Hospitals*, ViBIS (Knowledge Center for User Involvement in Health Care), 2014, Danish. http://www.danskepatienter.dk/sites/danskepatienter.dk/files/Rapporten.pdf.

[8] A. T. Johnsen, M. A. Petersen, L. Pedersen, L. J. Houmann, and M. Groenvold, "Do advanced cancer patients in Denmark receive the help they need? A nationally representative survey of the need related to 12 frequent symptoms/problems," *Psycho-Oncology*, vol. 22, no. 8, pp. 1724–1730, 2013.

[9] D. Blanch-Hartigan, N. Chawla, R. P. Moser, L. J. Finney Rutten, B. W. Hesse, and N. K. Arora, "Trends in cancer survivors' experience of patient-centered communication: results from the health information national trends survey (HINTS)," *Journal of Cancer Survivorship*, vol. 10, no. 6, pp. 1067–1077, 2016.

[10] A. A. Poulsen, J. Ziviani, K. Kotaniemi, and M. Law, "'I think I can': measuring confidence in goal pursuit," *British Journal of Occupational Therapy*, vol. 77, no. 2, pp. 64–66, 2014.

[11] D. M. Parker, *An Exploration of Client-Centred Practice in Occupational Therapy: Perspectives and Impact. A Thesis Submitted to the University of Birmingham for the Degree of Doctor of Philosophy*, School of Health and Population Sciences: University of Birmingham, 2013.

[12] K. G. Conceptual, *Foundations of Occupational Therapy Practice*, F.A. Davies, Philadelphia, 4th edition, 2009.

[13] E. M. Castro, T. Van Regenmortel, K. Vanhaecht, W. Sermeus, and A. Van Hecke, "Patient empowerment, patient participation and patient-centeredness in hospital care: a concept analysis based on a literature review," *Patient Education and Counseling*, vol. 99, no. 12, pp. 1923–1939, 2016.

[14] A. Kjellberg, I. Kåhlin, L. Haglund, and R. R. Taylor, "The myth of participation in occupational therapy: re-conceptualizing a client-centred approach," *Scandinavian Journal of Occupational Therapy*, vol. 19, no. 5, pp. 421–427, 2011.

[15] S. Rosewilliam, C. Sintler, A. D. Pandyan, J. Skelton, and C. A. Roskell, "Is the practice of goal-setting for patients in acute

stroke care patient-centred and what factors influence this? A qualitative study," *Clinical Rehabilitation*, vol. 30, no. 5, pp. 508–519, 2016.

[16] M. Law, S. Baptiste, A. Carswell, M. C. MA, H. Polatajko, and N. Pollock, *Canadian Occupational Performance Measure*, Ottawa, Ed., Ont.: CAOT Publications ACE, 5th edition, 2014.

[17] C. Donnelly, J. J. Eng, J. Hall et al., "Client-centred assessment and the identification of meaningful treatment goals for individuals with a spinal cord injury," *Spinal Cord*, vol. 42, no. 5, pp. 302–307, 2004.

[18] B. Kirsh and L. Cockburn, "The Canadian Occupational Performance Measure: a tool for recovery-based practice," *Psychiatric Rehabilitation Journal*, vol. 32, no. 3, pp. 171–176, 2009.

[19] A. Enemark Larsen and G. Carlsson, "Utility of the Canadian Occupational Performance Measure as an admission and outcome measure in interdisciplinary community-based geriatric rehabilitation," *Scandinavian Journal of Occupational Therapy*, vol. 19, no. 2, pp. 204–213, 2011.

[20] A. Carswell, M. A. McColl, S. Baptiste, M. Law, H. Polatajko, and N. Pollock, "The Canadian Occupational Performance Measure: a research and clinical literature review," *Canadian Journal of Occupational Therapy*, vol. 71, no. 4, pp. 210–222, 2004.

[21] D. M. Parker and C. H. Sykes, "A systematic review of the Canadian Occupational Performance Measure: a clinical practice perspective," *British Journal of Occupational Therapy*, vol. 69, no. 4, pp. 150–160, 2006.

[22] K. Fuller, "The effectiveness of occupational performance outcome measures within mental health practice," *British Journal of Occupational Therapy*, vol. 74, no. 8, pp. 399–405, 2011.

[23] H. L. Colquhoun, D. Levac, K. K. O'Brien et al., "Scoping reviews: time for clarity in definition, methods, and reporting," *Journal of Clinical Epidemiology*, vol. 67, no. 12, pp. 1291–1294, 2014.

[24] H. Arksey and L. O'Malley, "Scoping studies: towards a methodological framework," *International Journal of Social Research Methodology*, vol. 8, no. 1, pp. 19–32, 2005.

[25] D. Levac, H. Colquhoun, and K. K. O'Brien, "Scoping studies: advancing the methodology," *Implementation Science*, vol. 5, no. 1, p. 69, 2010.

[26] The Joanna Briggs Institute, "Joanna Briggs Institute Reviewers' Manual," in *Edition. The Joanna Briggs Institute*, The University of Adelaide, South Australia, 2014.

[27] U. H. Graneheim and B. Lundman, "Qualitative content analysis in nursing research: concepts, procedures and measures to achieve trustworthiness," *Nurse Education Today*, vol. 24, no. 2, pp. 105–112, 2004.

[28] A. Stevens, A. Beurskens, A. Köke, and T. van der Weijden, "The use of patient-specific measurement instruments in the process of goal-setting: a systematic review of available instruments and their feasibility," *Clinical Rehabilitation*, vol. 27, no. 11, pp. 1005–1019, 2013.

[29] S. D. Hannah, "Psychosocial issues after a traumatic hand injury: facilitating adjustment," *Journal of Hand Therapy*, vol. 24, no. 2, pp. 95–103, 2011.

[30] H. Tuntland, M. Aaslund, E. Langeland, B. Espehaug, and I. Kjeken, "Psychometric properties of the Canadian Occupational Performance Measure in home-dwelling older adults," *Journal of Multidisciplinary Healthcare*, vol. 9, pp. 411–423, 2016.

[31] S. T. B. Bjørkedal, A. M. B. Torsting, and T. Møller, "Rewarding yet demanding: client perspectives on enabling occupations during early stages of recovery from schizophrenia," *Scandinavian Journal of Occupational Therapy*, vol. 23, no. 2, pp. 97–106, 2015.

[32] J. M. Donovan, B. J. VanLeit, T. K. Crowe, and E. B. Keefe, "Occupational goals of mothers of children with disabilities: influence of temporal, social, and emotional contexts," *The American Journal of Occupational Therapy*, vol. 59, no. 3, pp. 249–261, 2005.

[33] L. Gustafsson, G. Mitchell, J. Fleming, and G. Price, "Clinical utility of the Canadian Occupational Performance Measure in spinal cord injury rehabilitation," *British Journal of Occupational Therapy*, vol. 75, no. 7, pp. 337–342, 2012.

[34] H. Colquhoun, L. Letts, M. Law, J. MacDermid, and M. Edwards, "Feasibility of the Canadian Occupational Performance Measure for routine use," *British Journal of Occupational Therapy*, vol. 73, no. 2, pp. 48–54, 2010.

[35] H. L. Colquhoun, L. J. Letts, M. C. Law, J. C. MacDermid, and C. A. Missiuna, "Administration of the Canadian Occupational Performance Measure: effect on practice," *Canadian Journal of Occupational Therapy*, vol. 79, no. 2, pp. 120–128, 2012.

[36] L. H. Engelbrecht, J. M. F. Casteleijn, and K. Uys, "Could health care workers determine the occupational performance priorities of people with disability living in a developing community?," *South African Journal of Occupational Therapy*, vol. 38, pp. 8–14, 2008.

[37] A. G. W. Anke and A. R. Fugl-Meyer, "Life satisfaction several years after severe multiple trauma–a retrospective investigation," *Clinical Rehabilitation*, vol. 17, no. 4, pp. 431–442, 2003.

[38] R. I. Cederlund, E. Ramel, H.-E. Rosberg, and L. B. Dahlin, "Outcome and clinical changes in patients 3, 6, 12 months after a severe or major hand injury - can sense of coherence be an indicator for rehabilitation focus?," *BMC Musculoskeletal Disorders*, vol. 11, no. 1, pp. 286–286, 2010.

[39] K. R. Whalley Hammell, "Client-centred practice in occupational therapy: critical reflections," *Scandinavian Journal of Occupational Therapy*, vol. 20, no. 3, pp. 174–181, 2013.

[40] M.-J. Drolet and M. Désormeaux-Moreau, "The values of occupational therapy: perceptions of occupational therapists in Quebec," *Scandinavian Journal of Occupational Therapy*, vol. 23, no. 4, pp. 272–285, 2016.

[41] Ergoterapeutforeningen [Danish Association of Occupational Therapy], "Professionsgrundlag for ergoterapi – En dokumentsamling om mission visioner værdier faglig etik og samarbejde," in *The Conceptual Foundation of the Occupational Therapy Profession - a Repository of Mission, Visions, Values, Professional Ethics and Collaboration*, Ergoterapeutforeningen, Denmark, 2015.

[42] World Federation of Occupational Therapists, WFOT, *Statement on Occupational Therapy*, 2010.

[43] W. M. M. Levack, S. G. Dean, R. J. Siegert, and K. M. McPherson, "Navigating patient-centered goal setting in inpatient stroke rehabilitation: how clinicians control the process to meet perceived professional responsibilities," *Patient Education and Counseling*, vol. 85, no. 2, pp. 206–213, 2011.

[44] D. Regioner and Den Tværregionale Task Force, "Styring efter værdi for patienten," *Danish Regions, the Interregional Task Force. Control by Value for the Patient*, 2015, http://regioner.dk/media/1313/afrapportering-styring-efter-vaerdi-for-patienten.pdf.

[45] W. B. Mortenson and I. Dyck, "Power and client-centred practice: an insider exploration of occupational therapists' experiences," *Canadian Journal of Occupational Therapy*, vol. 73, no. 5, pp. 261–271, 2006.

[46] M. Müller, R. Strobl, and E. Grill, "Goals of patients with rehabilitation needs in acute hospitals: goal achivement is an indicator for improved functioning," *Journal of Rehabilitation Medicine*, vol. 43, no. 2, pp. 145–150, 2011.

[47] M. K. Dekkers and K. Søballe, "Activities and impairments in the early stage of rehabilitation after Colles' fracture," *Disability and Rehabilitation*, vol. 26, no. 11, pp. 662–668, 2009.

[48] J. Tracey, "The emotional response to the injury and rehabilitation process," *Journal of Applied Sport Psychology*, vol. 15, no. 4, pp. 279–293, 2003.

[49] Y.-H. Chen, S. Rodger, and H. Polatajko, "Experiences with the COPM and client-centred practice in adult neurorehabilitation in Taiwan," *Occupational Therapy International*, vol. 9, no. 3, 184 pages, 2002.

13

Play, Playfulness, and Self-Efficacy: Parental Experiences with Children on the Autism Spectrum

Rosa Román-Oyola, Verónica Figueroa-Feliciano, Yoliannie Torres-Martínez, Jorge Torres-Vélez, Keyshla Encarnación-Pizarro, Samariz Fragoso-Pagán, and Luis Torres-Colón

University of Puerto Rico, Medical Sciences Campus, School of Health Professions, Occupational Therapy Program, PO Box 365067, San Juan, PR 00936-5067, USA

Correspondence should be addressed to Rosa Román-Oyola; rosa.roman2@upr.edu

Academic Editor: Karen Stagnitti

Background. Play serves as an essential medium for parent-child interaction; however, engaging children with ASD through play can be a challenge for parents. *Purpose.* The purpose of this phenomenological study was to explore the perspectives of parents with children on the autism spectrum regarding play experiences and self-efficacy during play encounters. *Method.* Semistructured interviews were administered to 8 parents of children 3–7 years of age with ASD. The analysis was guided by the constant comparison method. *Findings.* Parental narratives denoted playful experiences reflecting components of Skard and Bundy's model of playfulness. The facilitation of framing and suspension of reality were generally more challenging than facilitating intrinsic motivation and internal control. Participants associated self-efficacy during play with their perceived ability to interact with their child and with positive emotions experienced during play. Fathers generally derived a greater sense of self-efficacy from play encounters than mothers, and this was explained by differences in fathers' and mothers' motivations for playing. Mothers were motivated to play for outcome-oriented reasons (e.g., promote the child's progress) whereas fathers' motivations depicted greater emotional emphasis, reflecting a better match between motivation and perceived indicators of efficacy during play. *Conclusion.* The results suggest that a good match between motivation for playing and perceived indicators of efficacy during play is important for a parental sense of self-efficacy. Occupational therapists should utilize coaching strategies to increase parents' understanding of play and playfulness and how they can affect a sense of parental self-efficacy.

1. Introduction

Playing has an important and primary role in childhood. As a child's primary occupation [1], play is as natural as breathing [2]. Play involves a child's active participation in an activity or time spent with peers and involves agency and the ownership of ideas [3]. During play, children learn important motor, cognitive, and social skills as well as creativity and self-confidence, which are skills that are required throughout life [1, 4, 5].

Children approach play in different ways based on different motivations and dispositions. These motivations and dispositions form the subject's attitude during play, also known as playfulness. Skard and Bundy [6] proposed a model of playfulness that identifies four primary characteristics of play. The first characteristic is *framing*, which refers to behaviors used during play that identify the nature of the activity as play. Players give framing cues to others, and good players must be able to give and read cues. The second characteristic of play is that it is *intrinsically motivated*. This means that players engage in the play activity because they enjoy the activity and experience benefits as a result. The third characteristic of play is *internal control*; this characteristic allows players to decide what they want to play, who they want to play with, and how and when the play should end. The fourth and final characteristic is *freedom to suspend reality*, which determines how closely a play transaction resembles the objective reality. Different strategies are employed to facilitate the suspension of reality. A player can pretend that he is someone else or that an object is something other than what it really is (e.g., pretends to be a chef; pretends that a box is an airplane). Players can also suspend reality by teasing or telling jokes [6, 7].

According to Skard and Bundy's model [6], a child's level of playfulness is determined by the summation of all the aforementioned characteristics. Evidence indicates that playfulness can differ among children with various developmental challenges. Playfulness in children with autism spectrum disorders (ASD) is affected by behaviors inherently related to their condition; children with ASD tend to be less playful than their typically developing counterparts [8, 9]. Behavioral challenges for play in children with ASD include fixed interests, lack of flexibility, impaired social skills, engagement in ritual repetitive behaviors, low levels of pretend play, anger or frustration, hyper- or hyposensitivities, and difficulty understanding nonverbal cues [10, 11].

Evidence suggests that the inability of some children with ASD to fully engage in play has negative effects on parents' as well as the child's well-being and sense of self-efficacy [12, 13]. Bandura [14] defined self-efficacy as an individual's belief in their ability to achieve a goal or outcome. Parental self-efficacy refers to the confidence and expectations of a parent regarding their ability to perform the parental role competently and effectively [15]. Compared to parents of typically developing children, parents of children with ASD experience higher levels of stress, depression, and hopelessness [16–18]. Participation in and enjoyment of play have important benefits for both parents and children, especially in families of children with ASD. Adult playfulness is a significant predictor of emotional parental self-efficacy among parents raising children with ASD, more so than the degree of sensory processing impairment inherently related to the child's diagnosis [19].

Playfulness is a relationship-based phenomenon and an important factor for the development of social relationships between children and their main caregivers [2, 20, 21]. Given social and communication difficulties in children with ASD, their parents may feel incompetent in their ability to establish an emotional connection with them. Additionally, the quality of involvement of the parents is an important variable for the ability of children with ASD to participate in play [22–24] and can also benefit the parents. Parents of young children with ASD that actively participate in coaching processes or guided educational treatments based on the use of strategies to maximize engagement opportunities with their child exhibit increased competence and higher levels of effect [13, 25].

Available evidence supports a potential relationship between play, playfulness, and parental self-efficacy, especially in families raising young children on the autism spectrum. Yet few studies have examined the experiential components underlying this relationship. The purpose of this phenomenological study was to explore the perspectives of parents with children on the autism spectrum regarding play experiences and self-efficacy during play encounters. The study addressed two research questions: (1) How do parents' narratives about play encounters reflect the elements of a playful experience for their child (based on the model of Skard and Bundy)? (2) How efficient do fathers and mothers feel when playing with their child with ASD?

2. Methods

2.1. Study Design. This study was guided by a phenomenological design with an interpretative approach. Interpretative approaches within phenomenology allow ample examination of relationships and the significance of knowledge and contexts [26]. Interpretative approaches are philosophically associated with social constructivism, which emphasizes the subjective meaning of an individual's experiences [27]. Phenomenology studies these subjective meanings to explicate the structure or essence of the lived experience in search of the unity of meanings [28]. Our research involved a detailed examination of the significance of participant play experiences with their children with ASD, which we defined as the phenomenon under study.

2.2. Participants. All study procedures were reviewed and approved by the Institutional Review Board of the University of Puerto Rico, Medical Sciences Campus. Four couples of parents of children with ASD from different parts of Puerto Rico consented to participate in semistructured in-depth interviews. The inclusion criteria were as follows: (a) availability of both parents for participation, (b) parents ≥ 21 years of age, and (c) children 3–7 years of age with a diagnosis of ASD. Age range selections were made based on previous investigations of the importance of reciprocal interactions between parents and children [29]. Table 1 describes some characteristics of participant parental couples.

2.3. Recruitment. Participants were recruited through direct contact or by referral from occupational therapists of children with ASD. In cases of recruitment by referral, occupational therapists were asked to make the first contact with parents regardless of whether the children were currently receiving therapy. After parents communicated interest in the study, we personally delivered a participation package including two consent forms (one for each parent), a sociodemographic information data form and an instruction sheet. Interviews with participants were scheduled at the participants' convenience. To minimize the possibility of bias associated with social desirability and interviewers' gender in participant narratives [30, 31], fathers were interviewed by male researchers and mothers were interviewed by female researchers.

2.4. Data Collection and Analysis. Data were collected via in-depth semistructured interviews. Open-ended questions were employed to allow participants to interpret the meaning of the question and respond based on their personal feelings and perceptions. Probe questions were included as part of the protocol and used to enrich the discussion as needed. Examples are as follows:

TABLE 1: Description of participants.

Participants	Age	Gender and age of the child with ASD	Couple living together/apart	Additional members of the family
Mother 1	25	Female, 7	Together	2 sisters (5 and 3 y/o, respectively)
Father 1	31			
Mother 2	38	Female, 4	Together	No additional members
Father 2	43			
Mother 3	27	Male, 5	Apart	Child lives with mother but stays with father frequently. Has a brother (14 y/o) on his father's side, who lives with the father
Father 3	43			
Mother 4	40	Male, 5	Together	No additional members
Father 4	45			

Main question: how do you feel when playing with your son/daughter?

Possible probes: how satisfied do you feel with the way you play? Do you think that you interact effectively while playing? What makes you think that way? Is there anything you would change about those playing moments?

Interviewing researchers were trained in qualitative methods and use of the interview protocol. Prior to the study data collection, all researchers performed practice interviews with volunteer mothers and fathers of typically developing children using the study protocol. Mothers and fathers were interviewed separately. The length of each study interview varied by participant in accordance with their comments and experiences but generally lasted approximately 45 minutes to an hour. Interviews were audio-taped with the participants' consent for later transcription in Spanish. All identifying information was removed from transcripts, and the names mentioned during the interview were replaced with pseudonyms to protect the identities of the participants. Each parent received \$15.00 as compensation for their time.

The process of data analysis was guided by the principles of the constant comparison method [32], which allowed structural corroborations among members of the research team. The analysis steps included two cycles of coding as described by Saldaña [33]. For the purposes of the first coding cycle, each researcher was assigned to 1 of 2 analysis teams. The principal researcher and 2 other researchers participated in both teams. First, researchers thoroughly read the transcripts assigned to their respective team and individually identified initial categories. Then, individual researchers met with their respective teams to read transcripts as a group and discuss/agree upon emergent categories.

In the second coding cycle, portions of transcripts were organized into tables presenting mothers' and fathers' responses to the same questions side by side for intracouple comparisons of responses. Then, couples' responses were examined side by side for intercouple comparisons. During this cycle, researchers met several times to revise codes, share analytic memos, and reconfigure codes from the first cycle by linking interview chunks and/or initial codes. A total of four major patterns/themes were identified from the data: (1) general context of the playing experience; (2) playfulness in the context of parent-child interactions; (3) self-efficacy during play; and (4) motivations vs. benefits.

In qualitative studies, rigor is determined by the criteria of credibility, dependability, confirmability, and transferability [26]. Broad descriptions of the data collection and analysis process serve to reinforce credibility and dependability. Confirmability is achieved by showing that results are derived from a well-documented research process and through informants (e.g., participants' direct quotes) that support the results [34]. Transferability of the findings is demonstrated when practical implications derived from the findings are pertinent to other contexts [34].

3. Results

The following results include verbatim excerpts of participant narratives selected to exemplify the underlying themes. Identifying information has been removed from quotations. The verbatim texts were translated into English by the Translation Center, College of Humanities (University of PR), for the sole purpose of this article. Preservation of essential meaning, content, and, insofar as possible, general tone were the main goals of the translation. To enhance clarity and preserve the parents' anonymity, participants are identified with numbers 1 to 4 (e.g., mother number 1 and father number 1 form a parental couple). Each participant's number is shown at the beginning of each quotation.

3.1. General Context of the Play Experience. Prior to in-depth examination of the excerpts as they relate to the research questions, it is pertinent to contextualize participants' perspectives about play experiences with their children. In general, parents' play experiences were defined by codes related to emotions regarding play, relevance of play as part of a routine, and awareness of the child's diagnosis. All participants expressed positive emotions related to play experiences with their children. Satisfaction, happiness, and trust were among the most frequently expressed emotions. Participants also commented about the importance of playing with their children; their narratives reflected that moments for playing are specified as parts of the family routine. Generally, fathers indicated that they played with their children after arriving home from work.

In contrast, mothers more frequently commented about how they integrate play into household chores and child-care activities:

Mother 1: *We are playing from the moment we wake up, from the moment we are brushing our teeth we are already playing because it's a brushing teeth game, it's another one to get dressed, and that's how we move forward ...*

Father 1: *(We play) When I get home from work, before going to sleep... Like almost all of the time I am home, I try to spend it with my daughters and we are always playing*

Mother 3: *Look, I can be cooking, and he comes to the kitchen because he helps me a lot... He's very collaborative and he comes to the kitchen and wants to add sauce very carefully, right [... And while ...] the food is getting ready, we have a tickle or kiss game...*

Mother 4: *[...] When we get home, dad and I get turns. Dad makes dinner and mom helps with homework. I start playing with him while dinner is ready. After dinner, I make the next day's lunch and dad plays with him, that is to say, we switch.*

Narratives about the difficulty of incorporating play encounters into ordinary routines were also very common among the participants. Main reasons for this challenge were related to the time demands of complex daily routines as well as to the inherent social-emotional challenges faced by children with ASD:

Mother 1: *Sometimes it's complicated because she's not always in the mood to play or learn or to do things or every day activities such as getting dressed or whatever. But, that's why it's simpler with play, because there are moments in which [we lose control and] we start yelling and we see how agitated she is and truth is nothing will be solved that way. We have learned... we'll take it slowly, we'll take a breath, and we'll do it a different way, and playing, well, makes it simpler...*

Mother 4: *Well, we are not at home most of the day; we work from 8 (am) to 7 at night. So, he is in activities most of the day, but when we get home, dad and I take turns [to play].*

Father 4: *Obligations... like you have to do the laundry, you have to cook ... Here we both do the chores; my wife does some and I do some others. Sometimes my wife may be there (points to the dining room) working and I am over here making dinner for him and sometimes that moment, well, I am not dedicating it to him... Well, I do dedicate it to him because it's for him, but I am not playing with him. You get me?*

Mother 3: *Well look, in some aspect it is (easy for the boy to play), what happens is that there are moments where he wants to play and [...] I am a mom and I do not stop working and I still have responsibilities and, the truth is that, as a person, I get exhausted ...*

Participant narratives also denoted awareness of the challenges associated with their child's diagnosis. In the case of Mother 2, it was possible to perceive some frustration about the ways in which she was able or unable to play with her daughter:

Mother 2: *[...] When I notice we start playing (while moving a toy she's holding and acting like paying) "hi, how are you?" she hates that... when I grab a toy and [try imaginary play], she hates it. And the anxiety of not being able to accomplish it... It freezes me [...]. Because I get so anxious that "I must do it, and I have to do it" and that [anxiety] I need to control. It's something that "kills" me (laughs).*

Another way in which participants denoted consciousness about the child's diagnosis was by highlighting the importance of play interactions as a mean to promote and follow their child's progress:

Father 1: *Well, the moments I enjoy the most, sometimes are when, when she does something that surprises me. In other words, let us say, well, that she does not pay attention to some things or she's very reluctant to do so and so activity and in that moment, you are doing something, and she comes and starts doing what you are doing and we are getting along. (...) It's said that children [on the spectrum], do not let people hug them, that [they avoid] visual contact, that they do not let... And you can hug that girl! You can be with her, she comes to me when I get home, she jumps at me! I enjoy those things because I thought they would not happen.*

Mother 2: *Yes, (play has its benefits) because I can tell you that six months ago, we could not [play]. Then, as a mom and human being who has been there, I was very frustrated, right, over the diagnosis ... [But play] helps me to feel that we are moving forward, that it's worth the effort and it makes me feel that we are doing it right because we are seeing progress.*

3.2. Playfulness in the Context of Parent-Child Interactions. Analysis of participant narratives revealed the elements of playfulness embedded in parents' experiences. It was clear that play was often shaped by the child's preferences, indicating that parents sought interactions that were *intrinsically motivating* for their child. Most parents explained that the best way to play with their child was by immersing themselves in the type of play the child had already established, thus reflecting the element of motivation proposed in Skard and Bundy's model [6]. From parents' perspectives, parent-child interactions were more effective and enjoyable when play was intrinsically motivated rather than when the child's play preference was disrupted or when parents tried to impose their own choices on children during the play interaction:

Mother 2: *I try to play by her rules, and to not impose on her my way of playing. I can deal with her a little better when we play by her rules.*

Father 1: *... if you want to force the game she'll get difficult, but difficult as in she'll want to hit you and everything because she's doing something and you cannot interrupt what she's doing; because she'll start kicking at you and [yell] "I don't want to" and there will not be any break.*

Mother 4: *I try to play the same games he likes to encourage him.*

Father 2: *It's easy [to play]... The only thing I have to do is show her something she likes, and it's over. I show her the water bomb, and that's it, we start playing.*

Internal control was another element apparent in the narratives. Parents indicated that parent-child interactions were mainly arbitrated by the child, meaning that the child maintained overall control within play encounters. Although parents had some influence over some activities, they were mostly regulated by the child's preferences and feedback during the parent-child interaction. Parents indicated that children enjoyed play encounters and that interactions were reciprocal and occurred for longer periods of time when the child was in control. Both, mothers and fathers, denoted that when play preferences were forced, children tended to avoid play by displaying tantrums or trying to change play activities. This corresponds to Skard and Bundy's model [6]. When children feel in control and feel no constraints during play encounters, the outcomes of interactions are more effective, especially during parent-child interactions.

Father 4: *... it's easy [to play] as long as he likes the kind of play, it's easy. It's going to be very difficult if it's something he does not like...*

Father 2: *The hardest part, well, when the play is guided, you know there is free play and guided play [...] if it's a guided game, well, it is harder because setting a pattern with a structure is not so easy with her, but if it's a free activity you can spend the whole day playing.*

The element of *framing* was also noted in the narratives. Often, mothers and fathers indicated a desire to prolong play encounters. When the child's preference or interest during an activity was interrupted, parents resorted to framing or cueing the child to continue the play process. Main framing strategies included the presentation of preferred toys or games that the child would enjoy and the initiation of cues (or responses to child cues) for playing. These strategies prolonged attention and participation during play encounters.

Father 1: *I get one of her favorite toys or I take her blanket away from her to make her come after me because she loves blankets and she takes with her 4 or 6 blankets wherever she goes [...] Well, since I know she likes them, I take it away from her and I run to the bedroom and she comes looking for it. So, that's the moment I take to start playing. It's the same as with the little dolls [or other toys she love]... those are the little tricks I use [to play with her] (laughs)."*

Father 2: *She does not give up. When I get home, she tells me, "Seated" and then grabs me, pulls me by my arm, and takes me to the room and sits me on the floor (smiles) [saying:]. "Seated, let's play" and from there we start playing with anything that's available.*

Mother 2: *We are always having to create playtime in a way that gets her attention, whether cheering: "Yeah, Betsy, that's it, very good, we're going to play!" (lifting her arms in a cheering motion)... Very energetic, so it like grabs her attention and then she comes. That's what gets her.*

Furthermore, parents' descriptions of play encounters with their children reflected the element of *freedom to suspend reality*. It was relatively easy to observe simple forms of reality suspension such as teasing or rule stretching, especially among fathers. For example, Father 1 talked about play-wrestling with his daughter *("She knows the mood I have. She knows my attitude [...] Sometimes, she even knows what I want to do. You know if I pick her up and take her to bed, she knows that we're going to play wrestle or something like that... Then she gets excited, she gets motivated.")*. This brief excerpt from Father 1 denotes, not only the suspension of reality by stretching the rules (fathers do not typically wrestle with their daughters) but also the importance of his playful attitude ("*She knows the mood I have. She knows my attitude...*") to cue the daughter and frame the play experience. Another strategy for reality suspension was pretending to be an object (e.g., a doll or action figure); however, this was not effective for all participants. While Father 1 indicated the use of little dolls to maintain his daughter's attention during play, Mother 2 confessed that she would love to engage in more imaginary play with her daughter and suggested that this affected her sense of self-efficacy during play activities:

Mother 2 ... *I would like to make her playtime last longer. That's why, I do not feel a hundred percent satisfied, even though I feel happy that I am able to play with her... but it's really frustrating because you have to pull off this cooperative game and... I am like, "Here goes the car: beep beep." (Moving her hands like she's driving a car), but she does not like that. She does not like it to the point that she will even get rid of the toys, and take them away from me... She'll play with me; but it has to be dolling me up, putting makeup on me, doing my nails, but anything that has to do with grabbing toys or having conversations, she does not like it. That's where I am frustrated, I would love to be able to do that a little.*

3.3. Self-Efficacy during Play: Motivations vs. Benefits. All participants communicated feelings of efficacy and satisfaction regarding play experiences with their children. Perceived ability to interact with their child was the main aspect that made parents feel competent. Playing provided parents with an opportunity to relate to their children and strengthen parent-child bonds. Additionally, parents connected play efficacy with positive feelings experienced during play moments, such as the emotion of seeing a child participating in, completing, and enjoying a play activity:

Father 1: *I mean, I consider myself pretty effective. Any person can come along, even her mother, and tries to do what I do, and it will not work ... I mean, I have my way, my tricks... because it's a matter of motivating her to play, to take her the things she likes. If she likes dolls, or if you see on this day she woke up wanting her blanket or on that day she woke up wanting dolls... you already know which way to go to motivate her to play with you.*

Mother 1: *...For example, we were playing um ... bowling, and then, it happened that she knocked down the pins, and you see her joy... it's like "I did it!", like she feels successful.*

Overall, fathers verbalized feelings of better efficacy during play experiences with their children than did mothers. This observation is exemplified by the excerpt from Father 1 shown above. Indeed, mothers were more likely to identify aspects of the play process that they wanted to improve or change:

Mother 1: *[I would like to get better] as far more improvisation [...] and... I do not know maybe a little more athleticism, running harder.*

Mother 2: *I still need to learn a little more, how to get through to her, how to get her a little more interested, uh, work a little more in that area.*

Mother 3: *[How effective I feel] depends really on the game. There are games where like ... for example PlayStation: [He invites me] "Mommy come play with me." Now, there are other games, for example, painting... Surprisingly, that does not really get his attention. So, since I have to struggle a little bit for him to sit with me [...] it's a little challenging to get him interested and it's like (sighs) let me see what else I can do to get his attention.*

The analysis also identified different *motivations for playing* between fathers and mothers. It was notable that fathers' spontaneous responses about motivations for playing reflected a greater emphasis on emotional aspects such as seeing their children laughing, smiling, and happy, while mothers were motivated to play to promote progress and enhance their child's necessary skills. This difference is shown in the excerpts below, presented by a parental couple (e.g., Mother 1 followed by Father 1):

Mother 1: *[It motivates me] to see that you can accomplish a lot of things through playtime [for] example, writing, reading, colors, everything... Playing ... is the easiest way of teaching these children.*

Father 1: *Seeing her laugh, seeing that she's having a good time; also, we can learn too...*

Mother 4: *...Helping him, more than anything, to socialize, that when he sees the neighbors or his friends outside, he can be sociable [...] and that he spends time with them, that he does not become a shy person and above all, share with people.*

Father 4: *The first thing is the love I have towards him, as my son... that motivates me.*

Interestingly, when asked about the perceived *benefits* of playing experiences, an opposite trend was observed. Mothers' spontaneous responses tended to emphasize more emotional benefits of play (e.g., trust and bonding) while fathers were likely to identify aspects related to the child's progress or skill development.

Mother 3: *Aside from working on what we call quality time for both [...] Playing develops trust. He feels how we speak during playtime. So, he gets aware that: "Oh, I can speak with mommy", or "I can tell things to mommy", and since he's young now, it's important to develop this confidence and this communication with him... Playtime helps a lot with this. In addition, we have fun and we laugh together. So, when he gets older he's going to say: "I remember when mommy played that with me..."*

Father 3: *[...] Oh, yes, it [play]soothes him, it helps him to go to bed more relaxed.*

Mother 1: *Yes [play is beneficial]. As it pertains to confidence, I think my daughter pretty much trusts me ...*

Father 1: *Yes, because [in addition to strengthens the attachment], she develops a lot better, she accepts physical contact. If I had never played with her, if I had never become interested in playing with her, well, she would not want contact with anybody [...Also,] I think movement [coordination] is developed, I mean, before, she would trip over herself a lot. Sometimes, she did not even want to play. But now, not anymore. Now she's well-coordinated, very agile, and she has great equilibrium!*

4. Discussion

The purpose of this phenomenological study was to explore the play experiences of parents with children on the autism spectrum. First, we focused on parents' narratives reflecting playfulness while playing with their child. Consistent with previous research, there were characteristic differences in the contexts and types of play used by mothers and fathers [35–37]. Mothers tended to insert play moments into daily routines while fathers had opportunities for playing that were not necessarily embedded within other daily tasks.

We were able to identify elements of Skard and Bundy's model of playfulness [6] in participant comments. Mothers and fathers assigned importance to facilitating their child's *intrinsic motivation* and *internal control* and recognized that, by doing so, they were better able to engage the child in play. Skard and Bundy [6] stated that internal control requires that all participants in the play experience can make decisions regarding the details of the play encounter, thus implying a certain degree of negotiation. Yet we found that when parents, specifically fathers, wished to see the child's enjoyment during play moments, they opted to relinquish internal control to a substantial extent.

Parents' comments indicative of *framing* were generally efforts to offer "play cues" to children. The message "this is play" was deliberately linked to things that intrinsically motivated the child. The observed relationship between intrinsic motivation and framing is not surprising. Rather, we were interested in the "tangible quality" of the framing cues used by parents (or the child; e.g., the use of specific objects or a very energetic attitude). Although these types of cues can be used by any parent with any child, it is possible that tangible qualities have particular importance in families with children on the autism spectrum. Framing and scaffolding, although not equivalent, are conceptually related to one another. Various terms that refer to scaffolding strategies (e.g., prompting, modeling) can also be used as cues to portray a play situation to the child [38–40]. Social participation difficulties are thought to interfere with the development of complex play skills in children with ASD and might make it more difficult for parents to scaffold play [39]. Further, evidence suggests that children with ASD rely on others to generate novel ideas about how to play to a greater degree than do typically developing children [41].

Pretend play is the most common form of *suspension of reality* [7]. Children with ASD have a reduced preference for this type of play [42–44]. Experiences of participants in this study corroborated this idea and generally recounted less obvious suspensions of reality such as teasing (e.g., the father running with his daughter's blanket) or stretching the rules (e.g., the father play-wrestling with his daughter), especially in the narratives of fathers. We also recognized challenges related to engaging the child in pretend play situations. One mother verbalized significant frustration about not being able to actively engage her daughter in pretend play. This is consistent with previous evidence; in a cross-sectional study, Case-Smith and Kuhaneck [45] found that children with developmental delays tended to prefer rough-and-tumble play and object exploration and presented lower preferences for drawing and coloring, construction, and doll and action figurine play.

Our results indicated that, in terms of playfulness, facilitating the elements of framing and suspension of reality was more challenging than facilitating child's intrinsic motivation and internal control. This is in line with previous research stating that the number of imitated actions and amount of elaborate pretend play (both areas of difficulty for children with ASD) are positively associated with the suspension of reality and framing dimensions of playfulness, respectively [41]. Despite the difficulty of certain elements, it was perceived that participants assumed an important role in facilitating playful experiences with their children and that the playful attitude of parents was an important facilitator or barrier in this context.

The second question guiding our analysis in this study was how competent do fathers and mothers feel when playing with their child with ASD? Perceived ability to interact with the child and positive emotions experienced during play moments were among the main aspects that participants associated with self-efficacy during play. Fathers derived a greater sense of self-efficacy from play encounters while mothers were more likely to identify areas of their own performance that they wanted to improve. A key factor explaining differences in the perceived efficacy of mothers and fathers during play is their perceptions about the motivations for playing and the benefits associated with the play experience.

As stated, an ability to interact with children and the derivation of positive emotions from play interactions were identified by all participants as indicators of efficacy. The analysis of fathers' narratives reflected a better match between motivators for playing and the aforementioned indicators of efficacy. While fathers' motivations depicted a greater emotional emphasis (e.g., *"seeing her smiling"*), mothers' motivators were more outcome-oriented (i.e., more focused on promoting the child's development of skills; e.g., *"help him to socialize better"*). Interestingly, the opposite was observed when analyzing the benefits that parents derived from play moments. Fathers identified benefits that were more outcome- or task-oriented (e.g., ability to move more efficiently; a more relaxed state at sleeping time) while mothers identified more emotionally oriented benefits (e.g., own enjoyment and enhancement of the child's trust in them). Considering that fathers were more inclined to judge themselves as competent during play than mothers, the findings of this study suggest that a better match between motivators for playing and perceived indicators of efficacy during play are relevant to a parental sense of self-efficacy.

The present findings have several important implications. First, it may be useful to help parents to better understand the difference between play or playfulness and the elements of playfulness. A comprehensive understanding of the elements of playfulness can guide parents in equalizing the importance attributed to play as a means as well as an end. Too often, parents (in the case of this study, especially mothers) of children with ASD and other disabilities are so overwhelmed by delays in their child's development that they forget the importance of *playing playfully* and making play encounters a pleasurable experience for everyone involved. The enjoyment of these encounters not only addresses the child's challenges in social participation but also enhances parental self-efficacy [19].

Participants in this study cared about having opportunities to relate to and play with their children, but some (mothers more than fathers) were unable to derive a sensation of self-efficacy from playing. Education-based treatments may help parents like these to adjust their perceptions to improve consistency between definitions of efficacy during play and motivations to play, resulting in the enhanced perception of parental self-efficacy. Occupational performance coaching (OPC) can be an alternative. OPC is an educational treatment that uses collaborative problem-solving within a coaching relationship in which parents are guided to identify and apply effective solutions to occupational performance problems with their children [46].

This is particularly significant in the context of occupational therapists' family-centered interventions, since role competence is an important desired intervention outcome [47]. Occupational therapists have the opportunity to use coaching, especially when working with families with children in early childhood [48, 49]. In terms of play, important reflections include the following: How are we focusing coaching processes? Are we balancing teaching families about play as a means and as an end? Evidence indicates that there is still a long way to go; a study by Kuhaneck et al. [50] found that only 4% of 198 pediatric occupational therapists reported the use of play as an intervention outcome.

On the other hand, differences between parents in motivators for playing might be attributed to parents' perceptions about what is expected from them based on traditional gender roles [51]. Research suggests that gender roles are critical for defining the implicit objectives of parent-child interactions [52]. Further, evidence suggests that playfulness is a trait with likely ties to environmental and interactional characteristics [53]. Thus, it is pertinent to help parents to visualize playfulness not only simply as a personality trait but also as an environmental and interactional component. Parents themselves are a key part of the child's environment. Additionally, traditional gender roles are, to some extent, part of the parents' environment and can influence parents' expectancies about play encounters with their children. This concept merits further exploration in future studies. In summary, the results of this study suggest that parents' expectancies and attitudes affect not only the way in which they approach play encounters but also the way in which their children approach the play experience; this in turn has effects on parents' sense of self-efficacy during play.

4.1. Limitations. This study contributes to a body of knowledge about play and playfulness in families of children with ASD and the potential relevance of these constructs for parental self-efficacy. The profiles of couples that participated in this study were relatively diverse. This allowed the collection of information covering a broad spectrum of family contexts (e.g., parents living together with more than one child; parents living together with only one daughter with ASD; parents with one son with ASD not living together; and parents living together with very demanding workloads). While this can be considered a strength, it must be recognized that this was a phenomenological study with a limited number of participants (4 parental couples and therefore 8 participants). We understand that having a limited quantity of participant couples along with such diverse profiles entailed the main limitation of this study, because it impeded reaching saturation. For example, the narratives of Mother 2 (who had an only daughter) depicted substantial frustration regarding play interactions with her daughter with ASD (e.g., *when I grab a toy and [try imaginary play]... she hates it. And the anxiety of not being able to accomplish it... It freezes me [...]. Because I get so anxious...).* On the opposite, Mother 1 (who had two additional typically developing daughters) did not describe comparable frustrations with her daughter with ASD. Having additional participant mothers with similar family context (e.g., more mothers with an only daughter with ASD and mothers with additional neurotypical daughters) would have allowed us to verify if their experiences and perceptions were similar.

The abovementioned issues give rise to areas deserving additional exploration in future studies, such as play styles of parents of children with ASD in the context of families with multiple children, between dyads of mothers/fathers-daughters with ASD, among mothers/fathers-sons with ASD, and in the context of families in which parents do not live together or in which children are under the care of family members other than the parents. Additionally, it would be worthwhile to evaluate our findings against the narratives of parents with neurotypical children to verify whether the ability to sustain and enjoy play encounters with their children is linked in any way to their sense of self-efficacy. Finally, we recommended that future studies examining areas explored in this study utilize more comprehensive qualitative designs such as grounded theory.

5. Conclusion

The purpose of this study was to explore the perspectives of parents of children on the autism spectrum regarding play experiences and self-efficacy during play encounters with their children. Specific attention was given to elements of playfulness and parents' sense of self-efficacy during play encounters with their children. Participants' narratives indicated that facilitating framing and suspension of reality was more challenging than facilitating the child's intrinsic motivation and internal control during play. Finally, the results suggest that a better match between motivators for playing and perceived indicators of efficacy during play has a significant relevance for parental self-efficacy. Occupational therapists should employ coaching strategies to help parents increase their understanding of play and playfulness and how these elements can affect their sense of self-efficacy.

Conflicts of Interest

The authors declare that there are no conflicts of interest.

Acknowledgments

The preparation and publication of this article were partially funded by the Hispanic in Research Capability Endowment (HiREC), Universidad de Puerto Rico, Medical Sciences Campus.

References

[1] L. D. Parham and L. Fazio, *Play in Occupational Therapy for Children*, Mosby, St. Louis, MO, USA, 2nd edition, 2008.

[2] C. E. Schaefer and A. A. Drewes, "The therapeutic power of play and play therapy," in *Foundations of Play Therapy*, C. E. Schaefer, Ed., pp. 15–23, Wiley, Hoboken, NJ, USA, 2011.

[3] M. Theobald, S. Danby, J. Einarsdóttir et al., "Children's perspectives of play and learning for educational practice," *Education Sciences*, vol. 5, no. 4, pp. 345-362, 2015.

[4] E. P. Fisher, "The impact of play on development: a meta-analysis," *Play & Culture*, vol. 5, pp. 159–181, 1992.

[5] L. A. Barnett, "Characterizing playfulness: correlates with individual attributes and personality traits," *Play & Culture*, vol. 4, pp. 371–393, 1991.

[6] G. Skard and A. C. Bundy, "Test of playfulness," in *Play in Occupational Therapy for Children*, L. D. Parham and L. S. Fazio, Eds., pp. 71–93, Mosby, St. Louis, MO, USA, 2008.

[7] A. C. Bundy, "Children and play: can I play, too?," in *Kids Can Be Kids: A Childhood Occupation Approach*, S. J. Lane and A. C. Bundy, Eds., pp. 28–43, F. A. Davis, Philadelphia, PA, USA, 2012.

[8] R. P. Hobson, A. Lee, and J. A. Hobson, "Qualities of symbolic play among children with autism: a social-developmental perspective," *Journal of Autism and Developmental Disorders*, vol. 39, no. 1, pp. 12–22, 2009.

[9] N. Skaines, S. Rodger, and A. Bundy, "Playfulness in children with autistic disorder and their typically developing peers," *British Journal of Occupational Therapy*, vol. 69, no. 11, pp. 505–512, 2006.

[10] R. MacDonald, S. Sacramone, R. Mansfield, K. Wiltz, and W. H. Ahearn, "Using video modeling to teach reciprocal pretend play to children with autism," *Journal of Applied Behavior Analysis*, vol. 42, no. 1, pp. 43–55, 2009.

[11] J. Howard and K. McInnes, "The impact of children's perception of an activity as play rather than not play on emotional well-being," *Child: Care, Health and Development*, vol. 39, no. 5, pp. 737–742, 2013.

[12] T. W. Vernon, R. L. Koegel, H. Dauterman, and K. Stolen, "An early social engagement intervention for young children with autism and their parents," *Journal of Autism and Developmental Disorders*, vol. 42, no. 12, pp. 2702–2717, 2012.

[13] D. Keen, D. Couzens, S. Muspratt, and S. Rodger, "The effects of a parent-focused intervention for children with a recent diagnosis of autism spectrum disorder on parenting stress and competence," *Research in Autism Spectrum Disorders*, vol. 4, no. 2, pp. 229–241, 2010.

[14] A. Bandura, "Self-efficacy: toward a unifying theory of behavioral change," *Psychological Review*, vol. 84, no. 2, pp. 191–215, 1977.

[15] D. M. Teti and D. M. Gelfand, "Behavioral competence among mothers of infants in the first year: the mediational role of maternal self-efficacy," *Child Development*, vol. 62, no. 5, pp. 918–929, 1991.

[16] P. R. Benson and K. L. Karlof, "Anger, stress proliferation, and depressed mood among parents of children with ASD: a longitudinal replication," *Journal of Autism and Developmental Disorders*, vol. 39, no. 2, pp. 350–362, 2009.

[17] R. P. Hastings and T. Brown, "Behavior problems of children with autism, parental self-efficacy, and mental health," *American Journal on Mental Retardation*, vol. 107, no. 3, pp. 222–232, 2002.

[18] V. Totsika, R. P. Hastings, E. Emerson, D. M. Berridge, and G. A. Lancaster, "Prosocial skills in young children with autism, and their mothers' psychological well-being: longitudinal relationships," *Research in Autism Spectrum Disorders*, vol. 13-14, pp. 25–31, 2015.

[19] R. Román-Oyola, S. Reynolds, I. Soto-Feliciano, L. Cabrera-Mercader, and J. Vega-Santana, "Child's sensory profile and adult playfulness as predictors of parental self-efficacy," *American Journal of Occupational Therapy*, vol. 71, no. 2, 2017.

[20] G. L. Landreth, "Play therapy in elementary school settings," in *Handbook of Play Therapy*, C. E. Schaefer and K. J. O'Connor, Eds., pp. 202–212, Wiley, New York, NY, USA, 1983.

[21] B. Youell, "The importance of play and playfulness," *European Journal of Psychotherapy & Counselling*, vol. 10, no. 2, pp. 121–129, 2008.

[22] M. Flippin and L. R. Watson, "Fathers' and mothers' verbal responsiveness and the language skills of young children with autism spectrum disorder," *American Journal of Speech-Language Pathology*, vol. 24, no. 3, pp. 400–410, 2015.

[23] S. Y. Shire, A. Gulsrud, and C. Kasari, "Increasing responsive parent-child interactions and joint engagement: comparing the influence of parent-mediated intervention and parent psychoeducation," *Journal of Autism and Developmental Disorders*, vol. 46, no. 5, pp. 1737–1747, 2016.

[24] C. Kasari, A. C. Gulsrud, C. Wong, S. Kwon, and J. Locke, "Randomized controlled caregiver mediated joint engagement intervention for toddlers with autism," *Journal of Autism and Developmental Disorders*, vol. 40, no. 9, pp. 1045–1056, 2010.

[25] R. L. Koegel, A. Bimbela, and L. Schreibman, "Collateral effects of parent training on family interactions," *Journal of Autism and Developmental Disorders*, vol. 26, no. 3, pp. 347–359, 1996.

[26] Y. S. Lincoln and E. G. Guba, *Naturalistic Inquiry*, Sage Publications, Beverly Hills, CA, USA, 1985.

[27] J. Creswell, *Qualitative Inquiry and Research Design*, Sage Publications, Los Angeles, CA, USA, 2013.

[28] P. Rose, J. Beeby, and D. Parker, "Academic rigour in the lived experience of researchers using phenomenological methods in nursing," *Journal of Advanced Nursing*, vol. 21, no. 6, pp. 1123–1129, 1995.

[29] T. Keller, J. Ramisch, and M. Carolan, "Relationships of children with autism spectrum disorders and their fathers," *The Qualitative Report*, vol. 19, no. 33, pp. 1–15, 2014.

[30] B. Pini, "Interviewing men: gender and the collection and interpretation of qualitative data," *Journal of Sociology*, vol. 41, no. 2, pp. 201–216, 2005.

[31] A. Broom, K. Hand, and P. Tovey, "The role of gender, environment and individual biography in shaping qualitative interview data," *International Journal of Social Research Methodology*, vol. 12, no. 1, pp. 51–65, 2009.

[32] M. B. Miles, A. M. Huberman, and J. Saldaña, *Qualitative Data Analysis: A Methods Sourcebook*, Sage Publications, Thousand Oaks, CA, USA, 3rd edition, 2014.

[33] J. Saldaña, *The Coding Manual for Qualitative Researchers*, Sage Publications, Los Angeles, CA, USA, 2013.

[34] H. J. Streubert and D. R. Carpenter, *Qualitative Research in Nursing*, Wolters Kluwer Health, Philadelphia, PA, USA, 2011.

[35] R. Fletcher, J. StGeorge, and E. Freeman, "Rough and tumble play quality: theoretical foundations for a new measure of father–child interaction," *Early Child Development and Care*, vol. 183, no. 6, pp. 746–759, 2013.

[36] L. A. Newland, H. H. Chen, D. D. Coyl-Shepherd et al., "Parent and child perspectives on mothering and fathering: the influence of ecocultural niches," *Early Child Development and Care*, vol. 183, no. 3-4, pp. 534–552, 2013.

[37] D. Paquette, "Theorizing the father-child relationship: mechanisms and developmental outcomes," *Human Development*, vol. 47, no. 4, pp. 193–219, 2004.

[38] L. Fava, K. Strauss, G. Valeri, L. D'Elia, S. Arima, and S. Vicari, "The effectiveness of a cross-setting complementary staff- and parent-mediated early intensive behavioral intervention for young children with ASD," *Research in Autism Spectrum Disorders*, vol. 5, no. 4, pp. 1479–1492, 2011.

[39] J. M. Pierucci, "Mothers' scaffolding techniques used during play in toddlers with autism spectrum disorder," *Journal of Developmental and Physical Disabilities*, vol. 28, no. 2, pp. 217–235, 2016.

[40] L. A. Vismara, C. Colombi, and S. J. Rogers, "Can one hour per week of therapy lead to lasting changes in young children with autism," *Autism*, vol. 13, no. 1, pp. 93–115, 2009.

[41] Y. C. Lee, P. C. Chan, S. K. Lin, C. T. Chen, C. Y. Huang, and K. L. Chen, "Correlation patterns between pretend play and playfulness in children with autism spectrum disorder, developmental delay, and typical development," *Research in Autism Spectrum Disorders*, vol. 24, pp. 29–38, 2016.

[42] C. Jarrold, "A review of research into pretend play in autism," *Autism*, vol. 7, no. 4, pp. 379–390, 2003.

[43] K. Stagnitti and C. Unsworth, "The importance of pretend play in child development: an occupational therapy perspective," *British Journal of Occupational Therapy*, vol. 63, no. 3, pp. 121–127, 2000.

[44] K. Stagnitti, "Play therapy for school-age children with high-functioning autism," in *Play Therapy in Middle Childhood*, A. A. Drewes and C. E. Schaefer, Eds., pp. 237–255, American Psychological Association, Washington, DC, USA, 2016.

[45] J. Case-Smith and H. M. Kuhaneck, "Play preferences of typically developing children and children with developmental delays between ages 3 and 7 years," *Occupational Therapy Journal of Research*, vol. 28, no. 1, pp. 19–29, 2008.

[46] F. Graham, S. Rodger, and J. Ziviani, "Coaching parents to enable children's participation: an approach for working with parents and their children," *Australian Occupational Therapy Journal*, vol. 56, no. 1, pp. 16–23, 2009.

[47] American Occupational Therapy Association, "Occupational therapy practice framework: domain and process (3rd edition)," *American Journal of Occupational Therapy*, vol. 68, pp. S1–S48, 2017.

[48] C. T. Myers, J. Case-Smith, and J. Cason, "Early intervention," in *Occupational Therapy for Children and Adolescents*, J. Case-Smith and J. C. O'Brien, Eds., pp. 636–663, Elsevier, St. Louis, MO, USA, 2015.

[49] D. Simpson, "Coaching as a family-centred, occupational therapy intervention for autism: a literature review," *Journal of Occupational Therapy, Schools, & Early Intervention*, vol. 8, no. 2, pp. 109–125, 2015.

[50] H. M. Kuhaneck, K. J. Tanta, A. K. Coombs, and H. Pannone, "A survey of pediatric occupational therapists' use of play," *Journal of Occupational Therapy, Schools, & Early Intervention*, vol. 6, no. 3, pp. 213–227, 2013.

[51] K. Suwada, "Being a traditional dad or being more like a mum? Clashing models of fatherhood according to Swedish and Polish fathers," *Journal of Comparative Family Studies*, vol. 46, no. 4, pp. 467–481, 2015.

[52] J. M. StGeorge, J. C. Goodwin, and R. J. Fletcher, "Parents' views of father–child rough-and-tumble play," *Journal of Child and Family Studies*, vol. 27, no. 5, pp. 1502–1512, 2018.

[53] S. Pinchover, C. Shulman, and A. Bundy, "A comparison of playfulness of young children with and without autism spectrum disorder in interactions with their mothers and teachers," *Early Child Development and Care*, vol. 186, no. 12, pp. 1893–1906, 2016.

14

Loewenstein Occupational Therapy Cognitive Assessment to Evaluate People with Addictions

Gloria Rojo-Mota,[1,2] Eduardo J. Pedrero-Pérez,[1] José M. Ruiz-Sánchez de León,[3] Irene León-Frade,[1] Patricia Aldea-Poyo,[1] Marina Alonso-Rodríguez,[1] Jara Pedrero-Aguilar,[1] and Sara Morales-Alonso[1]

[1]*Institute of Addictions, Madrid Salud, Madrid City Council, Madrid, Spain*
[2]*King Juan Carlos University, Madrid, Spain*
[3]*Complutense University of Madrid, Madrid, Spain*

Correspondence should be addressed to Gloria Rojo-Mota; gloriaroj@yahoo.es

Academic Editor: Patricia Belchior

Background. The LOTCA (Loewenstein Occupational Therapy Cognitive Assessment) battery is a cognitive screening test which is widely used in occupational health. However, no work has been found that explores its use in addiction treatment. *Objectives of Study.* To explore the convergent validity of LOTCA with neuropsychological tests that assess related cerebral functional areas. *Methods.* The LOTCA, along with a battery of neuropsychological tests, was administered to a sample of 48 subjects who start a treatment by substance or gambling addictions. *Findings.* A correlational pattern was observed of a considerable magnitude between the effects of the LOTCA scales and those of some neuropsychological tests, but not with others. There is barely any convergence in measures with memory and executive function tests. *Relevance to Clinical Practice.* There is a lack of research applying test of occupational assessment to populations of patients treated by addictive behaviors. The LOTCA seems to be a reliable and valid test for preliminary screening of function in certain cognitive areas, easy, and quick to use (around 30 minutes). However, it must be supplemented with other tests for a full and ecological assessment of patients. *Limitations.* An incident, small-size sample. *Recommendations for Further Research.* New studies are needed to explore the applicability, diagnostic validity, and whole psychometric quality of the test in addiction-related treatment.

1. Introduction

Substance addiction is a health problem that affects all areas of individual functioning and their relation with environment. There are many ways to view addiction: from considering it a brain disease [1] to understanding it as a behavior more or less effective to cope with difficulties in life, which can be reversed even spontaneously without requiring medical treatment [2, 3]. In any case, is no doubt that "addictive behavior occurs within a social context, which can serve as a risk or protective factor as social contexts and individuals influence one another" ([4, p. 353]). Contrary to prior thinking, it has been recently suggested that addiction does not merely disrupt a person's occupational life; but rather, it constitutes a person's occupational life [5]. The establishment of habits and routines related to addiction impregnates a person's life in such way that only that which is related with drug use seems significant to them. The therapist's work lies in providing real life activities in a natural environment which have become dysfunctional throughout the addiction, abandoned, interrupted, or not accessed.

However, there is one significant difficulty in designing individual occupational treatments: the cognitive deficits which are often associated with the addiction. This happens in both cases of substance addictions [6] and cases of behavioral addictions [7]. Such deficits can represent preaddiction conditions and, therefore, vulnerabilities to developing the addiction, or effects deriving from the consumption of substances due to either the specific biochemical effects or the associated stress or restriction of stimulation or even a combination of both [8]. A comprehensive review found that certain cognitive deficits represent common addictive processes elements (deficits in episodic memory, emotional processing, and the executive components of updating and decision-making), while others are specifically associated with each substance (psychostimulants and alcohol use with impulsive action and cognitive flexibility, alcohol and MDMA with spatial processing, perceptual speed and selective attention, cannabis and methamphetamine on prospective memory deficits, and cannabis and MDMA on processing speed and complex planning) [9]. A change in habits involves cognitive and metacognitive skills that often reflect deficient performance in people with addictions [10], which is related to a "shut-down" of the prefrontal cortex, which stops exercising control over other cerebral areas [11]. Previous studies have shown that neuropsychological alterations are associated with reduced level of involvement and participation of drug dependent individuals in treatment programs and with a higher rate of dropping out of these programs [12], to the extent that individuals with addictive behaviors may have considerable difficulty in becoming aware of their own deficit, to understand and reason complex instructions, to inhibit impulsive responses, to plan their daily activities, and to make everyday decisions [13]. Their detection by cognitive assessment allows designing rehabilitation programs that are aimed to better use of other therapeutic resources available, such as cognitive therapy or therapy relapse prevention [14].

2. Literature Review

According to a recent review, occupational therapists have been participating in teams treating people with addictions for decades although their scientific production is quite scarce [15]. This review found a critical deficit in the availability of occupational assessment instruments, which have been validated in the field of addictions. Currently, they are only available nonreplicated works on the Executive Function Performance Test (EFPT) [16], the Assessment of Motor and Process Skills (AMPS) [17], the Allen Cognitive Level Screen-5 (ACLS-5) [18], and little more. The review concludes the need to validate occupational instruments in people with addictions who are undergoing treatment as an urgent need in order to promote and improve the scientific production of the profession in this clinical field.

One of the most widely used instruments in occupational health to assess cognitive performance is the Loewenstein Occupational Therapy Cognitive Assessment (LOTCA) battery [19]. It provides an assessment of basic cognitive skills required for everyday function, including orientation, visual perceptual and psychomotor abilities, problem-solving skills, and thinking operations. The results can also be used in treatment planning and to review progress over time. The test has been used in a large number of studies and its psychometric properties have proven satisfactory in many research projects and in very diverse populations and geographic areas. Just to mention a few of the most recent, it has been used in the geriatric population [20], for brain damage [21] and cases of schizophrenia [22], among others. It has also been used as a tool for measuring the effectiveness of treatments of stroke patients [23–26], in healthy individuals [27] and schoolchildren [28], among many other people [29]. No work has been found which uses LOTCA in a population of people with substance addiction undergoing treatment.

3. Study Objectives

The objective of this work is to apply LOTCA to a sample of people receiving treatment for substance addiction and to explore its convergent validity with other occupational and neuropsychological tests used to estimate cognitive deficits.

4. Methods

4.1. Participants and Procedures. The sample was obtained from a specific urban, public, and free center that treats people with substance addictions in the city of Madrid: the San Blas CAD Drug Addiction Care Center (Addiction Institute, Madrid Health, City of Madrid). The people access this service directly and are assessed using diagnostic interviews by a multidisciplinary team (doctors, nurses, psychologists, social workers, and occupational therapists). The criterion for inclusion in this study was complying with the requirements for being diagnosed with a Substance-Related Disorder, as per the DSM-5 [30]. The criteria for exclusion were having previously suffered any type of brain damage ($n = 0$), presenting some type of psychotic process in an active phase at the time of the initial assessment ($n = 0$), or presenting any condition that would prevent the proper comprehension of the instructions used to complete the tests such as language issues, illiteracy, and a state of confusion ($n = 1$). The time necessary in each case (generally between one and two weeks) for participants to be no longer under the effect of any non-prescribed substances was allowed to pass before the assessment. When necessary, this was confirmed with the visible ultraviolet spectrophotometry method to find metabolites of opiates, cocaine, cannabis, and benzodiazepines in the urine or breath alcohol testing (one subject was excluded due to active consumption upon assessment). The participants were informed of the two objectives of the assessment: to design an individualized treatment and to do research work. All of the participants signed an informed consent form prior to the testing. The study was authorized by the Research Unit of the Madrid Health Evaluation and Quality Department and was approved by the Addiction Institute Research Committee.

In order to do this study, the first 50 subjects beginning treatment with the service were recruited. The occupational tests were administered simultaneously by two occupational therapists (principal and observant evaluator) and the neuropsychological tests by three neuropsychologists (each patient was assigned to one of them). All of the participants underwent occupational testing and the battery of neuropsychology tests in a period of less than one week. Two of them did not finish the assessment because they did

TABLE 1: Descriptives of the sample.

	Gender		
	Male	Female	Total
n	38	10	48
%	79.2	20.8	100
		Age	
Mean	37.5	48.5	39.8
SD	12.2	10.7	12.6
Rank	18–62	32–67	18–67
		Academic level (%)	
Primary or less	23.4	30.0	25.0
Secondary (obligatory)	36.8	20.0	33.3
Secondary (advanced)	36.8	30.0	35.4
Universitary	2.6	20.0	6.3
		Main drug (%)	
Heroine	5.3	—	4.2
Cocaine	44.7	30.0	41.7
Alcohol	34.2	70.0	41.7
Cannabis	15.8	—	12.5

not want to, which means that the final sample was $n = 48$ subjects. The sample descriptors can be found in Table 1.

4.2. Instruments. The Loewenstein Occupational Therapy Cognitive Assessment (LOTCA) battery, which is a performance test, contains 20 items categorized into four subscales: orientation (2 items), perception (6 items), visuomotor organization (7 items), and thinking operations (5 items; the score for the pictorial sequence is obtained with the average of two tasks, A and B). The LOTCA kit contains testing materials (card decks, coloured blocks, pegboard set, and other materials) and a manual that includes definitions of the cognitive domains assessed, instructions for administration, and specific scoring guidelines. The scores were placed on a Likert-type scale ranging from 1 to 4 (with the exception of items 1–5 regarding categorization, unstructured Risk Object Classification [31], and structured ROC). The higher the scores were, the better the performance was. Because it is not meaningful to add up unrelated areas of cognitive and perceptual skills, we did not calculate a total score for the LOTCA. The time each participant took to complete the LOTCA was recorded as a proxy of the participant's information-processing speed. The LOTCA was administered and scored using the instructions in the test manual.

The Allen Cognitive Level Screen-5 (ACLS-5) [32] consists of a piece of leather perforated on all sides, leather laces, two types of needle, and a shoelace. Administration time is approximately 10 minutes. The assessment allows the clinician to evaluate the person's performance on three different leather-lacing tasks of varying challenge. The test consists of three visual motor learning tasks (stitching leather) with increased complexity in the activities. In order to complete the three tasks successfully, the person must pay attention to the verbal instructions and demonstration, understand and use sensory signals from the materials (leather, lace, and needles), and effectively use feedback from the motor actions during practice with the lacing materials. The test was applied with satisfactory results on subjects being treated for substance addiction and evidence was found of convergent validity with neuropsychology tests [32].

The battery of neuropsychology tests was based on prior suggestions for cognitive assessment among populations of people being treated for addiction [33]. Specifically, the following were administered in accordance with the standards found in each manual: the Brief Cognitive Status Exam (BCSE) [34] as a measure of one's overall mental state, the Wechsler Adult Intelligence Coding and Symbol Search to establish the Processing Speed Index (PSI), Digit Span and Symbol Span of the Wechsler Memory Scale [35] to assess working memory, the Rey-Osterrieth Complex Figure Test [36], and the Logic Memory Test to assess visual memory and verbal memory, as well as the Five-Digit Test [37], an alternative to the Stroop test, to assess inhibition and flexibility.

4.3. Data Analysis. The internal consistency of the test was studied using Cronbach's α. A confirmatory factor analysis was done on the theoretical structure of the survey using the unweighted least squares method since ordinal categorical items were used and normality was not expected in the distribution of the data. The indicators provided by the AMOS 18 program were used to study the adequacy of the theoretical model to the data: RMR = Root Mean Square Residual, with acceptable values below 0.06; GFI = General Fit Index; AGFI = Adjusted Goodness of Fit Index; NFI = Normed Fit Index; RFI = Relative Fit Index, all of which showed acceptable values above 0.90; PNFI = Parsimonious Normed Fit Index; PGFI = Parsimony Goodness of Fit Index, both acceptable with values above 0.7. Spearman's rho was used to study the correlations [38]. The comparisons between subgroups were made using nonparametric procedures. The statistical package SPSS 19 was used for these analyses.

5. Findings

Table 2 outlines the descriptors of the items obtained upon application to the sample. On the whole, the test showed reliability of Cronbach $\alpha = 0.854$. The confirmatory factor analysis showed suitable indicators of adequacy for the four-dimension theoretical model for the sample data (RMR = 0.05; GFI = 0.96; AGFI = 0.95; NFI = 0.94; RFI = 0.93; PNFI = 0.86; PGFI = 0.75).

Table 3 shows the correlations found between the LOTCA scales and the neuropsychology test scales. There were no significant differences between the scores obtained by men and women on the LOTCA scales ($0.44 < Z < 1.71$; $p > 0.05$ in all cases), or the primary drug ($0.92 < \chi^2_{(\text{d.f. }3)} < 4.01$; $p > 0.05$ in all cases). However, the difference in the time used by men and women to complete the test was significant: the men used less time (mean = 24.32; SD = 13.12) than the women (mean = 34.90; SD = 10.55). There were significant differences in relation to the education level of the participants: the higher the scores, the higher the education

Table 2: Scores obtained on the LOTCA scales and items.

	Score	Mean	Minimum	Maximum	SD
Orientation	2–8	7.73	6	8	0.50
Time	1–4	3.91	2	4	0.36
Place	1–4	3.82	3	4	0.39
Perception	6–24	22.52	18	24	2.09
Object identification	1–4	4.00	4	4	0.00
Shape identification	1–4	3.73	3	4	0.45
Overlapping figures	1–4	4.00	4	4	0.00
Object constancy	1–4	3.98	3	4	0.15
Spatial perception	1–4	3.91	2	4	0.36
Praxis	1–4	3.88	1	4	0.55
Visuomotor organization	7–28	24.18	15	28	3.59
Copying geometric forms	1–4	3.55	2	4	0.59
Reproducing a two-dimensional model	1–4	3.59	2	4	0.62
Constructing a pegboard design	1–4	3.66	1	4	0.71
Constructing a colored block design	1–4	3.66	1	4	0.81
Constructing a plain block design	1–4	3.20	1	4	1.00
Reproducing a puzzle	1–4	3.05	1	4	0.83
Drawing a clock	1–4	3.48	2	4	0.70
Thinking operations	5–23	18.26	11	23	3.51
Categorization	1–5	3.84	2	5	1.12
ROC: unstructured	1–5	3.64	1	5	1.24
ROC: structured	1–5	3.70	1	5	1.00
Pictorial sequence A	1–4	3.91	3	4	0.29
Pictorial sequence B	1–4	3.48	1	4	0.90
Geometrical sequence	1–4	3.39	1	4	0.97
Length of time (minutes)		29.84	14	55	10.52

level on all scales ($7.69 < \chi^2_{(\text{d.f. }3)} < 12.42$; $p > 0.05$ in all cases), except orientation ($\chi^2_{(\text{d.f. }3)} = 1.84$; $p = 0.61$), and in the time used to complete the test ($\chi^2_{(\text{d.f. }3)} = 3.12$; $p = 0.37$).

6. Discussion

LOTCA is a relatively systematic test that can be useful for initial assessments of people who are beginning treatment for addictive behaviors with or without substances. However, its use among this clinical population has never before been established. As a screening test of function areas, the results must show correlation with more demanding and systematic tests used in the field of neuropsychology. This work explored the existence of a relationship between both types of tests. The results are conclusive: there are correlations of a considerable size of effect with some tests, but not with others. Specifically, LOTCA does not seem to measure something related to executive functions given that it barely shows convergence in measurements with the 5-Digit Test.

However, there are correlations of a great effect size with other screening tests both in the field of occupational therapy (ACLS-5) and in the field of neuropsychology (BSCE). Specifically, the ACLS-5 is a motor test which includes comprehension of instructions, executive planning, and the ability to resolve conflicts that arise during its performance. These three abilities are measured by LOTCA and reflect considerable measurement convergence. The same occurs with the BCSE, which also explores these abilities, among others, although it is more aimed at the establishment of clinical cut-off points than differentiated estimation of the various abilities. To this end, LOTCA seems to be a good cognitive screening instrument.

There are also significant correlations with those obtained on the Rey Figure. This test, which is in the copy phase, involves visuomotor skills used to detect stimulus and their copying. In a second phase, it requires recent memory and maintaining copied sketches in the memory in addition to the motor skills.

There are also significant correlations with attention span tests as concerns both numbers and other types of symbols. However, the correlations shown are barely noticeable (and the fact that they appear due to a random effect cannot be discarded) when memory or executive function tests are involved.

The LOTCA orientation scale barely correlates with neuropsychology tests. This scale is likely useful in more serious cerebral function pathologies but not in addiction subjects, whose cognitive deficits are minor and do not affect such basic functions. Proof of this lies in the mean obtained by the sample studied being very close to the maximum possible (7.73 out of 8) which means that it is not related to

TABLE 3: Spearman correlations between the LOTCA scale scores and scale scores obtained with the neuropsychology battery of tests.

	LOTCA				
	Orientation	Visual perceptual abilities	Psychomotor abilities	Thinking operations	Execution time
ACLS-5	0.08	0.34**	0.53***	0.48***	−0.44***
BCSE	0.26*	0.55***	0.54***	0.51***	−0.58***
Rey Complex Figure					
Copy	0.33*	0.47***	0.55***	0.43**	−0.32*
Immediate recall	0.11	0.44***	0.56***	0.41**	−0.31*
WAIS-IV					
Coding	0.14	0.51***	0.59***	0.59***	−0.20
Symbol search	0.04	0.46***	0.64***	0.50***	−0.37**
Processing speed Index	0.10	0.54***	0.68***	0.60***	−0.17
Digit span	0.33*	0.68***	0.59***	0.51***	−0.41**
WMS-IV					
Symbol span	0.28*	0.50***	0.52***	0.54***	−0.31*
Logic memory I	0.27*	0.24	0.30	0.30*	−0.26
Logic memory II	0.24	0.27*	0.37**	0.34*	−0.30*
Five-Digit Test					
Reading	0.20	0.41**	0.33*	0.24	−0.21
Counting	0.15	0.25*	0.31*	0.16	−0.23
Choosing	0.06	0.35*	0.20	0.16	−0.11
Switching	−0.04	0.23	0.25*	0.23	−0.29*
Inhibition	−0.12	0.21	0.08	0.05	−0.23
Flexibility	−0.12	0.16	0.22	0.20	−0.15

Note: ***$p < 0.001$; **$p < 0.01$; *$p < 0.05$.

the performance level in the specific areas studied by other scales.

7. Limitations

This work has limitations that should be considered. The main limitation is the sample size, which is not sufficient enough to absolutely affirm the relationships observed. The method for obtaining the sample is merely incidental as the first subjects to arrive at the center's occupational therapy service were recruited which means that it is not possible to generalize the results obtained. Finally, there are newer versions of LOTCA than the one used which could provide all-new data not contemplated by this initial version.

8. Recommendations for Further Research

The nonexistence of research work where this test is applied to people with addictions means that this is a preliminary study that must be replicated on larger samples and with better sample selection methods. In conclusion, LOTCA is a cognitive screening test that allows for an approximation of some areas of cognitive function yet not all meaning that it must be supplemented with other tests that measure executive function and memory. As a screening test, it may be used ahead of others that are widely used in occupational therapy (i.e., ACLS-5) and neuropsychology (i.e., MMSE, MoCA, and BCSE) to the extent that, beyond estimating a general cut-off point of good or poor function, it explores the quality of execution in specific functional areas. In any case, this test does not make it possible to conduct a full neuropsychological assessment but rather simply quickly detects when and who should undergo it and in which areas more important deficits are detected. To this end, its use can encourage an understanding by a therapist of the more deficient areas of function, to refer patients to other professionals as necessary to conduct more in-depth assessments, to design intervention plans considering a patient's most important deficits, and to estimate the change generated after occupational intervention [39]. To this extent and with the precautions indicated in mind, its inclusion in the battery of tests administered by therapists participating in the treatment of people with addictions is recommended. New studies are needed to contribute more information on its potential and on the rest of the tests which must be used to supplement its use in order to provide a full occupational assessment that is adequate for people in rehabilitation processes for their addictive behaviors.

Competing Interests

No conflict of interests has been declared by the authors.

Authors' Contributions

Gloria Rojo-Mota is the principal investigator. Eduardo J. Pedrero-Pérez has made the psychometric data analysis. Gloria Rojo-Mota, Eduardo J. Pedrero-Pérez, and José M.

Ruiz-Sánchez de León have participated in study design, data processing, and article writing. José M. Ruiz-Sánchez de León has designed the battery of neuropsychological tests and has overseen the process of administration and processing data. Gloria Rojo-Mota and Irene León-Frade have administered occupational tests, have set up the database, and have corrected the tests and have obtained results. Patricia Aldea-Poyo, Marina Alonso-Rodríguez, Jara Pedrero-Aguilar, and Sara Morales-Alonso have administered the battery of neuropsychological tests, have set up the database, and have corrected the tests and have obtained results.

References

[1] N. D. Volkow, G. F. Koob, and A. T. McLellan, "Neurobiologic advances from the brain disease model of addiction," *The New England Journal of Medicine*, vol. 374, no. 4, pp. 363–371, 2016.

[2] S. Peele, "People control their addictions no matter how much the 'chronic' brain disease model of addiction indicates otherwise; We know that people can quit addictions—with special reference to harm reduction and mindfulness," *Addictive Behaviors Reports*, 2016.

[3] S. Peele, A. Brodsky, and M. Arnold, *The Truth About Addiction and Recovery*, Simon & Schuster, New York, NY, USA, 1992.

[4] E. Gifford and K. Humphreys, "The psychological science of addiction," *Addiction*, vol. 102, no. 3, pp. 352–361, 2007.

[5] S. Wasmuth, J. L. Crabtree, and P. J. Scott, "Exploring addiction-as-occupation," *British Journal of Occupational Therapy*, vol. 77, no. 12, pp. 605–613, 2014.

[6] A. Verdejo-García, A. Bechara, E. C. Recknor, and M. Pérez-García, "Executive dysfunction in substance dependent individuals during drug use and abstinence: an examination of the behavioral, cognitive and emotional correlates of addiction," *Journal of the International Neuropsychological Society*, vol. 12, no. 3, pp. 405–415, 2006.

[7] M. Brand, K. S. Young, and C. Laier, "Prefrontal control and Internet addiction: a theoretical model and review of neuropsychological and neuroimaging findings," *Frontiers in Human Neuroscience*, vol. 8, article 375, 2014.

[8] M. Yücel, D. I. Lubman, N. Solowij, and W. J. Brewer, "Understanding drug addiction: a neuropsychological perspective," *Australian and New Zealand Journal of Psychiatry*, vol. 41, no. 12, pp. 957–968, 2007.

[9] M. J. Fernández-Serrano, M. Pérez-García, and A. Verdejo-García, "What are the specific vs. generalized effects of drugs of abuse on neuropsychological performance?" *Neuroscience & Biobehavioral Reviews*, vol. 35, no. 3, pp. 377–406, 2011.

[10] S. L. Wasmuth, J. Outcalt, K. Buck, B. L. Leonhardt, J. Vohs, and P. H. Lysaker, "Metacognition in persons with substance abuse: findings and implications for occupational therapists," *Canadian Journal of Occupational Therapy*, vol. 82, no. 3, pp. 150–159, 2015.

[11] B. J. Everitt and T. W. Robbins, "Drug addiction: updating actions to habits to compulsions ten years on," *Annual Review of Psychology*, vol. 67, pp. 23–50, 2016.

[12] E. Aharonovich, D. S. Hasin, A. C. Brooks, X. Liu, A. Bisaga, and E. V. Nunes, "Cognitive deficits predict low treatment retention in cocaine dependent patients," *Drug and Alcohol Dependence*, vol. 81, no. 3, pp. 313–322, 2006.

[13] A. Verdejo-Garcia, N. Albein-Urios, J. M. Martinez-Gonzalez, E. Civit, R. de la Torre, and O. Lozano, "Decision-making impairment predicts 3-month hair-indexed cocaine relapse," *Psychopharmacology*, vol. 231, no. 21, pp. 4179–4187, 2014.

[14] W. Fals-Stewart and W. K. K. Lam, "Computer-assisted cognitive rehabilitation for the treatment of patients with substance use disorders: a randomized clinical trial," *Experimental and Clinical Psychopharmacology*, vol. 18, no. 1, pp. 87–98, 2010.

[15] G. Rojo Mota, Terapia ocupacional en adicciones: revisión de bases de datos internacionales. [Occupational therapy for addictions: Review of international databases]. Spanish. Terapia Ocupacional Galicia [online journal], vol. 18, 14 pages, http://www.revistatog.com/num18/pdfs/original3.pdf.

[16] E. Raphael-Greenfield, "Assessing executive and community functioning among homeless persons with substance use disorders using the executive function performance test," *Occupational Therapy International*, vol. 19, no. 3, pp. 135–143, 2012.

[17] G. Rojo-Mota, E. J. Pedrero-Pérez, J. M. Ruiz-Sánchez de León, and J. C. Miangolarra Page, "Assessment of motor and process skills in daily life activities of treated substance addicts," *Scandinavian Journal of Occupational Therapy*, vol. 21, no. 6, pp. 458–464, 2014.

[18] G. Rojo-Mota, E. J. Pedrero-Pérez, E. Huertas-Hoyas, B. Merritt, and D. MacKenzie, "Allen Cognitive Level Screen for the classification of subjects treated for addiction," *Scandinavian Journal of Occupational Therapy*, 2016.

[19] N. Katz, M. Itzkovich, S. Averbuch, and B. Elazar, "Loewenstein Occupational Therapy Cognitive Assessment (LOTCA) battery for brain-injured patients: reliability and validity," *The American Journal of Occupational Therapy*, vol. 43, no. 3, pp. 184–192, 1989.

[20] A. K. Mohd Natar, R. Nagappan, H. A. Ainuddin, G. Masuri, and C. K. K. Thanapalan, "Psychometric properties of the malay version of the loewenstein occupational therapy cognitive assessment for geriatrics (M-LOTCA-G) among the malaysian elderly population," *Educational Gerontology*, vol. 41, no. 1, pp. 27–40, 2015.

[21] Z.-Z. Yu, S.-J. Jiang, J. Li et al., "Clinical application of loewenstein occupational therapy cognitive assessment battery-second edition in evaluating of cognitive function of Chinese patients with post-stroke aphasia," *Chinese Medical Sciences Journal*, vol. 28, no. 3, pp. 167–171, 2013.

[22] C.-Y. Chou, M.-C. Ma, and T.-T. Yang, "Determinants of subjective health-related quality of life (HRQoL) for patients with schizophrenia," *Schizophrenia Research*, vol. 154, no. 1–3, pp. 83–88, 2014.

[23] A. Ávila, M. Durán, M. Peralbo, G. Torres, M. Saavedra, and I. M. Viana, "Effectiveness of an occupational therapy home programme in spain for people affected by stroke," *Occupational Therapy International*, vol. 22, no. 1, pp. 1–9, 2015.

[24] J.-H. Park and J.-H. Park, "The effects of a Korean computer-based cognitive rehabilitation program on cognitive function and visual perception ability of patients with acute stroke," *Journal of Physical Therapy Science*, vol. 27, no. 8, pp. 2577–2579, 2015.

[25] S. B. Shin, T. U. Kim, J. K. Hyun, and J. Y. Kim, "The prediction of clinical outcome using HbA1c in acute ischemic stroke of the deep branch of middle cerebral artery," *Annals of Rehabilitation Medicine*, vol. 39, no. 6, pp. 1011–1017, 2015.

[26] S.-Y. Wang, Z.-K. Gong, J. Sen, L. Han, M. Zhang, and W. Chen, "The usefulness of the Loewenstein Occupational Therapy Cognition Assessment in evaluating cognitive function in patients with stroke," *European Review for Medical and Pharmacological Sciences*, vol. 18, no. 23, pp. 3665–3672, 2014.

[27] A. H. Alghadir, S. A. Gabr, and E. S. Al-Eisa, "Effects of moderate aerobic exercise on cognitive abilities and redox state biomarkers in older adults," *Oxidative Medicine and Cellular Longevity*, vol. 2016, Article ID 2545168, 8 pages, 2016.

[28] F. Almomani, N. Josman, M. O. Al-Momani et al., "Factors related to cognitive function among elementary school children," *Scandinavian Journal of Occupational Therapy*, vol. 21, no. 3, pp. 191–198, 2014.

[29] A. H. Alghadir, S. A. Gabr, and E. S. Al-Eisa, "Assessment of the effects of glutamic acid decarboxylase antibodies and trace elements on cognitive performance in older adults," *Clinical Interventions in Aging*, vol. 10, pp. 1901–1907, 2015.

[30] American Psychiatric Association, *Diagnostic and Statistical Manual of Mental Disorders (DSM-5®)*, American Psychiatric Association, 2013.

[31] L. Williams Riska and C. K. Allen, "Research with non disabled population," in *Occupational Therapy for Psychiatric Diseases: Measurement and Management of Cognitive Disabilities*, C. K. Allen, Ed., vol. 68, pp. 315–338, Little, Brown & Co., Boston, Mass, USA, 1980.

[32] C. K. Allen, S. L. Austin, S. K. David, C. A. Earhart, D. B. McCraith, and L. Riska-Williams, *Manual for the Allen Cognitive Level Screen-5 (ACLS-5) and Large Allen Cognitive Level Screen (LACLS-5)*, CA-ACLS and LACLS Committee, Camarillo, Calif, USA, 2007.

[33] J. M. Ruiz-Sánchez de León, E. J. Pedrero-Pérez, G. Rojo-Mota, M. Llanero-Luque, and C. Puerta-García, "A proposal for a protocol of neuropsychological assessment for use in addictions," *Revista de Neurología*, vol. 53, no. 8, pp. 483–493, 2011.

[34] D. Wechsler, *Wechsler Memory Scale*, Pearson, San Antonio, Tex, USA, 4th edition, 2009.

[35] D. Wechsler, *Wechsler Adult Intelligence Scale*, Pearson, San Antonio, Tex, USA, 4th edition, 2008.

[36] A. Rey, "Lexamen psychologique dans les cas d'encephalopathies traumatique," *Archives de Psichologie*, vol. 28, pp. 286–340, 1941.

[37] M. A. Sedó, *FDT: Test de los Cinco Dígitos*, TEA, Madrid, Spain, 2007.

[38] L.-T. Hu and P. M. Bentler, "Cutoff criteria for fit indexes in covariance structure analysis: conventional criteria versus new alternatives," *Structural Equation Modeling*, vol. 6, no. 1, pp. 1–55, 1999.

[39] G. Rojo-Mota, "Occupational therapy in addiction: from theory to practice," *Revista Chilena de Terapia Ocupaciona*, vol. 16, pp. 159–171, 2016.

15

Evidence-Based Practice in Primary Care Occupational Therapy: A Cross-Sectional Survey in Sweden

Ann-Charlotte Lindström[1] and Susanne Bernhardsson[2,3]

[1]*Närhälsan Rehabilitation Sörhaga, Alingsås, Sweden*
[2]*Närhälsan Research and Development Primary Health Care, Region Västra Götaland, Gothenburg, Sweden*
[3]*Institute of Neuroscience and Physiology, Department of Health and Rehabilitation, Unit of Physiotherapy, University of Gothenburg, The Sahlgrenska Academy, Gothenburg, Sweden*

Correspondence should be addressed to Susanne Bernhardsson; susanne.bernhardsson@vgregion.se

Academic Editor: Jodie A. Copley

Introduction. Understanding of attitudes, knowledge, and behaviour related to evidence-based practice (EBP) and guidelines in Swedish occupational therapy is limited. The study aims were to investigate attitudes, knowledge, and behaviour related to evidence-based practice and guidelines of Swedish occupational therapists in primary care. *Methods.* A web-based survey of 94 Swedish primary care occupational therapists (response rate 53.7%). Data were analysed using logistic regressions. *Results.* Attitudes towards EBP and guidelines were highly positive (97%–98%). About half of the respondents reported confidence in finding and using evidence. Almost two-thirds reported being aware of guidelines and 47% knowing where to find guidelines. Four-fifths stated that they had easy access to guidelines and 75% that they used guidelines frequently. Men were more likely to feel confident to find research (OR 8.58, 95% CI 1.03 to 71.66; $p = 0.047$) and have easy access to guidelines (OR 9.10, 95% CI 1.94 to 42.83; $p = 0.005$). Occupational therapists older than 50 years were more likely to integrate patient preferences with guideline use (OR 6.44, 95% CI 1.14 to 36.57; $p = 0.035$). Few reported reading scientific articles, and many expressed uncertainty in finding research. The main barrier for using guidelines was reported to be lack of time. *Conclusion.* Although attitudes among primary care occupational therapists towards EBP are positive and a large proportion report using guidelines, many state that they want to learn more and improve their evidence-based practice skills. The findings suggest that education measures need to be taken to address the identified shortcomings.

1. Introduction

Evidence-based practice (EBP) means the integration of best available evidence from clinical research with clinical expertise and patients' preferences [1]. In recent years, EBP has become an expectation of most healthcare professionals and a vehicle to advance the profession and ensure that occupational therapists deliver quality services to their patients [2, 3]. Applying EBP ensures that clinicians use effective interventions to achieve desired outcomes and contributes to best quality care [4].

However, despite the spread of EBP during recent decades, research findings are not routinely used in occupational therapy practice [5–8]. To do so requires that clinicians have the necessary knowledge and skills to access, appraise, and apply research evidence in their clinical decision making, as well as sufficient time [9]. Applying EBP in occupational therapy is particularly challenging since research evidence for most interventions is limited [10]. Occupational therapy research has traditionally been more interpretive in approach, frequently involving case-based action with qualitative outcomes rather than effectiveness studies of interventions, and the profession has been slow to adopt research-informed practice [11]. Many factors affect whether occupational therapy practice is based on research evidence: individual factors such as attitude, preferences, educational level, context, knowledge, and skills, as well as organisational factors such as attitudes of managers and colleagues. Factors relating to both the individual and the organisation, e.g., support and time available to search for research evidence, are particularly important [10].

Knowledge and skills related to EBP vary among different countries, and various barriers for applying EBP have been identified [3–5, 9, 12]. A systematic review showed that attitudes toward EBP among occupational therapists in different countries vary [5]. While several of the included studies reported positive attitudes to various extents, some reported negative attitudes, particularly related to the perceived difficulty of understanding and applying EBP in clinical practice. In Sweden, hospital-employed occupational therapists have been shown to hold positive attitudes toward EBP, but lack of time is a key obstacle to integrating the research component of EBP into practice [13]. No study on EBP has been performed in a Swedish primary care occupational therapy context.

The use of clinical practice guidelines is a widely used strategy to implement EBP, and high quality guidelines provide evidence-based recommendations to support the clinician in choosing effective interventions. Over time, these types of guidelines have shifted from opinion-based to research-informed [14], thus constituting an excellent point of departure for integrating research findings with the other EBP components. An increasing number of guidelines are being produced that include recommendations for occupational therapy, for example, by the American Association of Occupational Therapists [15], the British Royal College of Occupational Therapists [16], and the Swedish National Association of Occupational Therapists [17]. However, implementation, uptake, and use of guidelines tend to vary based on different factors related to the guideline itself, the user/clinician, the patient, and the practice context [18].

There is a lack of knowledge about attitudes, access, knowledge, determinants, and use of EBP and clinical practice guidelines in primary care occupational therapy in Sweden, and whether any associations exist with demographic characteristics. Knowledge about these factors is important so that current trends in occupational therapy practice can be identified [12]. This knowledge also provides a basis for developing effective implementation strategies for clinical practice guidelines in order to increase the extent to which occupational therapy practice is evidence-based. Primary care occupational therapists in Sweden treat a wide variety of conditions and practice autonomously, without need for a doctor's referral, and applying EBP and using guidelines in everyday patient work are important so that patients are treated with effective methods and receive equal care. Therefore, the aim of this study was to investigate attitudes, knowledge, and behaviour related to EBP and guidelines among Swedish occupational therapists in primary care.

2. Methods

2.1. Participants and Setting. Eligible participants in this survey were occupational therapists employed in primary care by the Region Västra Götaland and currently practicing occupational therapy ($n = 193$). This is Sweden's second largest county council, providing healthcare services to nearly 1.7 million inhabitants in western Sweden. Individuals on parental leave and long-term sick leave ($n = 16$) and those involved in development of regional clinical practice guidelines ($n = 2$) were excluded. Data were collected during November–December 2016.

2.2. Data Collection. Eligible participants were invited to respond to the web-based survey, using the survey software esMaker® (Entergate AB, Halmstad, Sweden). Three reminder notices were sent via e-mail during a two-month period. A statement in the survey informed the respondents that their response was assumed as informed consent. The survey was filled out anonymously, and responses could not be traced back to the respondents. According to Swedish law, ethical approval for this type of research was not required.

Questions for the survey were drawn from a validated EBP questionnaire, originally developed by Jette et al. [19] to examine EBP and guideline variables among American physiotherapists. The questionnaire had been previously translated, adapted, and validated for a Swedish primary care context [20] and used to survey Swedish physiotherapists [21]. It was for the present study minimally modified for use with occupational therapists in the same context. The questionnaire comprised eight items on participant characteristics and 23 items reflecting various aspects of EBP and guidelines in the following domains: attitudes, knowledge, behaviour, and prerequisites and barriers related to EBP resources and guidelines. Most items were rated on 5-point Likert type scales ranging from "strongly disagree" to "strongly agree," with a "neutral" category in the middle. The item on frequency of use of guidelines ranged from "very infrequently" to "very frequently." The items on awareness that guidelines exist and knowing how and where to find them were answered with "yes," "to some extent," or "no."

2.3. Data Analysis. Frequencies and distributions were analyzed with descriptive statistics. Bivariate logistic regression analyses were performed to explore associations with demographic variables. Associations between attitudinal, knowledge, and behavioural variables and frequent guideline use were also explored. Variables identified as significant in univariate analyses were tested for correlation against a criteria of Spearman's rho < 0.7 to qualify for inclusion in a multivariable model. They were entered in a multivariable model, using the stepwise forward conditional method. Interaction effects were tested at the 1% level.

Before analysis, response categories for the dependent variable "use of guidelines" were dichotomised into "frequent use" versus "infrequent use" (including "sometimes") and for independent variables into "agree" versus "disagree." Responses for the items with 3-point scales were dichotomised into "yes" versus "no/to some extent." The significance level was set to 0.05. Missing data were handled with listwise deletion. Statistical analyses were performed using IBM SPSS version 22.0.

3. Results

3.1. Respondents. Of the 175 occupational therapists invited to participate, 94 responded: response rate 53.7%. Participant characteristics are shown in Table 1. Internal missing values ranged from 0 to 5 (0% to 5.3%).

3.2. Attitudes, Knowledge, and Behaviour Related to EBP. Response frequencies for all variables are presented in Table 2. Most respondents agreed that EBP is necessary to practice (97%) and helps in decision making (92%). Approximately half of the respondents disagreed that EBP creates unreasonable demands (51%). Most (97%) agreed to wanting to improve their skills to apply EBP in their practice. Fifty-two percent agreed to feeling confident in their ability to find relevant research for their clinical questions, and 56% reported feeling confident about treating patients according to current best evidence.

Fifty percent stated that they agreed that the use of research was encouraged at their workplace, whereas 32% disagreed. Forty-six percent agreed that they knew how to access databases through the electronic library, whereas 45% disagreed.

Eighty-two percent of the respondents reported reading fewer than two articles and the rest of the respondents (19%) read 2–5 articles in an average month. Ninety percent reported performing fewer than two, 9% 2–5, and 1% 6–10 database searches per month on average.

Table 1: Participant characteristics ($n = 94$).

Characteristic	n	%
Sex		
Women	85	90.4
Men	9	9.6
Age (years)		
20–29	7	7.4
30–39	29	30.9
40–49	22	23.4
50–59	24	25.5
>60	12	12.8
Education level/degree		
Lower level degree	16	17.0
Bachelor's degree	74	78.7
Master's degree	4	4.3
PhD student or PhD	0	0.0
Certified specialist	8	8.6
Years of experience in primary care occupational therapy		
<3	31	33.0
3–5	11	11.7
6–10	13	13.8
11–15	12	12.8
16–20	11	11.7
>20	16	17.0

3.3. Attitudes, Knowledge, and Behaviour Related to Guidelines. All of the respondents agreed that it is important to use guidelines. Sixty-five percent stated that they were aware of guidelines relevant to their work and 32% that they were partially aware. Nearly half of the respondents (47%) knew where to find guidelines on the Internet, and 44% knew this to some extent. Eighty-one percent agreed to having easy access to relevant guidelines at their workplace. Seventy-five percent reported knowing how to integrate patient preferences with guidelines.

All of the respondents agreed that guidelines are important for the patient to get the best treatment possible. Ninety-five percent agreed that guidelines facilitate their work, and 99% agreed that guidelines are important so that patients receive equal treatment. Seventy-five percent of the respondents reported using guidelines frequently or very frequently, 21% sometimes, and 3% infrequently or never.

Therapists who perceived that they had easy access to guidelines, as well as those who felt confident in their ability to treat patients according to evidence, were more likely to use guidelines frequently (Table 3). Other variables that were associated with frequent guideline use in univariate analyses did not remain significant in the final multiple regression model. No significant interaction effects between those variables and demographic variables were found.

Reported barriers for using guidelines are shown in Figure 1. The most important barrier was lack of time, cited by 72% of the respondents. This was followed by a perceived paucity of guidelines relevant for primary care occupational therapy, that it takes too much time to read guidelines, and that guidelines are too general and unspecific. The category "too much recipe" represents the perception that many patients do not fit a specific guideline, e.g., due to comorbidity or other complex situations.

3.4. Associations with Demographic Variables. Few demographic characteristics were associated with EBP and guideline variables. Men were more likely than women to report self-efficacy in finding research (OR 8.58, 95% CI 1.03 to 71.66; $p = 0.047$) and having easy access to guidelines (OR 9.10, 95% CI 1.94 to 42.83; $p = 0.005$). Occupational therapists older than 50 years were more likely to report knowing how to integrate patient preferences with guideline use than younger therapists (OR 6.44, 95% CI 1.14 to 36.57; $p = 0.035$). No significant association was found between EBP variables and therapist experience.

4. Discussion

The study provides new knowledge on EBP and guideline use among primary care occupational therapists. Key findings of this study are that attitudes toward EBP and guidelines were highly positive and that a large majority of the respondents were aware of relevant guidelines and knew where to find them. Four-fifths reported having easy access to guidelines, and three quarters claimed to use guidelines frequently. The largest barrier for using guidelines was lack of time. Two factors were found to predict frequent guideline use: feeling able to treat patients according to evidence and having easy access to guidelines.

TABLE 2: Distribution of questionnaire responses.

Variable	n	Response frequencies*				
Attitudes to EBP		*Strongly disagree*	*Disagree*	*Neutral*	*Agree*	*Strongly agree*
EBP is necessary to practice	94	0 (0.0%)	0 (0.0%)	3 (3.2%)	45 (47.9%)	46 (48.9%)
EBP creates unreasonable demands	94	12 (12.8%)	36 (38.3%)	19 (20.2%)	26 (27.7%)	1 (1.1%)
EBP helps decision making	94	0 (0.0%)	0 (0.0%)	8 (8.5%)	53 (56.4%)	33 (35.1%)
Want to learn/improve skills	92	0 (0.0%)	0 (0.0%)	3 (3.3%)	34 (37.0%)	55 (59.8%)
Strong evidence is lacking for most treatments	90	6 (6.7%)	27 (30.0%)	12 (5.2%)	38 (42.2%)	7 (7.8%)
Self-efficacy to find research	94	8 (8.5%)	25 (26.6%)	12 (12.8%)	39 (41.5%)	10 (10.6%)
Self-efficacy to treat patients according to evidence	93	2 (2.2%)	18 (19.4%)	21 (22.6%)	48 (51.6%)	4 (4.3%)
Knowledge about EBP		*Strongly disagree*	*Disagree*	*Neutral*	*Agree*	*Strongly agree*
Know how to access databases	92	25 (27.2%)	16 (17.4%)	9 (9.8%)	31 (33.7%)	11 (12.0%)
Behaviour related to EBP		*≤1/month*	*2–5/month*	*6–10/month*	*11–15/month*	*16+/month*
Read articles, no. of articles per month	92	75 (81.5%)	17 (18.5%)	0 (0.0%)	0 (0.0%)	0 (0.0%)
Search databases, no. of searches per month	93	84 (90.3%)	9 (8.6%)	1 (1.1%)	0 (0.0%)	0 (0.0%)
Prerequisites for EBP		*Strongly disagree*	*Disagree*	*Neutral*	*Agree*	*Strongly agree*
EBP encouraged at workplace	94	10 (10.6%)	20 (21.3%)	17 (18.1%)	35 (37.2%)	12 (12.9%)
Attitudes to guidelines		*Strongly disagree*	*Disagree*	*Neutral*	*Agree*	*Strongly agree*
Important that guidelines exist	93	0 (0.0%)	2 (2.2%)	0 (0%)	12 (12.9%)	79 (84.9%)
Important to use guidelines	91	0 (0.0%)	0 (0%)	0 (0%)	26 (28.6%)	65 (71.4%)
Guidelines are important to facilitate practice	94	0 (0.0%)	1 (1.1%)	3 (3.2%)	41 (43.6%)	49 (52.1%)
Knowledge about guidelines		*Strongly disagree*	*Disagree*	*Neutral*	*Agree*	*Strongly agree*
Know how to integrate pat. pref. w/ guidelines	92	0 (0.0%)	0 (0.0%)	23 (25.0%)	59 (64.1%)	10 (10.9%)
		No	*To some extent*	*Yes*		
Aware that guidelines exist	93	3 (3.2%)	30 (32.3%)	60 (64.5%)		
Know where to find guidelines	93	8 (8.6%)	41 (44.1%)	44 (47.3%)		
Prerequisites for use of guidelines		*Strongly disagree*	*Disagree*	*Neutral*	*Agree*	*Strongly agree*
Have easy access to guidelines	92	3 (3.3%)	5 (5.4%)	10 (10.9%)	54 (58.7%)	20 (21.7%)
Behaviour related to guidelines		*Very infrequently or never*	*Infrequently*	*Sometimes*	*Frequently*	*Very frequently or always*
Use guidelines	93	2 (2.2%)	1 (1.1%)	20 (21.5%)	51 (54.8%)	19 (20.4%)

*Data are numbers (percentages).

TABLE 3: Significant associations in univariate analyses and in the final multiple logistic regression model. Dependent variable: frequent use of guidelines.

Independent variable	Level	n	Univariate associations Odds ratio (95% CI)	p	B (SE)	Multiple associations Odds ratio (95% CI)	p
Strong evidence is lacking for most interventions	Disagree	89	3.43 (1.05–11.25)	0.042			
	Agree		Reference				
Self-efficacy to treat patients according to evidence	Agree	92	3.30 (1.23–8.87)	0.018	1.93 (0.71)	6.91 (1.73–27.60)	0.006
	Disagree		Reference			Reference	
Know where to find guidelines	Yes	92	6.57 (1.43–30.25)	0.016			
	No		Reference				
Easy access to guidelines	Agree	91	11.27 (3.50–36.36)	<0.001	2.92 (0.73)	18.57 (4.40–78.26)	<0.001
	Disagree		Reference			Reference	
Know how to integrate patient preferences with guidelines	Agree	91	4.28 (1.53–11.97)	0.006			
	Disagree		Reference				

[b]Nagelkerke $R^2 = 0.42$, overall correctly predicted = 75.3%, B = unstandardised regression coefficient, SE = standard error, CI = confidence interval.

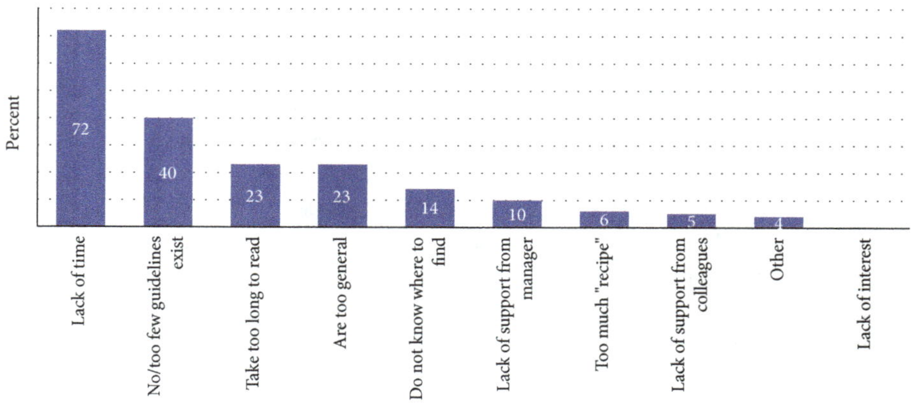

FIGURE 1: Reported barriers for using guidelines.

Although the vast majority of the occupational therapists had very positive attitudes to both EBP and guidelines, EBP-related behaviour did not reflect these attitudes. Only a small proportion said that they searched the literature and read scientific articles. These findings may be related to EBP not being taught consistently at undergraduate occupational therapy programs. The reported high awareness of guidelines, knowledge of where to find them, and easy access to them were likely related to a guideline project that had been ongoing within the county council over the past few years. That project involved the development of several practice guidelines that were published on a dedicated website, in order to make the guidelines easily accessible. Awareness and access are important prerequisites of guideline use, which in fact also was quite high; three quarters of the respondents reporting using guidelines frequently, with another fifth using guidelines sometimes.

The finding that men were more likely than women to report self-efficacy to find research and having easy access to guidelines needs to be interpreted with caution, because gender distribution of the sample was quite skewed, less than one-tenth were men. In addition, the confidence intervals for the odds ratios were quite wide. The finding that older occupational therapists were more likely to know how to integrate patient preferences with guideline use may be understandable, in that younger therapists did not have as much experience with different kinds of patients and therefore may not be skilled in incorporating their preferences into therapy.

Only two variables, self-efficacy to treat patients according to evidence and having easy access to guidelines, remained significantly associated with frequent use of guidelines in the final regression model. While easy access to guidelines is an obvious prerequisite of using them, feeling confident in one's ability to treat patients according to evidence is an interesting finding and less easily explainable. The opposite would have been more logical—feeling confident to treat according to evidence would reduce the need for guidelines. However, the link may be more easily understood when considering that those who are keen on and able to treat according to evidence are probably also more likely to want to rely on guidelines that include evidence-based recommendations.

The findings of positive attitudes toward EBP but limited perceived knowledge and skills are supported by research from other countries. McCluskey [9] reported that half of the occupational therapists in an Australian survey rated their level of EBP knowledge and skills as low. Lyons et al. [4] reported positive attitudes towards research among Australian paediatric occupational therapists, but poor confidence in research knowledge and in how to implement research findings into practice. In South Africa, Buchanan [22] showed positive perceptions toward EBP among occupational therapists but poor confidence in EBP skills, attributed primarily to limited knowledge and skills.

In our study, most respondents estimated their EBP knowledge from moderate to high; yet nearly all expressed a desire to learn more about EBP. Similar findings were shown in the study by Lyons et al. [4], where the respondents held positive attitudes toward research and wanted to access new information to guide practice.

Our study suggests a gap between positive attitudes towards EBP and sufficient knowledge to apply EBP by searching for and reading scientific literature. This gap was also identified by Upton et al. [5], who found that occupational therapists across several countries generally hold positive attitudes toward EBP but that these attitudes do not necessarily translate into practice. Salls et al. [8] showed that although a large majority of American occupational therapists considered EBP important to their practice, use of research findings to inform practice remained limited.

Our study, like most studies on EBP in occupational therapy, was conducted among practicing clinicians. In students, it is likely that search and appraisal skills are taught already in undergraduate training and that both attitudes and behaviours related to EBP therefore are more positive than those of practicing therapists. Stronge and Cahill [3] found that students in Ireland had a clear understanding of EBP and were willing to practice EBP in their future and that many accessed evidence on a weekly basis. However, Crabtree et al. [23] showed that although a master-level EBP training program improved basic EBP skills and knowledge among Canadian students, those skills were not retained after eight weeks of fieldwork. To support both students and recent graduates entering clinical practice, those findings, as well as the findings of our study, underscore the importance of continued training of clinicians in EBP skills.

Occupational therapists are expected to base their practice on the best available evidence [24, 25]. In our study, half of the respondents disagreed that applying EBP in daily practice is an unreasonable requirement, representing a positive attitude to EBP. However, nearly one-third considered it an unreasonable requirement. The reason for this negative attitude is not known, but a plausible explanation is a perceived lack of time, which was identified as a major barrier to EBP.

The multiple barriers identified for using EBP and guidelines are consistent with previous research. Lack of time was by far the most important barrier, and a quarter of the respondents also stated that it took too much time to read guidelines. Upton et al. [5] identified lack of time, availability and accessibility to research, and limited research skills as main barriers for applying EBP among occupational therapists. Lyons et al. [4] reported lack of time to read research and to implement new ideas as the greatest barriers for applying EBP in clinical practice among Australian occupational therapists. Lack of skills to understand statistics and to evaluate research quality was also among the top perceived barriers. Among South African occupational therapists, reported barriers include lack of time, knowledge, and convenient access to evidence [22]. In US occupational therapists, lack of time, high continuing education costs, weak research analysis skills, and placing higher value on clinical experience than on research have been reported as import barriers [26]. In Sweden, Heiwe et al. [13] identified lack of time, statistical knowledge, and research and appraisal skills as important barriers for EBP among hospital-based occupational therapists. Similar barriers have also consistently been reported in other healthcare professions, for example, physiotherapists [21, 27, 28], physicians [29, 30], and nurses [31].

The finding that some therapists felt that guideline use was too "recipe-like" may be indicative of the complexity of clinical reasoning and decision making and why therapists may not be using research evidence as the predominant method of achieving EBP. Planning individual therapy requires integration of research evidence with a range of different information sources such as the patient and their circumstances and experiences and the setting, in order to be both evidence-based and client-centred. Clinical reasoning, involving the thinking process of planning, conducting, and reflecting on clinical practice [32], is an essential part of making decisions about occupational therapy service delivery. It often draws on factual knowledge, tacit and practical know-how, and gut response to clients and their situations in an attempt to synthesize these different modes through metacognition [33]. Clinical reasoning is a skill that evolves with experience and has been suggested to differ between novice and experienced occupational therapists [34]. Even though our study failed to show any differences related to age or experience, it is likely that older and more experienced therapists rely more on their experience and less on research evidence than do their younger colleagues. Integrating the three EBP components is not self-evident. The research evidence component is conceptually different from the other two components; it denotes published, collective evidence, whereas clinical expertise and patient preferences mostly relate to the individual level [35]. Viewed in this light, the level of guideline use showed in this study forms a solid basis for integration with the other components. Treatment decisions should be made jointly with the patient, and their preferences and values should be elicited as part of this dialogue so that treatment can be adequately individualised and person-centred. This is particularly important in occupational therapy where several treatment options may be appropriate and research evidence for some treatments remains limited [36]. Communication and a good patient-therapist dialogue then become even more important and lay the ground for collaborative rehabilitation [37].

The history and tradition of occupational therapy is another barrier that may impede EBP. Occupational therapy is a profession that tends to rely on professional craft and personal knowledge which may reduce the importance attached to EBP [38]. Welch and Dawson [38] found that research knowledge was not included in British occupational therapists' construct of a good practitioner and that they lacked confidence in EBP. However, they also showed that practice-embedded collaborative learning was a way to develop this confidence and facilitate the therapists' use of research knowledge in their clinical reasoning. Furthermore, as suggested by Miller and Willis [11], the occupational therapy profession has produced less research in comparison to other health professionals such as physicians, nurses, and physiotherapists, which may constitute a significant barrier for occupational therapists to adopt and apply EBP. The low volume of research produced likely contributes to the low evidence grade for many occupational therapy interventions, the paucity of clinical practice guidelines, and to the fairly high proportion of respondents in our survey who did not feel confident in finding and using evidence to treat their patients.

In our study, nearly half of the respondents reported that guidelines were lacking for their specific patient population. Many also perceived that existing guidelines were too general in their recommendations. These are barriers related to guideline development that can and should be addressed by policy makers and guideline development teams, who could make further efforts to ensure that more relevant guidelines are developed and that they are specific in scope and recommendations.

4.1. Strengths and Limitations. Study limitations include a relatively low response rate and the lack of nonresponse analysis. With the exception of gender, we had no data on characteristics or outcome variables for those who did not respond to the survey. Men were overrepresented among respondents (10%) vs. nonrespondents (3%). Perhaps, those who responded to the survey were more positive toward EBP than those who did not respond. A further limitation is that, as in all questionnaire-based surveys, data were self-reported. Only publically employed occupational therapists were surveyed; attitudes and behaviour among private practitioners may differ.

A strength of the study is the use of a validated and reliable EBP questionnaire [20], which has previously been used among physiotherapists in Sweden [21]. Advantages of this questionnaire is that it targets practicing clinicians rather than students and that it, in addition to EBP variables, includes items on guidelines. Its forerunner, an EBP questionnaire developed by Jette et al. [19], has been used in a multitude of studies, particularly in physiotherapy [13, 39–42].

The study participants are likely to be similar in characteristics, attitudes, and behaviours to the national population of occupational therapists in primary care in Sweden; the findings can therefore probably be generalised to the rest of Sweden and possibly other countries with similar healthcare systems and practices. Still, the relatively low sample size calls for caution on an overly broad generalisation of the findings.

4.2. Implications for Practice and Research. The study findings have several implications for both clinicians and researchers in primary care occupational therapy. The prerequisites for applying EBP to a greater extent create high demands for the coming years, on both practicing therapists, their managers, as well as students and recent graduates who are entering the job market. Because today's occupational therapy, students learn EBP skills in their undergraduate training, efforts on improving EBP skills, and behaviour should focus on continued professional development efforts among practicing occupational therapists in primary care. Such practitioner training should be comprehensive, contextually relevant, and collaborative to help practitioners implement and integrate EBP into clinical practice and is more likely to change practice patterns if conducted in workplace settings [43]. The importance of integrating different sources of evidence into clinical reasoning should be emphasised.

The insight provided by this study into the reported attitudes towards knowledge of and barriers for EBP and guidelines can facilitate the development of strategies for increasing the use of EBP among occupational therapists. The identified barriers related to EBP could be addressed in several ways. The barriers related to the use of guidelines would be particularly relevant to address in guideline development work: making the guidelines brief, specific, and with clear links to the underpinning evidence.

The major barrier of perceived time constraints, which could be both a personal and a contextual or organisational barrier, needs to be addressed. This barrier is not likely to be reduced without organisational or managerial support, for instance, by provision of protected work time for searching and appraising literature and other EBP activities. One such activity that may be both effective and cost-effective, in that it requires minimal resources, could be the organisation of journal clubs. This is a form of EBP teaching that allows participants to keep up-to-date with current, clinically relevant, research evidence as well as to improve their research appraisal skills. Journal clubs have been shown to be acceptable to occupational therapists and other allied health professionals and to be likely to be used with enthusiasm to achieve EBP [44].

4.3. Future Research. To minimise bias from self-reported data, there is a need to develop objective measures for assessing implementation of EBP. For a deeper understanding of EBP behaviours, as well as barriers and facilitators for applying EBP, a qualitative approach using individual interviews or focus groups is suggested. Furthermore, research is needed to address the remaining knowledge gaps with regard to occupational therapy interventions. Many of the interventions that occupational therapists use have yet to be underpinned by substantial research evidence, due to the limited number of studies performed as well as problems with research design.

5. Conclusions

This study provides new knowledge about attitudes, knowledge, behaviour, prerequisites, and barriers to EBP and guidelines among Swedish primary care occupational therapists that are likely to be transferable to other countries with similar healthcare systems. In spite of very positive attitudes and a fairly high use of clinical guidelines, the large proportion of occupational therapists who wanted to learn more about EBP, the small proportion who searched for and read scientific articles, and the fairly poor self-efficacy in finding research and in treating patients according to research evidence sends a signal to managers and decision makers that measures need to be taken to address these shortcomings. The study findings highlight the importance of continual professional development and training in EBP skills, with focus on search and appraisal of literature as well as on integrating different sources of evidence into clinical reasoning. In addition, more research is needed to address knowledge gaps that remain with regard to occupational therapy interventions.

Conflicts of Interest

The authors declare no conflicts of interest.

Acknowledgments

This work was partially supported by the Research and Development Centre of Gothenburg and Södra Bohuslän. The authors wish to thank all the occupational therapists in primary care in the region of Västra Götaland for participating in the study and for taking the time to answer the questionnaire.

References

[1] D. L. Sackett, W. M. C. Rosenberg, J. A. M. Gray, R. B. Haynes, and W. S. Richardson, "Evidence based medicine: what it is and what it isn't," *BMJ*, vol. 312, no. 7023, pp. 71-72, 1996.

[2] P. A. Crist, "Adapting research instruction to support the scholarship of practice: practice-scholar partnerships,"

Occupational Therapy In Health Care, vol. 24, no. 1, pp. 39–55, 2010.

[3] M. Stronge and M. Cahill, "Self-reported knowledge, attitudes and behaviour towards evidence-based practice of occupational therapy students in Ireland," *Occupational Therapy International*, vol. 19, no. 1, pp. 7–16, 2012.

[4] C. Lyons, T. Brown, M. H. Tseng, J. Casey, and R. McDonald, "Evidence-based practice and research utilisation: perceived research knowledge, attitudes, practices and barriers among Australian paediatric occupational therapists," *Australian Occupational Therapy Journal*, vol. 58, no. 3, pp. 178–186, 2011.

[5] D. Upton, D. Stephens, B. Williams, and L. Scurlock-Evans, "Occupational therapists' attitudes, knowledge, and implementation of evidence-based practice: a systematic review of published research," *British Journal of Occupational Therapy*, vol. 77, no. 1, pp. 24–38, 2014.

[6] K. A. V. Cameron, S. Ballantyne, A. Kulbitsky, M. Margolis-Gal, T. Daugherty, and F. Ludwig, "Utilization of evidence-based practice by registered occupational therapists," *Occupational Therapy International*, vol. 12, no. 3, pp. 123–136, 2005.

[7] D. B. Philibert, P. Snyder, D. Judd, and M. M. Windsor, "Practitioners' reading patterns, attitudes, and use of research reported in occupational therapy journals," *American Journal of Occupational Therapy*, vol. 57, no. 4, pp. 450–458, 2003.

[8] J. Salls, C. Dolhi, L. Silverman, and M. Hansen, "The use of evidence-based practice by occupational therapists," *Occupational Therapy In Health Care*, vol. 23, no. 2, pp. 134–145, 2009.

[9] A. McCluskey, "Occupational therapists report a low level of knowledge, skill and involvement in evidence-based practice," *Australian Occupational Therapy Journal*, vol. 50, no. 1, pp. 3–12, 2003.

[10] A. Thomas and M. Law, "Research utilization and evidence-based practice in occupational therapy: a scoping study," *American Journal of Occupational Therapy*, vol. 67, no. 4, pp. e55–e65, 2013.

[11] E. Miller and M. Willis, "The Cochrane Collaboration and occupational therapy: an emerging partnership," *British Journal of Occupational Therapy*, vol. 63, no. 6, pp. 288–290, 2000.

[12] S. Mulligan, B. P. White, and S. Arthanat, "An examination of occupation-based, client-centered, evidence-based occupational therapy practices in New Hampshire," *OTJR: Occupation, Participation and Health*, vol. 34, no. 2, pp. 106–116, 2014.

[13] S. Heiwe, K. N. Kajermo, R. Tyni-Lenne et al., "Evidence-based practice: attitudes, knowledge and behaviour among allied health care professionals," *International Journal for Quality in Health Care*, vol. 23, no. 2, pp. 198–209, 2011.

[14] T. Kredo, S. Bernhardsson, S. Machingaidze et al., "Guide to clinical practice guidelines: the current state of play," *International Journal for Quality in Health Care*, vol. 28, no. 1, pp. 122–128, 2016.

[15] The American Association of Occupational Therapists, "Practice guidelines," Bethesda, MD, USA, August 2018, https://www.aota.org/Practice/Researchers/practice-guidelines.aspx.

[16] Royal College of Occupational Therapists, "RCOT practice guidelines," London, UK, August 2018, https://www.rcot.co.uk/practice-resources/rcot-practice-guidelines.

[17] Arbetsterapeuterna, "Riktlinjer," The National Association of Occupational Therapists, Stockholm, Sweden, August 2018, https://www.arbetsterapeuterna.se/Min-profession/riktlinjer/.

[18] M. Stergiou-Kita, "Implementing clinical practice guidelines in occupational therapy practice: recommendations from the research evidence," *Australian Occupational Therapy Journal*, vol. 57, no. 2, pp. 76–87, 2010.

[19] D. U. Jette, K. Bacon, C. Batty et al., "Evidence-based practice: beliefs, attitudes, knowledge, and behaviors of physical therapists," *Physical Therapy*, vol. 83, no. 9, pp. 786–805, 2003.

[20] S. Bernhardsson and M. E. H Larsson, "Measuring evidence-based practice in physical therapy: translation, adaptation, further development, validation, and reliability test of a questionnaire," *Physical Therapy*, vol. 93, no. 6, pp. 819–832, 2013.

[21] S. Bernhardsson, K. Johansson, P. Nilsen, B. Oberg, and M. E. H. Larsson, "Determinants of guideline use in primary care physical therapy: a cross-sectional survey of attitudes, knowledge, and behavior," *Physical Therapy*, vol. 94, no. 3, pp. 343–354, 2014.

[22] H. Buchanan, *Evidence-Based Practice in Occupational Therapy in South Africa and the Western Cape, [Ph.D. thesis]*, University of Cape Town, Cape Town, South Africa, 2011.

[23] J. L. Crabtree, M. Justiss, and S. Swinehart, "Occupational therapy master-level students' evidence-based practice knowledge and skills before and after fieldwork," *Occupational Therapy In Health Care*, vol. 26, no. 2-3, pp. 138–149, 2012.

[24] *Code of Ethics for Occupational Therapists*, Swedish Association of Occupational Therapists, Nacka, Sweden, 2012, https://www.arbetsterapeuterna.se/Global/Forlag/Etisk%20kod/CodeofEthics2012_final2016.pdf.

[25] W. Coster, "International conference on evidence-based practice: a collaborative effort of the American Occupational Therapy Association, the American Occupational Therapy Foundation, and the Agency for Healthcare Research and Quality," *American Journal of Occupational Therapy*, vol. 59, no. 3, pp. 356–358, 2005.

[26] A. MacEwan Dysart and G. S. Tomlin, "Factors related to evidence-based practice among U.S. occupational therapy clinicians," *American Journal of Occupational Therapy*, vol. 56, no. 3, pp. 275–284, 2002.

[27] L. Scurlock-Evans, P. Upton, and D. Upton, "Evidence-based practice in physiotherapy: a systematic review of barriers, enablers and interventions," *Physiotherapy*, vol. 100, no. 3, pp. 208–219, 2014.

[28] T. M. da Silva, L. da Cunha Menezes Costa, A. N. Garcia, and L. O. P. Costa, "What do physical therapists think about evidence-based practice? A systematic review," *Manual Therapy*, vol. 20, no. 3, pp. 388–401, 2015.

[29] H. Sadeghi-Bazargani, J. S. Tabrizi, and S. Azami-Aghdash, "Barriers to evidence-based medicine: a systematic review," *Journal of Evaluation in Clinical Practice*, vol. 20, no. 6, pp. 793–802, 2014.

[30] S. Zwolsman, E. te Pas, L. Hooft, M. W. D. Waard, and N. van Dijk, "Barriers to GPs' use of evidence-based medicine: a systematic review," *British Journal of General Practice*, vol. 62, no. 600, pp. e511–e521, 2012.

[31] F. Sadoughi, T. Azadi, and T. Azadi, "Barriers to using electronic evidence based literature in nursing practice: a systematised review," *Health Information & Libraries Journal*, vol. 34, no. 3, pp. 187–199, 2017.

[32] J. C. Rogers, "Teaching clinical reasoning for practice in geriatrics," *Physical & Occupational Therapy In Geriatrics*, vol. 1, no. 3, pp. 29–37, 1982.

[33] C. Unsworth and A. Baker, "A systematic review of professional reasoning literature in occupational therapy," *British Journal of Occupational Therapy*, vol. 79, no. 1, pp. 5–16, 2016.

[34] D. Gibson, B. Velde, T. Hoff, D. Kvashay, P. L. Manross, and V. Moreau, "Clinical reasoning of a novice versus an experienced occupational therapist: a qualitative study," *Occupational Therapy In Health Care*, vol. 12, no. 4, pp. 15–31, 2000.

[35] J. Rycroft-Malone, K. Seers, A. Titchen, G. Harvey, A. Kitson, and B. McCormack, "What counts as evidence in evidence-based practice?," *Journal of Advanced Nursing*, vol. 47, no. 1, pp. 81–90, 2004.

[36] M. P. Dijkers, S. L. Murphy, and J. Krellman, "Evidence-based practice for rehabilitation professionals: concepts and controversies," *Archives of Physical Medicine and Rehabilitation*, vol. 93, no. 8, pp. S164–S176, 2012.

[37] S. Bernhardsson, K. S. Samsson, K. Johansson, B. Öberg, and M. E. H. Larsson, "A preference for dialogue: exploring the influence of patient preferences on clinical decision making and treatment in primary care physiotherapy," *European Journal of Physiotherapy*, 2018.

[38] A. Welch and P. Dawson, "Closing the gap: collaborative learning as a strategy to embed evidence within occupational therapy practice," *Journal of Evaluation in Clinical Practice*, vol. 12, no. 2, pp. 227–238, 2006.

[39] N. M. Salbach, S. B. Jaglal, N. Korner-Bitensky, S. Rappolt, and D. Davis, "Practitioner and organizational barriers to evidence-based practice of physical therapists for people with stroke," *Physical Therapy*, vol. 87, no. 10, pp. 1284–1303, 2007.

[40] R. Iles and M. Davidson, "Evidence based practice: a survey of physiotherapists' current practice," *Physiotherapy Research International*, vol. 11, no. 2, pp. 93–103, 2006.

[41] R. Ramirez-Velez, M. C. Bagur-Calafat, J. E. Correa-Bautista, and M. Girabent-Farres, "Barriers against incorporating evidence-based practice in physical therapy in Colombia: current state and factors associated," *BMC Medical Education*, vol. 15, no. 1, p. 220, 2015.

[42] T. M. Silva, L. C. M. Costa, and L. O. P. Costa, "Evidence-based practice: a survey regarding behavior, knowledge, skills, resources, opinions and perceived barriers of Brazilian physical therapists from São Paulo state," *Brazilian Journal of Physical Therapy*, vol. 19, no. 4, pp. 294–303, 2015.

[43] C. T. Myers and J. Lotz, "Practitioner training for use of evidence-based practice in occupational therapy," *Occupational Therapy In Health Care*, vol. 31, no. 3, pp. 214–237, 2017.

[44] L. M. Lizarondo, K. Grimmer-Somers, and S. Kumar, "Exploring the perspectives of allied health practitioners toward the use of journal clubs as a medium for promoting evidence-based practice: a qualitative study," *BMC Medical Education*, vol. 11, no. 1, p. 66, 2011.

Identification of Sensory Processing and Integration Symptom Clusters

Lucy Jane Miller,[1] Sarah A. Schoen,[1] Shelley Mulligan,[2] and Jillian Sullivan[3]

[1]*STAR Institute, 5420 S. Quebec Street, Suite 105, Greenwood Village, CO 80111, USA*
[2]*Department of Occupational Therapy, 4 Library Way, University of New Hampshire, Durham, NH 03824, USA*
[3]*Northeastern University, 312E Robinson Hall, 360 Huntington Ave., Boston, MA 02115, USA*

Correspondence should be addressed to Sarah A. Schoen; sarah.schoen@spdstar.org

Academic Editor: Claudia Hilton

Rationale. This study explored subtypes of sensory processing disorder (SPD) by examining the clinical presentations of cluster groups that emerged from scores of children with SPD on the Sensory Processing 3-Dimension (SP-3D) Inventory. *Method.* A nonexperimental design was used involving data extraction from the records of 252 children with SPD. Exploratory cluster analyses were conducted with scores from the SP-3D Inventory which measures sensory overresponsivity (SOR), sensory underresponsivity (SUR), sensory craving (SC), postural disorder, dyspraxia, and sensory discrimination. Scores related to adaptive behavior, social-emotional functioning, and attention among children with different sensory modulation patterns were then examined and compared. *Results.* Three distinct cluster groups emerged from the data: High SOR only, High SUR with SOR, and High SC with SOR. All groups showed low performance within multiple domains of adaptive behavior. Atypical behaviors associated with social-emotional functioning and attention varied among the groups. *Implications.* The SP-3D Inventory shows promise as a tool for assisting in identifying patterns of sensory dysfunction and for guiding intervention. Better characterization can guide intervention precision and facilitate homogenous samples for research.

1. Introduction

Current estimates indicate that 5% to 16.5% of the general population [1, 2] have symptoms associated with sensory processing challenges and these estimates are higher for clinical populations such as autism spectrum disorder (ASD) [3] and attention deficit hyperactivity disorder (ADHD) [4]. Sensory processing is part of normal development and reflects one's ability to interpret and respond to daily sensory experiences [5]. The integration of sensory information contributes to successful functioning in daily life reflected in our ability to self-regulate, interact socially [2], and develop adaptive behavioral skills/abilities [6]. Thus, sensory processing is only considered a problem when it interferes with functioning in daily life. In fact, the autism literature has been recently characterized as a form of atypical sensory processing that enhances daily life called enhanced perception linked to superior sensory acuity [7]. However, some subtypes of sensory processing have been associated with impairments in activities of daily living [6] and with other kinds of behavioral problems [8]. An increase in recognition of sensory processing challenges [7] supports the need to articulate patterns of dysfunction and associated functional deficits across clinical populations. Clinically meaningful descriptions will facilitate increased understanding of the clinical presentation, which can provide more specificity for guiding intervention and greater homogeneity of samples for research.

Interest in understanding and defining the patterns of sensory processing dysfunction has been prevalent since Ayres first developed the Southern California Sensory Integration Tests [9], followed by the Sensory Integration and Praxis Tests [SIPT] [10]. With the publication of the sensory profile [11], responsivity patterns characteristic of individuals with sensory modulation challenges were included. Davies and Tucker [12] summarized the evidence from 1986 to 2006, and they found that the literature was limited by the specific assessment tools used because no single study included a comprehensive assessment of sensory function and sensory-based motor performance. Thus, it is difficult to arrive at a consensus regarding factors or cluster groups across studies due to the varied constructs evaluated by different assessment tools, as well as due to heterogeneity and comorbidities in the samples studied [13].

Sensory processing dysfunction includes a heterogeneous set of symptoms that affects the manner in which individuals use sensory information for emotion regulation, motor performance, social interaction, and daily life functioning at home, at school, and in the community [14–16]. Some research to date has described the neurodevelopmental, behavioral, and functional characteristics and correlates of children who present with sensory processing challenges. For example, a systematic review by Koenig and Rudney [17] found that children with sensory overresponsive (SOR) patterns and sensory-related motor dysfunction have more difficulty with social participation and performance of activities of daily living than children with sensory underresponsivity (SUR). Reynolds and Lane [18] also found SOR to be associated with poor performance of activities of daily living. Elbasan et al. [19] associated disruption in performance in activities of daily living with visual and tactile discrimination problems, postural problems, and dyspraxia.

SOR in the tactile and auditory domains has been given the most attention in the literature. SOR has been associated with anxiety in children and adolescents previously classified as Asperger's syndrome (e.g., high functioning autism) [20] as well as with problems acquiring a number of adaptive behavior and functional skills [18, 21, 22]. SOR has also been associated with children who have attention deficit disorders [17, 22–24]. Although we are beginning to understand the clinical presentations of each sensory processing pattern in various clinical conditions, there is a need for further clarification of relations among patterns and differential association with occupational performance in children without comorbid diagnoses [12].

This study fills the gap in research elucidated by Davies and Tucker [25] by using a comprehensive assessment of sensory processing functions including sensory modulation, sensory discrimination, and sensory-based motor abilities, called the Sensory Processing 3-Dimension Inventory [26], previously called the Sensory Processing Scale [27]. We use a more homogeneous sample, since samples with different diagnoses and comorbidities may present differently, and our investigation of patterns includes constructs related to functioning in everyday life. Thus, the present study expands upon previous studies by examining characteristics within sensory modulation dysfunction related to adaptive behavior, social-emotional functioning, and inattention/overactivity; the study by Mailloux and colleagues [28] examined patterns of dyspraxia and sensory discrimination and the study by Mailloux and colleagues [28, 29] only examined sensory modulation. Knowledge of the patterns of dysfunction and associated functional impairments provides greater homogeneity of samples in research studies which allows for comparisons of results across studies [12]. Clinicians also need this information to increase treatment specificity and communication among parents, teachers, and other professionals.

Cluster analysis was used to determine whether a sample of children with known sensory processing challenges could be organized into clinically meaningful groups based on similarities and differences. Cluster analyses are exploratory, multivariate data reduction strategies that are commonly used to discover groupings of individuals across a variety of clinical conditions that tend to be heterogeneous in nature [30]. Cluster analysis facilitates the identification of patterns within groups and is useful in evaluating diagnostic taxonomies [31, 32]. Information regarding patterns of dysfunction is helpful so that interventions can be tailored to meet specific sensory processing and associated functional challenges of each group identified. Researchers can also use information from cluster analyses to form more homogeneous samples in treatment effectiveness studies and when investigating the underlying neurological mechanisms of a disorder. The following research questions were addressed: (a) what distinct and clinical meaningful cluster groups emerge based on scores from the SP-3D Inventory? and (b) what are the characteristics of children within each of the cluster groupings with respect to dimensions adaptive behavior, social-emotional functioning, and inattention/overactivity?

2. Method

2.1. Procedures and Participants. The study was conducted at Sensory Therapies And Research (STAR) Institute for Sensory Processing Disorder in Greenwood Village, CO, and involved retrospective data extraction from the charts of clients with SPD seen from 2007 to 2013. The data collected were from caregiver report measures used in routine clinical care. Chart review and data entry of deidentified information were completed by research assistants, supervised by a senior researcher following procedures approved by the Rocky Mountain University of Health Professions Institutional Review Board.

The sample consisted of data from 252 children ages 4 to 14 years ($M = 6.9$ years, SD = 2.05) who did not meet criteria for an autism spectrum disorder, a neurologic or orthopedic syndrome, or a mental health diagnosis based on parent report of medical history from a community pediatrician. Males made up 180 of the 252 participants (71.4%) and 80% of the sample were Caucasian. Socioeconomic status was based on parent education, with 61% of parents reporting that they had a high school education and 39% a college education or above. All participants completed a 2-hour, comprehensive performance-based occupational therapy evaluation including a standardized assessment of motor functioning, norm-referenced parent-rating scales of sensory, adaptive, and problem behaviors, and clinical observations of sensory processing, postural control, and motor performance. Only those children who had complete data on the Sensory Processing Three-Dimension Inventory were included. This sample was representative of a clinical sample of children with SPD referred to the STAR Institute for sensory and behavioral challenges that significantly interfered with daily functioning at home, at school, and/or in the community.

2.2. Instrumentation

Sensory Processing Three-Dimension Inventory. The Sensory Processing Three-Dimension (SP-3D) Inventory [33, 34] utilizes parent report to measure all subtypes of SPD based on the nosology [13], with six subscales: sensory overresponsivity (SOR), sensory underresponsivity (SUR), sensory craving (SC), postural disorder (PD), dyspraxia (DYS), and sensory discrimination disorder (SDD). For the three modulation subscales (SOR, SUR, and SC) and one sensory discrimination subscale, items address behaviors believed to be associated with the processing of the input from the visual, tactile, vestibular, proprioception, auditory, gustatory, and olfactory sensory domains. Scoring utilizes a binary system which requires the informant to indicate whether any of the behavioral descriptions/items apply to their child (applicable = 1; not applicable = 0). The SP-3D Inventory takes approximately 20 minutes to complete and consists of 182 items. Total scores reflect the sum of items endorsed by the parent on each subscale or SPD subtype, and higher scores suggest greater impairment. Scores for this study were transformed into percentages of total items endorsed to account for the variability in total number of items on each subscale, which were as follows: SOR-47 items; SUR-21 items, SC-28 items, SDD-26 items; posture disorder-23 items; and dyspraxia-37 items. Previous research demonstrates acceptable internal consistency reliability (α = .63–.75) and discriminative validity (Cohen's d = .56–1.53 [33, 35]. Principal axis factor analysis also confirmed the internal structure of the modulation subscales [33]. For this sample, internal consistency reliability for the subscales ranged from α = .80 to α = .92).

Adaptive Behavior Assessment Scale-II. The Adaptive Behavior Assessment Scale (ABAS-II) [36] is a norm-referenced, caregiver rating scale for individuals from birth to 21 years. The ABAS-II provides a comprehensive assessment of a child's adaptive behavior including functioning in ten related adaptive skill areas: communication, community use, functional academics, school/home living, health and safety, leisure, self-care, self-direction, social, and work. Three composite scores, conceptual, social, and practical, make up the General Adaptive Composite (GAC). Higher scores reflect *better* adaptive functioning. Internal consistency reliability for the GAC and all adaptive skill areas was found to be high for all age groups (α = .79–.99). Data in the test manual supports the tool's reliability and validity.

Behavior Assessment System for Children-2. The Behavior Assessment System for Children-2 (BASC-2) [26] is a norm-referenced measure of emotional and behavioral disorders for children 4 to 18 years. The parent-rating measure assesses a child's problem behaviors in the community and at home, including hyperactivity, aggression, conduct problems, anxiety, depression, somatization, attention problems, learning problems, atypicality, and withdrawal. The four composite scores are externalizing problems, internalizing problems, adaptive skills, and behavioral symptoms index. Higher scores indicate *greater* impairment. For this study, the adaptive subscale was not used because the content is similar to the ABAS-II, and the conduct disorder subscale score was not reported because the age range was limited to children 6 years and older. Reliability and validity data are reported to be strong including internal consistency reliability of the scales with Cronbach α values ranging from .38 to .94 [26].

The Swanson, Nolan, and Pelham Parent-Rating Scale. The Swanson, Nolan, and Pelham Parent-Rating Scale (SNAP-IV) [27] is an 18-item, parent report used to characterize ADHD features. It has two subscales characterizing each of the ADHD subtypes; 9 items represent the hyperactive/impulsive subtype, and 9 items represent the inattentive subtype. A 4-point Likert scale is used to rate behaviors from 0, not at all, to 3, very much. Internal consistency reliability for the parent report form is high α = .94 [30] with Cronbach α values for the inattentive and hyperactive/impulsive subscales .90 and .79, respectively [30]. Studies of predictive validity, sensitivity, and specificity support the tool as an acceptable measure of behaviors associated with ADHD [30].

2.3. Data Analysis. A Ward's agglomerative hierarchical cluster analysis was first conducted using the items from all subscales of the SP-3D Inventory to identify potential cluster solutions based on squared Euclidean values in a distance matrix [37]. Next, a K-means clustering algorithm based on the results from the hierarchical analysis (as described by [38]) was conducted to derive the final clusters. No meaningful cluster groupings emerged using all six of the SP3D Inventory subscales. Cluster analysis is considered an exploratory and somewhat subjective technique which evaluates children's scores on all variables by how close or distant they are from other children [39]. A lack of meaningful cluster groups may have occurred because of the inherent heterogeneity of children with SPD, that is, children having many different combinations of the various subtypes. To explore the data further with less variability, cluster analysis was repeated using only the scales representing sensory modulation behaviors. When there appears to be no interpretable solution, the literature suggests carefully considering the variables that are included in the analysis [39, 40]. Since sensory modulation has a strong theoretical foundation and is a common sensory processing symptomatology, cluster analysis was rerun using the three modulation subscales. A 3-cluster solution which grouped children based on the scoring of items on the SOR, SUR, and SC subscales best fit the data (based on effect size attributed to each cluster variable). Subsequent analyses then examined the specific characteristics of each cluster group, and differences in their scores from the ABAS-II, BASC-2, and SNAP-IV as well as from the other three SP3D Inventory subscales (e.g., posture, dyspraxia, and sensory discrimination).

One-way ANOVAs were performed to assess cluster group differences. Games-Howell post hoc tests were used when the Brown-Forsythe test for robustness of the median was significant. Due to the exploratory nature of this investigation, and to minimize the potential for Type II errors, an alpha level of $p < 0.05$ was used to determine statistical

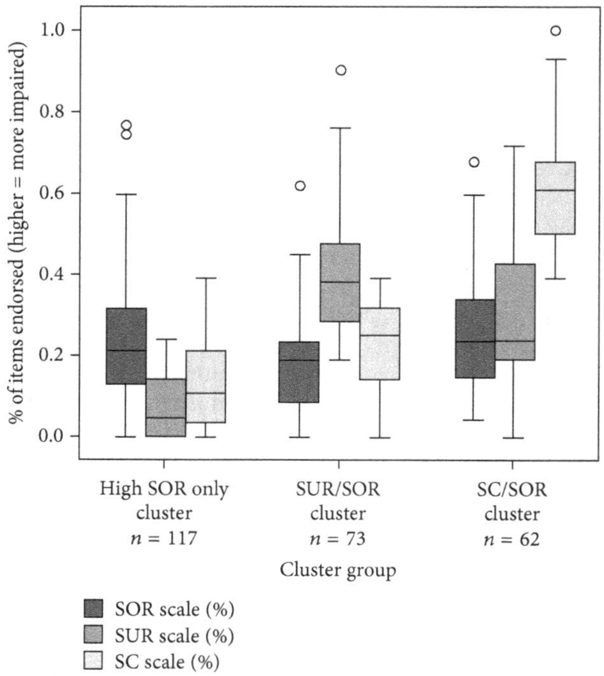

FIGURE 1: Cluster groupings.

differences despite multiple comparisons, as suggested by [41].

3. Results

The distance matrix from the hierarchical cluster analysis provided support for a three-cluster solution: (a) High SOR only cluster ($n = 117$); (b) High SUR plus SOR cluster ($n = 73$); and (c) High SC plus SOR cluster ($n = 62$) (see Figure 1).

In terms of demographics, the High SOR only group was 70.9% male with a mean age of 7.28 (SD = 2.23). The High SUR plus SOR (SUR/SOR) cluster group was 64.4% male with a mean age of 6.78 (SD = 1.92), and the High SC plus SOR (SC/SOR) cluster group was 80.6% male with a mean age of 6.37 (SD = 1.67). A one-way ANOVA confirmed cluster group differences for age, F (2, 249) = 4.37, $p = 0.014$, with the High SOR only cluster group being significantly older than the SC cluster group ($p = 0.004$) but not significantly different from the SUR cluster group ($p = 0.099$). Chi-square analysis showed no significant differences in gender distribution among the groups, χ^2 (2) = 4.37, $p = 0.11$.

The three-cluster solution in the K-means analysis produced groups that significantly differed in their SP-3D Inventory SOR subscale score, F (2, 249) = 3.45, $p = 0.033$; $\eta^2 = .011$, SUR subscale score, F (2, 249) = 142.89, $p < 0.001$, $\eta^2 = .376$, and SC subscale score F (2, 249) = 326.93, $p < 0.001$, $\eta^2 = .724$. Games-Howell post hoc tests showed that the High SC/SOR cluster group had more SOR behaviors than was found in the High SUR/SOR cluster group ($p = 0.028$) although the High SOR only cluster group did not significantly differ from the other cluster groups on their SOR subscale scores ($p > 0.05$). Thus, all cluster groups had some behaviors related to overresponsivity. Sensory craving behaviors were much more prevalent in the High SC/SOR cluster group and sensory underresponsivity subscale behaviors were more prevalent in the High SUR/SOR cluster group ($p < 0.01$). Table 1 summarizes the findings for the SP-3D Inventory by cluster group.

Using one-way ANOVAs, significant group differences among the three-cluster groups were found on the SP-3D Inventory postural subscale, F (2, 249) = 7.33, $p < 0.01$; praxis subscale, F (2, 249) = 23.96, $p < 0.001$; and sensory discrimination subscale, F (2, 249) = 28.21, $p < 0.001$. Post hoc tests revealed that, in comparison with the High SOR only cluster group, the High SC/SOR and High SUR/SC groups showed significantly higher (more impairment) scores on the postural, praxis, and sensory discrimination disorder subscales ($p < 0.01$ for all). The High SUR/SOR and High SC/SOR cluster groups did not significantly differ from each other on the total scores for the postural, praxis, or discrimination subscales.

Data from the SP3D Inventory was available from a previous study [26] for a nonrepresentative typically developing sample of children ($n = 140$) for comparison to the clinical sample. All subscale scores for the High SUR/SOR and High SC/SOR cluster groups are more than two standard deviations above the typical mean. Subscale scores for the High SOR only group were most elevated for sensory overresponsivity. See Table 1.

An exploratory analysis was conducted of frequency of item endorsement across the three-cluster groups to discover trends within the data. Significant or near significant differences were identified for several items. The High SUR/SOR cluster group had more problems with dressing and undressing ($p = 0.019$) such as placing arm or leg correctly in clothing ($p = 0.044$), completing fasteners ($p = 0.066$), and tending to look disheveled ($p = 0.012$). They also tended to prefer sedentary activities ($p < 0.001$) and had difficulty climbing on or over objects ($p = 0.010$) and licking an ice cream cone ($p = 0.067$). The High SC/SOR cluster group tended to crave tactile stimuli (examining toys by touching and feeling; $p = 0.082$) and had more problems grading force needed for a task ($p = 0.079$), maintaining or copying rhythmical movements ($p = 0.149$), and differentiating printed figures that appear similar ($p = 0.011$).

The Adaptive Behavior Assessment System-II (ABAS-II) scores were available for 170 (67% of the sample) children, and they are summarized in Table 2. A one-way ANOVA showed no group differences on the General Adaptive Composite (GAC) nor any of the other composite scores ($p > 0.1$ for all). However, the mean GAC score was more than one standard deviation below the mean suggesting below-average functioning in adaptive behavior for all cluster groups. Scores on the conceptual composite (i.e., self-direction, functional academics, and communication) and the social composite (i.e., social skills and leisure activities) were at or below one standard deviation for the High SUR/SOR and High SC/SOR cluster groups and within normal limits for the High SOR only cluster group. The communication subscale of the ABAS-II showed significant differences F (2, 167) = 3.41,

Table 1: Mean scores from SP3D Inventory group.

Variable	SOR only group Mean (SD)	SUR/SOR group Mean (SD)	SC/SOR group Mean (SD)	Typical group Mean (SD)
SP3D Inventory	*n = 117*	*n = 73*	*n = 62*	*n = 140*
SOR scale	10.6 (6.9)	8.89 (6.48)	11.95 (7.07)	2.25 (2.43)
SUR scale	1.73 (1.61)	8.42 (3.08)	6.35 (3.94)	0.96 (2.13)
SC scale	3.53 (3.18)	6.33 (3.05)	17.03 (4.1[illegible])	0.58 (1.14)
Posture scale	4.09 (4.29)	6.22 (5.05)	6.6 (5.35)	0.64 (1.91)
Praxis scale	7.49 (6.26)	14.23 (8)	12.15 (6.4[illegible])	1.57 (3.36)
Discrimination scale	1.87 (2.16)	4.1 (3.25)	4.74 (2.91)	0.48 (1.65)

Table 2: Mean scores from the ABAS II by cluster group.

Variable	SOR only group Mean (SD)	SUR/SOR group Mean (SD)	SC/SOR group Mean (SD)
ABAS II	*n = 72*	*n = 49*	*n = 49*
General Adaptive Composite	82.1 (16.2)	79.0 (17.1)	77.8 (12.6)
Conceptual composite	87.2 (15.4)	83.7 (15.9)	83.1 (12.7)
Communication	8.8 (3.2)	7.4 (3.3)	7.6 (3.3)
Functional academic	8.5 (3.3)	8.3 (3.5)	8.3 (2.6)
Self-direction	6.3 (3.6)	6.3 (3.1)	5.7 (2.5)
Social composite	88.3 (16.6)	82.9 (18.1)	84.7 (14.1)
Leisure	8.6 (3.0)	7.6 (3.3)	7.9 (2.8)
Social	7.1 (3.3)	6.6 (3.5)	6.9 (3.0)
Practical composite	79.6 (16.9)	75.9 (17.5)	75.9 (12.1)
Community use	7.6 (3.5)	7.1 (3.3)	6.9 (3.1)
Home living	6.4 (3.5)	5.9 (3.2)	5.8 (2.5)
Health and safety	8.3 (3.5)	6.6 (3.6)	6.9 (2.9)
Self-care	5.1 (2.7)	5.1 (2.9)	4.8 (2.0)

Note. Atypical on ABAS-II composite scores is ≤85. Atypical on ABAS-II subscales is ≤7.

$p = 0.035$; among the groups with the High SUR/SOR cluster group scoring lower than the High SOR only group ($p = 0.05$). On the health and safety subscale, the High SUR/SOR group ($p = 0.034$) and High SC/SOR group ($p = 0.06$) had lower scores than the High SOR only group. Subscale mean scores for each of the three-cluster groups on self-direction, home living, and self-care were more than one standard deviation below the mean, while functional academics, communication, and leisure mean scores fell within the typical range for all three-cluster groups.

The Behavior Assessment System for Children-2 (BASC-2) scores were available for 188 of the subjects (74.6% of the total sample) and are presented in Table 3. For composite scores, one-way ANOVAs confirmed cluster group differences for externalizing behavior: $F(2, 185) = 19.74$, $p < 0.001$; internalizing behavior: $F(2, 185) = 5.22$, $p = 0.006$; and for the behavioral symptoms index: $F(2, 185) = 15.63$, $p < 0.001$. For externalizing, post hoc tests revealed that the High SC/SOR cluster group had more symptoms than the High SOR only and High SUR/SOR groups ($p < 0.001$; <0.002, resp.). For internalizing and externalizing composites, High SC/SOR cluster was the only cluster whose mean score fell in the clinically significant range, and this group had greater symptoms than both the High SUR/SOR group ($p = 0.008$) and the High SOR only group ($p = 0.041$). For the behavioral index composite, the High SUR/SOR and High SC/SOR cluster group's means fell in the clinically significant range. Both the High SUR/SOR cluster ($p = 0.003$) and the High SC/SOR cluster ($p < 0.001$) groups had greater symptoms than the High SOR only cluster group.

At the subscale level, Games-Howell post hoc tests revealed that hyperactivity showed the biggest difference between groups, with the High SC/SOR cluster showing the most symptoms compared to the High SUR/SOR cluster ($p < 0.001$) and the High SOR only group ($p < 0.001$). The High SOR only and High SUR/SOR groups differed but only marginally ($p = 0.06$). On the aggression subscale, only the High SC/SOR cluster group was in the clinically significantly range, while both the High SUR/SOR and High SC/SOR cluster groups had hyperactivity scores falling in the clinically significant range. The BASC-2 anxiety subscale showed that the High SC/SOR cluster group had the most symptoms, reaching statistical significance when compared to the High SUR cluster group ($p = 0.006$). The High SUR/SOR and High SOR only cluster groups did not differ on this subscale ($p = 0.32$). On the depression subscale, the High SC/SOR

Table 3: Mean scores from BASC-2 by cluster group.

Variable	SOR only group Mean (SD)	SUR/SOR group Mean (SD)	SC/SOR group Mean (SD)
BASC-2	*n = 78*	*n = 57*	*n = 53*
Externalizing composite	54.1 (10.5)	58.9 (11.4)	66.4 (11.5)
Hyperactivity	56.9 (11.3)	61.4 (11.2)	72.7 (12.0)
Aggression	52.6 (10.1)	56.7 (12.4)	61.2 (21.1)
Conduct problems	49.3 (13.1)	55.0 (11.9)	53.0 (9.3)
Internalizing composite	57.0 (11.9)	55.3 (11.6)	62.4 (12.8)
Anxiety	56.8 (13.0)	52.6 (11.5)	60.4 (14.2)
Depression	57.4 (11.9)	58.2 (11.4)	64.8 (13.4)
Somatization	51.9 (13.0)	52.7 (12.2)	53.8 (12.2)
Behavioral index composite	58.1 (10.2)	64.2 (10.4)	68.7 (12.2)
Atypicality	55.5 (11.1)	65.7 (14.3)	65.4 (16.0)
Withdrawal	58.1 (13.9)	60.2 (15.3)	56.5 (15.1)
Attention	56.0 (10.9)	62.4 (7.5)	64.6 (8.6)

Note. Atypical on BASC-2 is ≥60.

group again showed the most symptoms, with significant differences between the High SC/SOR group and the SUR ($p = 0.018$) and SOR ($p = 0.004$) groups. On the behavior atypicality and attention subscales, the High SOR only group had scores falling in the typical range, which was significantly different than the High SUR/SOR and High SC/SOR groups ($p < 0.001$ for both). The High SC/SOR and High SUR/SOR cluster groups did not significantly differ from each other on these scales. Withdrawal was in the clinically significant range for the High SUR/SOR cluster group only, and none of the groups had atypical conduct problems or somatization symptoms.

The SNAP-IV scores were available for 78 (31%) children in the sample with the results showing cluster group differences on the SNAP-IV total score, $F(2, 76) = 24.49$, $p < 0.001$. The High SC/SOR group had more symptoms on the SNAP-IV than the High SOR only ($p < 0.001$) and the High SUR/SOR ($p = 0.009$) groups, and the High SUR/SOR cluster had more symptoms than the High SOR only group ($p = 0.002$). In examining specific ADHD behaviors, post hoc tests indicated that the High SC/SOR cluster group had more hyperactivity symptoms than either the High SUR/SOR cluster group ($p < 0.001$) or the High SOR only cluster group ($p < 0.001$), but the High SC/SOR cluster group was not significantly different from the High SUR/SOR group on inattention ($p = 0.942$). The High SOR only group had fewer hyperactivity and inattention symptoms than the High SUR/SOR group ($p = 0.044$; $p = 0.008$, resp.) and fewer than the High SC/SOR group ($p < 0.001$; $p = 0.003$, resp.). Only fifty-five percent of this sample qualified for an ADHD diagnosis.

4. Discussion

Clusters that emerged from the analysis partially support the sensory modulation patterns, described by Miller et al. [13]. Although all three groups had symptoms of sensory overresponsivity, SUR and SC seemed to suggest distinct groups with the third group differentiated by elevated SOR symptoms only and fewer other sensory and motor symptoms, while distinct groups representing postural disorder, dyspraxia, and sensory discrimination disorder did not emerge from the analyses. Other methodology that has been used to examine sensory processing constructs was conducted by Su and Parham [42] using the Sensory Processing Measure [43], a similar measure of sensory processing challenges. In this study, Su and Parham used confirmatory factor analysis to test whether sensory questionnaire items represent distinct sensory processing constructs using a sample of 454 children from 2 to 10 years of age. They found that items associated with individual sensory systems, tactile, vestibular-proprioceptive, visual, and auditory systems, formed distinct factors rather than patterns of sensory processing such as sensory over- or underresponsivity and sensory discrimination.

Previous research has suggested that postural disorder and dyspraxia may be a single construct [44] and perhaps there is too much overlap in the SP-3D Inventory items from these two subscales to form distinct cluster groupings. Moreover, underlying sensory discrimination problems such as tactile discrimination has commonly been associated with motor planning deficits (called somatopraxis; see [28, 45]) which may be an explanation for the lack of sensory-based motor clusters emerging from this SP-3D Inventory data.

Upon examination of the characteristics of each of the sensory modulation cluster groups that did emerge, some differences were found related to postural, praxis, and sensory discrimination functions, adaptive behavior, and social-emotional and attention/hyperactivity behaviors. The High SOR only group had elevated overresponsivity scores but fewer symptoms related to postural disorder, dyspraxia, and sensory discrimination and all scores falling within normal limits on the BASC-2. The High SOR only group did have atypical scores on scales measuring performance in activities of daily living and self-direction. The High SUR/SOR group had many atypical adaptive behavior scores, with the lowest social composite score, similar delays in daily living skills and self-direction, and additional delays in health and safety and community use. Dyspraxia and postural symptoms were common in this group especially with a preference for sedentary activities and poor participation in dressing, undressing, and climbing. Inattention and withdrawal also scored high in this group. The High SC/SOR group had the greatest number of adaptive behaviors and behavioral symptoms and was differentiated from the other groups by clinically significant externalizing and internalizing behaviors, specifically hyperactivity, aggression, depression, and anxiety. The High SC/SOR cluster showed problems related to grading force, performing rhythmical movements, and visual discrimination. In adaptive behavior, the High SC/SOR group showed symptoms within all three composite scores measuring social, conceptual, and practical daily living skill domains.

A previous study of sensory modulation dysfunction phenotypes by James et al. [29] supported two of the cluster groups, SC and SUR, that were found in our study. Similarly, defining characteristics of the SC cluster included aggression, inattention, and many externalizing behaviors. Additionally, SOR was present in both clusters identified by James et al. [29] as it was in this study. Our results also support the coexistence of sensory modulation symptoms with motor problems, building on findings in previous studies [28, 29]. Clinically, it is not surprising that the SUR and SC cluster groups had associated motor difficulties as children who crave sensory input tend to engage in a great deal of nonproductive, nonpurposeful movement.

The finding that children fitting the High SC/SOR cluster also often have praxis problems may dispel the notion that sensory craving is just a compensatory behavioral strategy that is employed to counteract sensory over- or underresponsivity. Other evidence supporting our results [18, 46] suggests that SC comprises its own symptom cluster which can be associated with sensory-based motor challenges and externalizing behaviors. For the High SUR/SOR cluster, we suggest that the lack of awareness to body sensations coupled with a reduced or slowed reactivity to external environmental sensory demands affects their motor skill acquisition and motor planning.

The High SUR/SOR and High SC/SOR cluster groups had more symptoms in social-emotional and fewer adaptive behavior abilities than the High SOR only cluster group, although all three-cluster groups had challenges in adaptive behavior. Individuals in the High SC/SOR cluster group tended to be more aggressive, hyperactive, anxious, and depressed than individuals in the other two cluster groups. We found more attention problems in the High SUR/SOR and High SC/SOR cluster groups unlike a previous study that found an association between inattention and only sensory overresponsivity [28, 29].

Of interest is that children in the High SC/SOR cluster were slightly younger than the other two cluster groups. One possibility is that individuals with SC tend to be more disruptive and thus may be identified at an earlier age. Children with SUR are usually quiet and passive and may not be identified until daily life requirements (functions) at school or at home become intolerable. Another possibility is that sensory craving or externalizing behavior tends to decline as children with age, similar to the decline in hyperactivity that tends to occur in children with ADHD as they get older [47].

Sensory processing challenges are increasingly recognized as a component of other disorders such as ADHD [24, 48] and ASD [49, 50]. Studies aiming to describe phenotypic characteristics may assist in differentiating clinical conditions. Research describing sensory patterns in ASD suggest cluster groups based on sensory domain involvement such as tactile, auditory, and movement sensitivity [32]. Other studies suggest patterns based on severity of symptoms as well as reflecting the cooccurrence of hyperresponsiveness (e.g., SOR) and hyporesponsiveness (e.g., SUR) responsivity possibly similar to the SUR/SOR cluster group identified in this study [51, 52]. Furthermore, behavioral manifestations of sensory symptoms in ASD have been shown to be more severe than those in individuals without a comorbid diagnosis [53].

This study suggests that ADHD and children with sensory processing challenges have some characteristics in common but also may differ. Research examining ADHD symptoms within individuals with sensory processing challenges shows an overlap with behaviors such as hyperactivity, inattention, and motor incoordination cooccurring with sensory issues [54]. In this study, many children who did not meet criteria for an ADHD diagnosis fell within each of the clusters. Similarly, Ben-Sasson et al. [55] identified a group of children with elevated ADHD symptoms *only* as well as a group with elevated SOR symptoms *only*, thus supporting the independence and uniqueness of each disorder.

Delineation of patterns of sensory processing dysfunction will help to facilitate outcomes research because in order to compare the effectiveness of intervention approaches, homogenous samples are necessary [12]. The clusters identified in this study represent different symptom presentations which likely require differing intervention strategies, so a greater understanding of the distinguishing characteristics of children within each pattern will help guide intervention. Finally, clarifying various patterns of dysfunction sets the stage for the study of the neuroanatomical and neurophysiological underpinnings of these cluster groups [56].

Limitations within the study design must be considered in the interpretation of findings. First, data were collected retrospectively from just one private clinic in Colorado and therefore may not be representative of all clinical samples of children with sensory processing challenges. The BASC-2, ABAS-II, and SNAP-IV were available only for a subset of the participants resulting in smaller samples of children with data from these questionnaires. These findings should be replicated in other clinic settings and with different samples. The age range in this study was broad, so that if developmental changes exist within sensory symptom presentation, an examination of scores by age may yield different outcomes. Finally, the SP-3D Inventory is a new tool, and extensive study of its reliability and validity is needed to support its use as a comprehensive parent report measure of sensory processing. Future studies should focus on delineation of sensory domain characteristics of overresponsivity within the cluster groups to determine if this helps to further define the cluster groupings. Additionally, correlational studies are suggested to help determine if having both SUR and SOR or both SC and SOR put children at greater risk for behavioral and adaptive behavior problems compared to SUR or SC alone.

5. Conclusions and Implications for Occupational Therapy Practice

This study provides information to the categorization of patterns of children with sensory processing challenges who do not meet criteria for other clinical diagnoses. This work assists in enhancing the clarity of communication used to describe children with sensory processing challenges both within and outside the occupational therapy profession. The results supported three distinct groups all with symptoms of sensory overresponsivity (e.g., High SOR only, High SUR/SOR cluster, and High SC/SOR cluster), and within these patterns, differing symptoms related to motor challenges and sensory discrimination challenges were found. All three-cluster groups had some challenges in occupational performance with individuals in the High SUR/SOR and High SC/SOR clusters displaying more challenges than children in the High SOR only group. This study builds on previous work by further elucidating patterns of sensory processing dysfunction and associated functional and behavioral symptoms that characterize each group. A greater understanding of the strengths and challenges inherent within each pattern is useful for guiding the delivery of appropriate occupational therapy interventions and for selecting homogenous participants for research.

Conflicts of Interest

The authors declare that there are no conflicts of interest regarding the publication of this paper.

Acknowledgments

The authors thank the children and families who participated in the study. They also wish to thank their research assistants Andrea Valdez, Shannon Hampton, and Aryanna Wiggins for their tireless effort on this manuscript. Primary funding for this work was provided by the Wallace Research Foundation. Additional support was provided by the National Institutes of Health Grant R21 HD41614-01 to Lucy Jane Miller and by the National Institutes of Health Grant T32MH15442 to the University of Colorado Denver in support of Sarah A. Schoen.

References

[1] A. Ben-Sasson, L. Hen, R. Fluss, S. A. Cermak, B. Engel-Yeger, and E. Gal, "A meta-analysis of sensory modulation symptoms in individuals with autism spectrum disorders," *Journal of Autism and Developmental Disorders*, vol. 39, no. 1, pp. 1–11, 2009.

[2] R. R. Ahn, L. J. Miller, S. Milberger, and D. N. McIntosh, "Prevalence of parents' perceptions of sensory processing disorders among kindergarten children," *American Journal of Occupational Therapy*, vol. 58, no. 3, pp. 287–293, 2004.

[3] S. D. Tomchek and W. Dunn, "Sensory processing in children with and without autism: a comparative study using the short sensory profile," *The American Journal of Occupational Therapy*, vol. 61, no. 2, pp. 190–200, 2007.

[4] S. J. Lane, S. Reynolds, and L. Thacker, "Sensory over-responsivity and ADHD: Differentiating using electrodermal responses, cortisol, and anxiety," *Frontiers in Integrative Neuroscience*, vol. 4, no. 8, 2010.

[5] L. J. Miller, *Sensational kids: Hope and help for children with sensory processing disorder*, Penguin Group (USA) Inc., New York, NY, USA, 2014.

[6] T. Bar-Shalita, J.-J. Vatine, and S. Parush, "Sensory modulation disorder: A risk factor for participation in daily life activities," *Developmental Medicine & Child Neurology*, vol. 50, no. 12, pp. 932–937, 2008.

[7] L. Mottron, M. Dawson, I. Soulières, B. Hubert, and J. Burack, "Enhanced perceptual functioning in autism: an update, and eight principles of autistic perception," *Journal of Autism and Developmental Disorders*, vol. 36, no. 1, pp. 27–43, 2006.

[8] S. G. Hofmann and S. Bitran, "Sensory-processing sensitivity in social anxiety disorder: Relationship to harm avoidance and diagnostic subtypes," *Journal of Anxiety Disorders*, vol. 21, no. 7, pp. 944–954, 2007.

[9] A. J. Ayres, *Southern California Sensory Integration Tests manual*, Western Psychological Services, Las Angeles, CA, USA, 1972.

[10] A. J. Ayres, *Sensory Integration and Praxis Tests (SIPT)*, Western Psychological services, California, calif, USA, 1989.

[11] W. Dunn, *The Sensory Profile*, Psychological Corporation, San Antonio , TX, USA, 1999.

[12] P. L. Davies and R. Tucker, "Evidence review to investigate the support for subtypes of children with difficulty processing and integrating sensory information," *American Journal of Occupational Therapy*, vol. 64, pp. 391–402, 2010.

[13] L. J. Miller, M. E. Anzalone, S. J. Lane, S. A. Cermak, and E. T. Osten, "Concept evolution in sensory integration: A proposed nosology for diagnosis," *American Journal of Occupational Therapy*, vol. 61, no. 2, pp. 135–142, 2007.

[14] A. Ben-Sasson, T. W. Soto, F. Martínez-Pedraza, and A. S. Carter, "Early sensory over-responsivity in toddlers with autism spectrum disorders as a predictor of family impairment and parenting stress," *Journal of Child Psychology and Psychiatry and Allied Disciplines*, vol. 54, no. 8, pp. 846–853, 2013.

[15] A. S. Carter, A. Ben-Sasson, and M. J. Briggs-Gowan, "Sensory over-responsivity, psychopathology, and family impairment in school-aged children," *Journal of the American Academy of Child and Adolescent Psychiatry*, vol. 50, no. 12, pp. 1210–1219, 2011.

[16] L. Gourley, C. Wind, E. M. Henninger, and S. Chinitz, "Sensory Processing Difficulties, Behavioral Problems, and Parental Stress in a Clinical Population of Young Children," *Journal of Child and Family Studies*, vol. 22, no. 7, pp. 912–921, 2013.

[17] K. P. Koenig and S. G. Rudney, "Performance challenges for children and adolescents with difficulty processing and integrating sensory information: A systematic review," *American Journal of Occupational Therapy*, vol. 64, no. 3, pp. 430–442, 2010.

[18] S. Reynolds and S. J. Lane, "Diagnostic validity of sensory over-responsivity: A review of the literature and case reports," *Journal of Autism and Developmental Disorders*, vol. 38, no. 3, pp. 516–529, 2008.

[19] B. Elbasan, H. Kayihan, and I. Duzgun, "Sensory integration and activities of daily living in children with developmental coordination disorder," *Italian Journal of Pediatrics*, vol. 38, no. 1, article no. 14, 2012.

[20] B. Pfeiffer, M. Kinnealey, C. Reed, and G. Herzberg, "Sensory modulation and affective disorders in children and adolescents with Asperger's disorder," *American Journal of Occupational Therapy*, vol. 59, no. 3, pp. 335–345, 2005.

[21] S. J. Rogers, S. Hepburn, and E. Wehner, "Parent Reports of Sensory Symptoms in Toddlers with Autism and Those with Other Developmental Disorders," *Journal of Autism and Developmental Disorders*, vol. 33, no. 6, pp. 631–642, 2003.

[22] S. Reynolds and S. J. Lane, "Sensory overresponsivity and anxiety in children with ADHD," *American Journal of Occupational Therapy*, vol. 63, no. 4, pp. 433–440, 2009.

[23] R. Iwanaga, H. Ozawa, C. Kawasaki, and R. Tsuchida, "Characteristics of the sensory-motor, verbal and cognitive abilities of preschool boys with attention deficit/hyperactivity disorder combined type," *Psychiatry and Clinical Neurosciences*, vol. 60, no. 1, pp. 37–45, 2006.

[24] A. Ghanizadeh, "Sensory processing problems in children with ADHD, a systematic review," *Psychiatry Investigation*, vol. 8, no. 2, pp. 89–94, 2011.

[25] P. L. Davies and R. Tucker, "Evidence review to investigate the support for subtypes of children with difficulty processing and integrating sensory information," *American Journal of Occupational Therapy*, vol. 64, no. 3, pp. 391–402, 2010.

[26] C. R. Reynolds and R. W. Kamphaus, *Behavior Assessment System for Children-2*, AGS Publishing, Circle Pines, MN, USA, 2003.

[27] J. M. Swanson, SNAP-IV Scale, 1995, Irvine, CA: University of California Development Center.

[28] Z. Mailloux, S. Mulligan, S. S. Roley et al., "Verification and clarification of patterns of sensory integrative dysfunction," *American Journal of Occupational Therapy*, vol. 65, no. 2, pp. 143–151, 2011.

[29] K. James, L. J. Miller, R. Schaaf, D. M. Nielsen, and S. A. Schoen, "Phenotypes within sensory modulation dysfunction," *Comprehensive Psychiatry*, vol. 52, no. 6, pp. 715–724, 2011.

[30] R. Bussing, M. Fernandez, M. Harwood et al., "Parent and teacher SNAP-IV ratings of attention deficit hyperactivity disorder symptoms: psychometric properties and normative ratings from a school district sample," *Assessment*, vol. 15, no. 3, pp. 317–328, 2008.

[31] A. S. Carter, M. J. Briggs-Gowan, and N. O. Davis, "Assessment of young children's social-emotional development and psychopathology: recent advances and recommendations for practice," *Journal of Child Psychology and Psychiatry and Allied Disciplines*, vol. 45, no. 1, pp. 109–134, 2004.

[32] A. E. Lane, R. L. Young, A. E. Z. Baker, and M. T. Angley, "Sensory processing subtypes in autism: association with adaptive behavior," *Journal of Autism and Developmental Disorders*, vol. 40, no. 1, pp. 112–122, 2010.

[33] S. A. Schoen, L. J. Miller, and J. Sullivan, "The development and psychometric properties of the Sensory Processing Scale Inventory: A report measure of sensory modulation," *Journal of Intellectual and Developmental Disability*, pp. 1–10, 2016.

[34] S. A. Schoen, L. J. Miller, and J. Sullivan, "The development and psychometric properties of the Sensory Processing Scale Inventory: A report measure of sensory modulation," *Journal of Intellectual and Developmental Disability*, vol. 42, no. 1, pp. 12–21, 2017.

[35] S. A. Schoen, L. J. Miller, and K. E. Green, "Pilot study of the sensory over-responsivity scales: Assessment and inventory," *American Journal of Occupational Therapy*, vol. 62, no. 4, pp. 393–406, 2008.

[36] P. L. Harrison and T. Oakland, *Adaptive Behavior Assessment System-II*, Psychological Corporation, San Antonio , TX, USA, 2003.

[37] P. A. J. Gore, "Handbook of applied multivariate statistics and mathematical modeling," in *Handbook of applied multivariate and mathematical modeling*, H. E. A. Tinsley and and S. D. Brown, Eds., pp. 298–318, Academic Press, Cambridge, MA, USA, 2000.

[38] J. Mandara, "The typological approach in child and family psychology: A review of theory, methods, and research," *Clinical Child and Family Psychology Review*, vol. 6, no. 2, pp. 129–146, 2003.

[39] M. Norusis, "IBM SPSS* statistics 19," in *Advanced Statistical Procedures Companion*, pp. 375–404, Addison Wesley, Boston, Mass, USA, 2011.

[40] O. Yim and K. T. Ramdeen, "Hierarchical Cluster Analysis: Comparison of Three Linkage Measures and Application to Psychological Data," *The Quantitative Methods for Psychology*, vol. 11, no. 1, pp. 8–21, 2015.

[41] R. Bender and S. Lange, "Adjusting for multiple testing—when and how?" *Journal of Clinical Epidemiology*, vol. 54, no. 4, pp. 343–349, 2001.

[42] C.-T. Su and L. D. Parham, "Validity of sensory systems as distinct constructs," *American Journal of Occupational Therapy*, vol. 68, no. 5, pp. 546–554, 2014.

[43] L. D. Parham and C. Ecker, *Sensory Processing Measure (SPM): Manual*, Western Psychological Services, Los Angeles, CA, USA, 2007.

[44] J. Lai, A. G. Fisher, L. C. Magalhães, and A. C. Bundy, "Construct Validity of the Sensory Integration and Praxis Tests," *The Occupational Therapy Journal of Research*, vol. 16, no. 2, pp. 75–97, 2016.

[45] A. van Jaarsveld, "Patterns of sensory integration dysfunction in children from South Africa," *South African Journal of Occupational Therapy*, p. 44, 2014.

[46] M. Liss, C. Saulnier, D. Fein, and M. Kinsbourne, "Sensory and attention abnormalities in autistic spectrum disorders," *Autism*, vol. 10, no. 2, pp. 155–172, 2006.

[47] S. V. Faraone, J. Biederman, and E. Mick, "The age-dependent decline of attention deficit hyperactivity disorder: a meta-analysis of follow-up studies," *Psychological Medicine*, vol. 36, no. 2, pp. 159–165, 2006.

[48] B. Pfeiffer, B. P. Daly, E. G. Nicholls, and D. F. Gullo, "Assessing sensory processing problems in children with and without attention deficit hyperactivity disorder," *Physical & Occupational Therapy in Pediatrics*, vol. 35, no. 1, pp. 1–12, 2015.

[49] A. Ben-Sasson, S. A. Cermak, G. I. Orsmond et al., "Extreme sensory modulation behaviors in toddlers with autism spectrum disorders," *The American Journal of Occupational Therapy*, vol. 61, no. 5, pp. 584–592, 2007.

[50] A. E. Z. Baker, A. Lane, M. T. Angley, and R. L. Young, "The relationship between sensory processing patterns and behavioural responsiveness in autistic disorder: A pilot study," *Journal of Autism and Developmental Disorders*, vol. 38, no. 5, pp. 867–875, 2008.

[51] K. Ausderau, J. Sideris, M. Furlong, L. M. Little, J. Bulluck, and G. T. Baranek, "National survey of sensory features in

children with ASD: Factor structure of the sensory experience questionnaire (3.0)," *Journal of Autism and Developmental Disorders*, vol. 44, no. 4, pp. 915–925, 2014.

[52] K. K. Ausderau, M. Furlong, J. Sideris et al., "Sensory subtypes in children with autism spectrum disorder: Latent profile transition analysis using a national survey of sensory features," *Journal of Child Psychology and Psychiatry and Allied Disciplines*, vol. 55, no. 8, pp. 935–944, 2014.

[53] S. A. Schoen, L. J. Miller, B. A. Brett-Green, and D. M. Nielsen, "Physiological and behavioral differences in sensory processing: A comparison of children with Autism Spectrum Disorder and Sensory Modulation Disorder," *Frontiers in Integrative Neuroscience*, vol. 3, article no. 29, 2009.

[54] A. Yochman, O. Alon-Beery, A. Sribman, and S. Parush, "Differential diagnosis of sensory modulation disorder (SMD) and attention deficit hyperactivity disorder (ADHD): Participation, sensation, and attention," *Frontiers in Human Neuroscience*, vol. 7, 2013.

[55] A. Ben-Sasson, T. W. Soto, A. E. Heberle, A. S. Carter, and M. J. Briggs-Gowan, "Early and Concurrent Features of ADHD and Sensory Over-Responsivity Symptom Clusters," *Journal of Attention Disorders*, vol. 21, no. 10, pp. 835–845, 2014.

[56] L. F. Koziol, D. E. Budding, and D. Chidekel, "Sensory integration, sensory processing, and sensory modulation disorders: Putative functional neuroanatomic underpinnings," *The Cerebellum*, vol. 10, no. 4, pp. 770–792, 2011.

17

Exploring the Influence of an E-Learning Sensory Processing-Based Module for Graduate Level Occupational Therapy Students on Clinical Reasoning

Bryan M. Gee,[1] Jane Strickland,[1] Kelly Thompson,[1] and Lucy Jane Miller[2,3]

[1] *Idaho State University, Pocatello, ID, USA*
[2] *STAR Institute for Sensory Processing Disorder, Greenwood Village, CO, USA*
[3] *Department of Pediatrics, University of Colorado, Denver, CO, USA*

Correspondence should be addressed to Bryan M. Gee; geebrya@isu.edu

Academic Editor: Lynette A. MacKenzie

The purpose of this study was to explore the effectiveness of a series of online, module-based instructional reusable learning objects (RLOs) targeted at entry-level, 1st year, Master of Occupational Therapy students. The content of the RLOs addressed knowledge and implementation of A SECRET, a parental reasoning approach for children with a sensory processing disorder, specifically sensory over responsiveness. Nine RLOs were developed and embedded within a commonly used learning management system. Participants ($n = 8$) were evaluated regarding their ability to discriminate between appropriate and inappropriate A SECRET strategies using a selected-response assessment. The participants' overall average score was 68%, a positive finding given the novelty of the instruction, assessment, and the content.

1. Introduction

Occupational therapy (OT) educators train entry-level OT students to identify, evaluate, and treat children with sensory processing difficulties and disorders [1]. This charge originates from the American Occupational Therapy Association's (AOTA) 2011 educational standards for Accreditation Council of Occupational Therapy Education (ACOTE) and AOTA's Blue Print for the Future of Entry Level Education [2]. According to both AOTA's accreditation standards and ACOTE's blueprint, entry level occupational therapists should demonstrate competency in assessing sensory needs and providing stimulation and environmental self-management strategies to those with sensory processing deficits [3].

It has been reported that 83–90% of occupational therapists working with pediatric populations provide interventions to address their clients' sensory processing deficits [4]. Green et al. [5] reported that a sensory processing approach was the third most frequent strategy in intervention with children with ASD. Furthermore, ACOTE requires students to "demonstrate an understanding of health literacy and the ability to educate and train the client, caregiver, family and significant others, and communities to facilitate skills in areas of occupation as well as prevention, health maintenance, health promotion, and safety" [3, p. 25] and "apply the principles of the teaching–learning process using educational methods to design experiences to address the needs of the client, family, significant others, colleagues, other health providers, and the public." (p. 25).

Based upon the literature, it is evident that a wide array of children demonstrate sensory processing disturbances and that occupational therapists incorporate sensory processing approaches to address those difficulties [6–8]. The type of sensory processing frame of reference (e.g., Dunn's Model of Sensory Processing, Ayres Sensory Integration Intervention®, Nosology of Sensory Processing), type of comprehensive intervention strategy (e.g., Ayres Sensory Integration Intervention, Sensory Treatment and Research Center Sensory

Processing Approach), specialized sensory based intervention (e.g., sound-based interventions, therapy ball chairs, weighted vests, deep pressure vests, Wilbarger Deep Pressure Brushing Protocol, and the Astronaut Training Program), and sensory motor intervention (e.g., therapeutic horseback riding, therapy balls) are taught in entry-level occupational therapy programs [1]. However, teaching a clinical reasoning process (e.g., A SECRET) to entry-level occupational therapy students as part of their defined curriculum has not been widely reported in the literature.

Occupational therapy has been employing diverse instructional technologies from hybrid (online/face-to-face) courses to exclusively online offerings for several years [9]. Furthermore, other health professions have used instructional technology and distributed learning as part of their entry-level programs, including pharmacy, nursing, physician assistant, speech language pathology, and physical therapy [10–12].

Interestingly, nursing, pharmacy, and physician assistant programs in the United Kingdom have been using learning objects (LOs) and/or reusable learning objects (RLOs) to bridge knowledge gaps due to content/course removal or to enhance skills and abilities without additional class time [11, 12]. Currently, however, there is limited information regarding the use of RLOs in occupational therapy entry-level education as mechanisms to enhance face-to-face or hybrid instruction with the exception of Gee et al. [13] who reported favorable opinions among occupational therapy students who used an RLO related to goal writing for existing and future coursework/clinical rotations.

In general, RLOs are "any digital resource that can be used and reused to support learning" [14, p. 6]. Reusable learning objects typically are small, discrete, self-contained digital objects that may be sequenced, combined, and used within a variety of instructional activities [14] including integration into formal lectures or as stand-alone elements for remediation or background knowledge development [11, 15]. Much like the educational handouts, manipulatives, and "objects" classroom teachers have always created and then shared with learners, RLOs afford even greater transportability beyond the confines of place and time.

Though RLOs within some of the health science education or professional programs [11, 12], there is a lack of published literature documenting the implementation of RLOs into the broader rehabilitation sciences for entry-level professional education, especially in occupational therapy. There are several characteristics distinguishing RLOs from other pedagogical tools and resources, including reusability, accessibility, interoperability, durability, granularity, sequencing, framing, stringing, and combinability.

The RLOs that were designed and developed related to A SECRET in this study intentionally employed these characteristics to increase the likelihood they would be instructionally sound. A SECRET is a mnemonic for (A) Attention, (S) Sensation, (E) Emotional Regulation, (C) Culture/Context/Condition, (R) Relationships, (E) Environment, and (T) Task [16] (see Figure 1). A SECRET [16, 17] is a problem-solving framework developed for parents and caregivers to enhance problem-solving abilities for their child/client's challenging

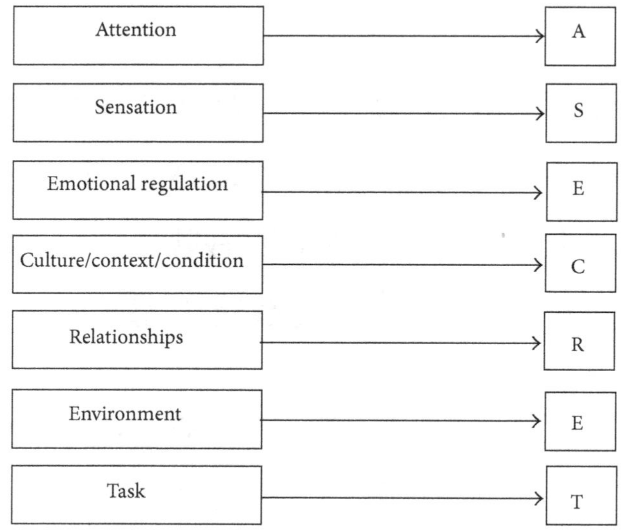

Figure 1: A SECRET framework.

sensory related behaviors. The framework attempts to capture how clinicians think about sensory related behaviors and the questions to ask that may lead to the design and implementation of strategies to reduce duration, frequency, and/or intensity of episodes for a child with SPD (sensory processing disorder) [16, 17].

The A SECRET framework is targeted to address sensory related behaviors among children who are diagnosed with SPD or have sensory processing difficulties that may comorbidly occur with other medical, behavioral, or developmental conditions [16, 17]. The A SECRET approach is grounded in the theoretical Ecological Model of Sensory Modulation [18]. The purpose of the study was to track student performance on a selected response, case based scenario after completing instructional modules and RLOs related to sensory processing and A SECRET.

2. Method

2.1. Participants. The participants of this study were eight MOT students between the ages of 20 and 50 years, who were in the first 12 months of the program (a three-year Master of Occupational Therapy degree) at an intermountain west public university. All the participants met the minimum criteria for admission into the MOT program and have a bachelor's degree in an associated area (University Studies, Psychology, Sociology, Exercise Science, etc.).

2.2. Inclusion/Exclusion Criteria. Individuals who took part met the following inclusion criteria. Specifically, they were 1st year occupational therapy students who (a) had no formal coursework related to sensory processing disorders and A SECRET problem solving strategies; (b) had access to an internet-capable computer; (c) could complete the online foundational instruction for sensory processing and sensory processing disorders from Sensory Processing Disorder University (SPDU); and (d) could complete the A SECRET instructional RLO modules via the Moodle LMS (learning management system) during the designated two-week time frame.

2.3. Method of Subject Recruitment. Upon institutional IRB approval, the participants were obtained through purposeful sampling methods at the targeted university. A total of 12 subjects were recruited from the first year MOT class. Of these initial 12, there were eight participants who completed the study. The remaining four withdrew for various reasons (lack of time or semester workload issues).

2.4. Design. A case study research design [19] was used to better understand the learners' experience with specific interaction events with the e-learning system, multimedia case scenarios, and researcher-created RLOs. The primary research question addressed in the investigation was what is the level of occupational therapy (OT) students' problem-solving performance for A SECRET after viewing a simulation case study of a child with Sensory Over-Responsiveness (SOR) as measured by a postsimulation selected response assessment?

2.5. Procedures Applied to Participants. Once the researcher obtained participants' signed informed consent, they were instructed to complete the sequenced instructional modules with content related to (a) sensory processing, (b) sensory modulation, (c) sensory processing difficulties, and (d) sensory over responsiveness via the SPDU modules. Upon completion of this foundational knowledge, participants began the nine RLOs (strung together) related to A SECRET organized into an instructional module and accessed within a learning management system at the targeted university. Subjects were then presented with a multimedia (video, audio, and text) simulated case scenario followed by a multiple-choice assessment (i.e., a quiz within the LMS) pertaining to each of the seven elements of A SECRET, one question for each element. Within the quiz, participants were required to rank-order (i.e., 1 = appropriate to 6 = inappropriate) a list of six predetermined strategies for each element and provide a rationale/justification for the strategies ranked as 1 and 2 and 5 and 6, considered by the participant to be appropriate (a rating of 1 or 2) and justification for why they chose the ranking of "inappropriate" (a position of 5 or 6). Finally, participants were directed to move to the next element within the assessment. They could move back and forth to different questions within the assessment; however, access to the previously viewed client history or video vignette while completing the assessment was prohibited by design. This was done in order to simulate clinical observation challenges found within existing clinical experiences in pediatric practice.

2.6. Description of the Measure. Given the unique nature of the content and delivery of the A SECRET instructional modules and the targeted participants for this study (1st year MOT students) a novel measurement tool was designed and developed as a part of the instructional design process of the overall project in order to capture the student performance and reasoning, specifically, to determine if 1st year MOT students could discriminate between predetermined A SECRET strategies that were categorized as appropriate, adequate, and inappropriate using the content learned from the instruction and contextual information gleaned within a case scenario.

Fourteen occupational therapy practitioners who had experience with evaluating and treating children with SPD and/or implementing the A SECRET reasoning approach assisted with the process of developing the measure. The measure included a client history/evaluation (diagnostics, evaluation findings, and parental report) and a five-minute video vignette documenting his occupational performance deficits rooted in sensory processing. The initial rounds of strategy generation, included six occupational therapy practitioners who reviewed the case scenario and generated a list of viable strategies for each element of A SECRET. Grammatical revisions and a finalization of the initial strategy list were made to the measure. Eight additional expert reviewers then ranked each of the six strategies for each element of A SECRET. The strategies were grouped into three categories, appropriate, adequate, and inappropriate, based upon a minimum of 80% consensus of the 8 expert reviews. A second review and finalization were conducted to incorporate the ratings and other comments/corrections made by the expert reviewers. Please refer to Figures 2–4 for an example of the measure (presented in a learning management system).

A total of 6 points were possible for each element category on the assessment with a total of 42 points. However, based upon how the assessment was developed, the participant could receive 100% by getting all 6 of the rankings in the correct order. They could receive 67% by getting up to 4 ranked correctly, but they were unable to get 83% with five of the rankings correct because each strategy was assigned a ranking and participants had to provide a different ranking for each strategy; thus, making an error with one strategy actually produced two errors.

During the instructional design process, it was estimated that, generally, a 70% overall on the A SECRET Case Scenario Assessment would constitute a "good" score given the limitations of the ranking system and the novelty of the pilot implementation for this kind of assessment process.

3. Findings

All eight participants completed the A SECRET Case Scenario assessment, which required identification and ranking of the two most appropriate strategies for that element (signified by the number 1 or 2); ranking the two strategies that were inappropriate (designated as 5 or 6) and the remaining two categorized as adequate (identified as 3 or 4) from a predetermined list of six strategies for each element. Participants' rankings were compared to the grading key, in which one point was given for each ranking that fell within the correct category of appropriate, inappropriate, or adequate. If the participant ranked a strategy in the wrong order but in the correct category, it was still considered accurate. Descriptive statistics (mean, mode, median, standard deviation, range, and sum) were calculated for each category of the assessment using SPSS 23.0 [20] for the participants' aggregate scores on

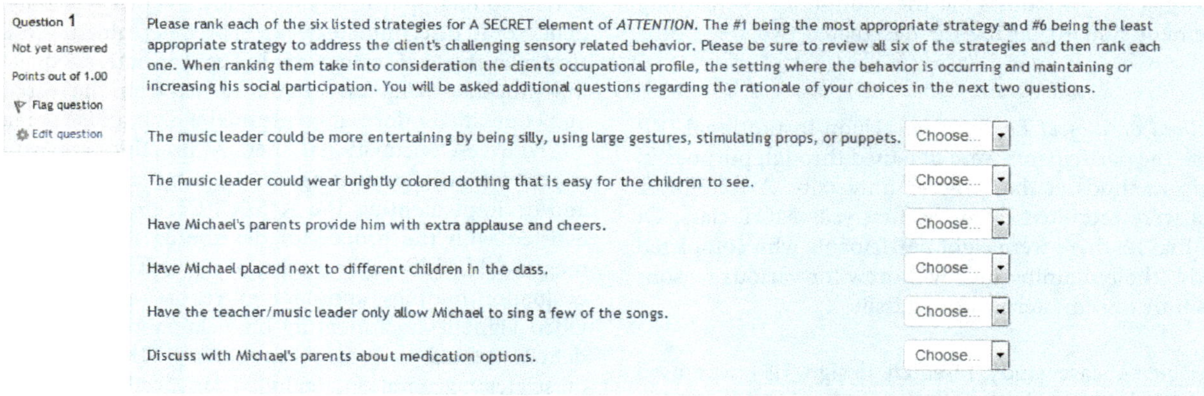

FIGURE 2: Sample A SECRET selected response question.

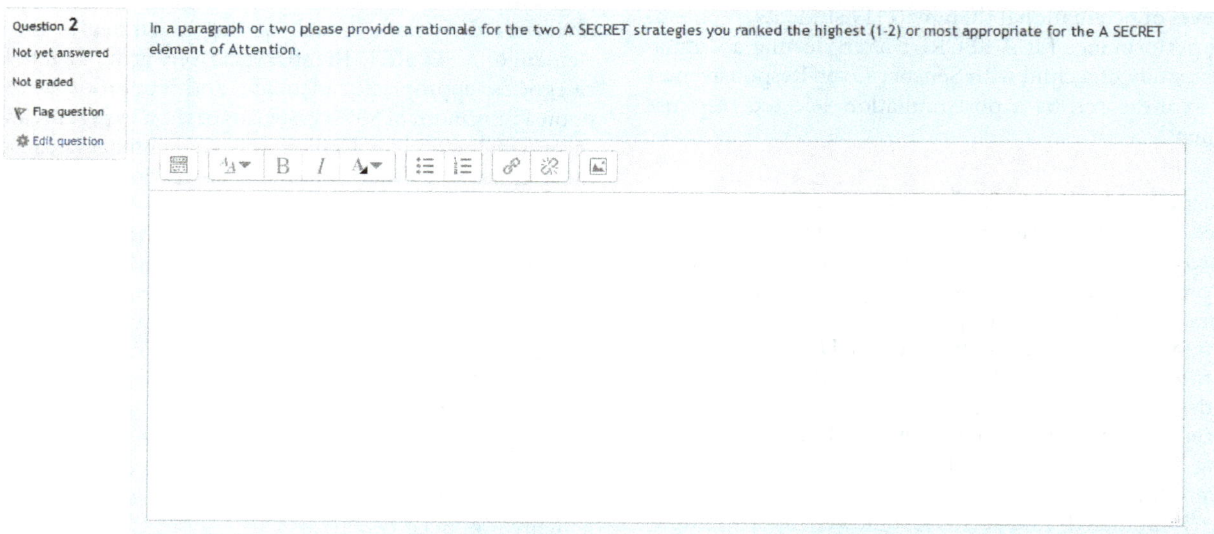

FIGURE 3: Sample A SECRET rationale of appropriate strategy ratings.

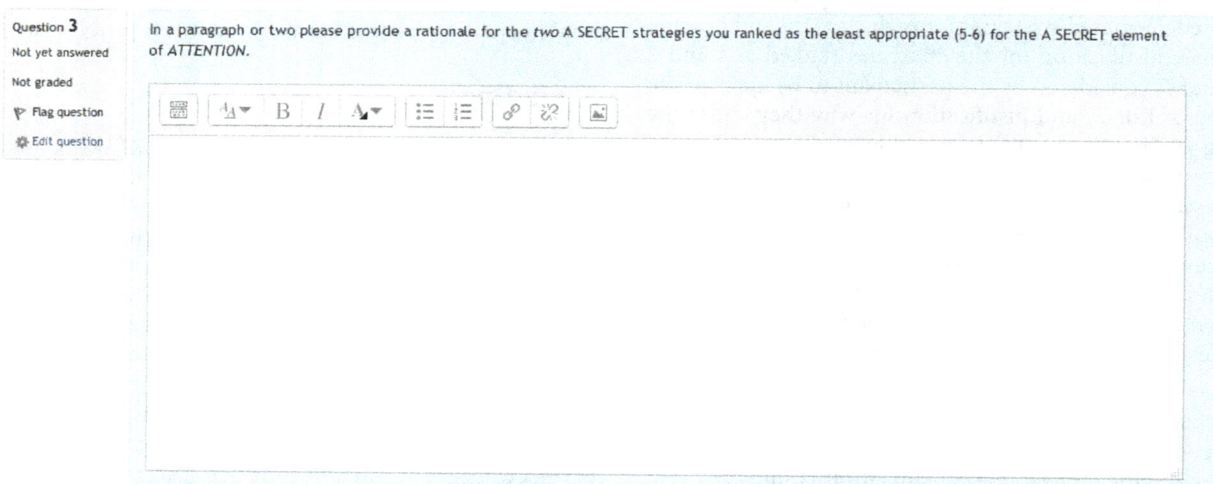

FIGURE 4: Sample A SECRET rationale of inappropriate strategy ratings.

TABLE 1: Descriptive statistics for the ASECRET case scenario assessment.

Statistics	Attention	Sensation	Emotion regulation	Culture	Relation	Environment	Task
			A SECRET category				
N	8	8	8	8	8	8	8
M	4.12	3	3.37	3.12	6	2.37	4
Mdn	3.5	3	3.5	3.5	6	2	4
Mode	3	2	2	4	6	2	4
Std dev.	1.64	0.92	1.40	1.72	0	0.91	1.51
Range	4	2	4	5	0	3	4
Sum	33	24	27	25	48	19	32

TABLE 2: A SECRET case scenario raw scores.

Participant	Attention total	Sensation total	Emotional regulation total	Culture total	Relationships total	Environment total	Task total	Overall score
01	4	4	3	2	4	2	4	23
02	2	4	2	1	4	1	2	16
03	4	2	3	4	4	1	2	20
04	2	2	2	1	4	1	4	16
05	3	2	3	3	4	2	3	20
06	3	3	3	3	4	0	2	18
07	2	3	2	2	4	1	2	16
08	4	2	4	3	4	3	3	23
Element sum score	*24*	22	22	19	*32*	11	*22*	**152**
% of correct appropriate versus inappropriate strategy rankings	*75%*	68%	68%	60%	***100%***	34%	68%	**68%**

the selected response portion of the A SECRET case scenario assessment (refer to Table 1).

When looking at the aggregate performance, participants scored the lowest in the category of *environment* (M = 2.37, SD = 0.91) while 100% obtained full credit in the category of *relationships* (M = 6, SD = 0), as depicted in Table 2. The overall research question was to determine if students could discriminate between and correctly rank the appropriate (two strategies) and inappropriate (two strategies) A SECRET strategies, where tracking performance on the neutral strategies was not scored. The cohort of participants attained an overall score of 68% which was 2% shy of the predetermined threshold of 70% established during the design of the measure and instructional intervention.

4. Discussion

This is the first study of its kind exploring the effectiveness of an e-learning module to influence knowledge and reasoning of OT students. Previous research that have been conducted within the OT profession has focused on using e-learning technologies to augment level II clinical rotations [21–26], which typically occur at the end of a student's courses of study.

The results from this study indicated the overall participant performance ($n = 8$) on the A SECRET selected-response assessment were two percentage points away from the initial achievement criterion (70%) established by the researcher during the Analyze phase of the premodule instructional design. This indicates a positive finding regarding the instructional influence of the researcher's A SECRET module, given that participants were MOT students in their first year of study who had not completed any courses related to OT interventions (e.g., psychosocial or behavioral dysfunction in adults and/or children). Without implementing the A SECRET case scenario as both a pre- and a postmeasure, it was difficult to determine how much the RLOs could have impacted the participants' knowledge and application of A SECRET.

The participants' specific performances with the *attention* and *relationship* elements exceeded the predetermined threshold and indicate these RLOs were effective in informing them of the content and the process related to these portions of A SECRET. It is further argued the participants' overall performance on the assessment (i.e., approaching the targeted threshold of 70%) adds merit to the effectiveness of the RLOs in teaching the MOT students to logically reason through challenging behaviors related to sensory processing through a simulated format.

Additionally, these participants had taken a course during the second semester in the curriculum that focused on the task (activity) analysis procedure. This may be why they scored well on the *task* subtest on the assessment. However, it is difficult to ascertain why each participant accurately ranked each item on the *relationship* subtest. It may be assumed that the items were too easy or that the items ranked as appropriate versus inappropriate were too obvious to the participants. However, it is also likely the relationship RLO was the most effective at conveying the information through the use of quality multimedia, content, case examples, and instructional design strategies.

The participants' overall mean of correct rankings of strategies was 68% on the selected-response portion of the A SECRET case scenario. This is below the 70% targeted criterion established by the researcher as part of the instructional design process for the A SECRET module. This original threshold was determined due to several factors: (1) the novelty of the instruction; (2) the uniqueness of the content; and (3) the lack of in-depth exposure to the intervention process for specific conditions and populations at this point in the program. The participants were able to reach, or exceed, the 70% criterion for two elements of A SECRET: *attention* and *relationship*. It is difficult to ascertain why the participants performed well with these two elements but not on the other five. The participants scored less than 70% on the latter four elements (*sensation*, *emotional regulation*, *culture*, *environment*, and *task*). The participants scored within two percentage points on *sensation* and *emotional regulation*, which is promising given the novelty of the instruction and the measure. However, of those five, Miller et al. [27] have reported that the element of *culture* is the most difficult to teach and for clients/caregivers to understand.

Culture as a part of the A SECRET process was difficult to define, especially in the context of the A SECRET reasoning approach, as it was poorly operationalized. Culture may be interpreted differently by therapists, parents, or caregivers. In future studies, the RLO containing the element *culture* could be enhanced with additional video-based examples incorporating diverse applications of strategies with different sensory problem difficulties or different ages of children.

To date, there is one published study using RLOs within occupational therapy entry-level education [28] and one in OT clinical practice [13]. The findings from the Gee et al. [28] and the Gee et al. [13] investigations indicated the value of RLOs as an adjunctive instructional resource to support student learning. In this current research investigation, given that this was the participants' first exposure to the A SECRET reasoning process, their performance should be considered promising. Furthermore, this is the first study of its kind exploring the use of RLOs to instruct students related to structured, prescriptive reasoning process and, specifically, the A SECRET reasoning approach.

4.1. Limitations and Recommendations for Future Research. The nature of the case study approach that was used had inherent limitations, including the inability to generalize, limited opportunity to conduct analysis beyond descriptive statistics, and a narrower focus of questioning and discovery. Therefore, it is recommended that additional research be conducted using the same instructional content and delivery, but with an approach that permits a larger sample size and includes using control and experimental groups.

An increased sample size would allow for the exploration of relationships between the four constructs on the attitudinal survey and/or different demographic profiles of the participants. The above-mentioned design recommendations could be accomplished using MOT students enrolled in their first year from ISU as well as students from larger academic institutions.

Using cohorts of students within the ISU MOT program could result in varying types of opportunities for further research and development. Assessing student performance across the three different cohorts within the ISU MOT program to evaluate their performance with the selected-response case scenario, as well as tracking differences with how each cohort approached the case scenario would provide insight. Performance of participants who took part in the A SECRET module as a stand-alone instructional activity versus those who had the module imbedded within a formal course relevant to the A SECRET process (e.g., pediatric practice courses) could also be examined.

Another possibility would be to determine if the ISU A SECRET module could be implemented within courses that address adults diagnosed with mental illness who also exhibit symptoms related to sensory processing disturbances. A case study could be conducted assessing the attitudes of students regarding the existing content and the difficulty or ease of aligning the content to adult populations within *Psychosocial Dysfunction in Occupation*.

For this study, the A SECRET instructional module was developed to target a variety of learners, although it was tested using 1st year MOT students. The module could be implemented in a different instructional context with caregivers, parents, and teachers of children with sensory processing disturbances. This could be conducted within the context of the Sensory Processing Disorder University to evaluate performance within the instructional content module and then the long-term outcomes (three, six, and 12 months after instruction) in order to assess retention as well as performance in implementing it with their own child in addressing behaviors that are rooted in sensory processing.

4.2. Implications for Occupational Therapy Education. The procedures used in this design and development of the RLOs and instructional module in preparation for the study provide examples that may enhance occupational therapy education. The authors used a formal instructional design process and procedure as a mechanism to design and develop the instruction, specifically, the ADDIE model of instructional design [29]. Approaching instructional problems and/or opportunities using a formal approach may ensure that the instruction designed is of higher quality and is meeting the needs of the targeted population [29]. Using simulated case studies, which are paired with specific content, may support the students understanding of content and also the application of some types of clinical reasoning such as procedural and conditional reasoning. Providing instruction that supports structured reasoning early in a curriculum may also support student learning experiences during clinical rotations, as they arrive with specific tools instead of muddied pragmatic approaches often employed by practicing clinicians. Instructional technology such as RLOs sequenced as an instructional module may enhance clinical reasoning strategies such as those employed by the A SECRET reasoning approach to challenging behavior related to sensory processing.

Competing Interests

The authors declare that there is no conflict of interests regarding the publication of this paper.

References

[1] S. Reynolds, R. Watling, A. L. Zapletal, and T. May-Benson, "Sensory integration in entry-level occupational therapy education," *Sensory Integration Special Interest Section Quarterly Newsletter*, vol. 35, no. 4, pp. 1–4, 2012.

[2] Accreditation Council for Occupational Therapy Education, "Blueprint for the future of entry-level education in occupational therapy," *American Journal of Occupational Therapy*, vol. 64, no. 1, pp. 186–203, 2010.

[3] American Occupational Therapy Association, "2011 Accreditation Council for Occupational Therapy Education (ACOTE®) Standards," *American Journal of Occupational Therapy*, vol. 66, pp. S6–S74, 2012.

[4] American Occupational Therapy Association, *2010 Occupational Therapy Compensation and Workforce Study*, AOTA Press, Bethesda, Md, USA, 2010.

[5] V. A. Green, K. A. Pituch, J. Itchon, A. Choi, M. O'Reilly, and J. Sigafoos, "Internet survey of treatments used by parents of children with autism," *Research in Developmental Disabilities*, vol. 27, no. 1, pp. 70–84, 2006.

[6] J. P. Owen, E. J. Marco, S. Desai et al., "Abnormal white matter microstructure in children with sensory processing disorders," *NeuroImage: Clinical*, vol. 2, no. 1, pp. 844–853, 2013.

[7] S. D. Tomchek, R. A. Huebner, and W. Dunn, "Patterns of sensory processing in children with an autism spectrum disorder," *Research in Autism Spectrum Disorders*, vol. 8, no. 9, pp. 1214–1224, 2014.

[8] A. C. Wickremasinghe, E. E. Rogers, B. C. Johnson, A. Shen, A. J. Barkovich, and E. J. Marco, "Children born prematurely have atypical Sensory Profiles," *Journal of Perinatology*, vol. 33, no. 8, pp. 631–635, 2013.

[9] J. S. Jedlicka, S. W. Brown, A. E. Bunch, and L. E. Jaffe, "A comparison of distance education instructional methods in occupational therapy," *Journal of Allied Health*, vol. 31, no. 4, pp. 247–251, 2002.

[10] H. Blake, "Computer-based learning objects in healthcare: the student experience," *International Journal of Nursing Education Scholarship*, vol. 7, no. 1, pp. 1–15, 2010.

[11] J. S. Lymn, F. Bath-Hextall, and H. J. Wharrad, "Pharmacology education for nurse prescribing students—a lesson in reusable learning objects," *BMC Nursing*, vol. 7, article 2, 2008.

[12] R. J. Windle, D. McCormick, J. Dandrea, and H. Wharrad, "The characteristics of reusable learning objects that enhance learning: a case-study in health-science education," *British Journal of Educational Technology*, vol 42, no. 5, pp. 811–823, 2011.

[13] B. M. Gee, K. Moholy, K. Lloyd, and A. Seikel, "Field-testing reusable learning objects related to sensory over-responsiveness," *The Open Journal of Occupational Therapy*, vol. 3, no. 2, article 4, 2015.

[14] D. Wiley, *The Instructional Use of Learning Objects*, AIT/AECT, Bloomington, Ind, USA, 2002.

[15] P. Delich, K. Kelly, and D. McIntosh, *Emerging Technologies in E-Learning in Education for a Digital World: Advice, Guidelines, and Effective Practice from Around the Globe*, BCcampus and Commonwealth of Learning, Vancouver, British Columbia, 2008.

[16] L. Miller, *Sensational Kids: Hope and Help for Children with Sensory Processing Disorder (SPD)*, Perigee Books, 2006.

[17] D. S. Bialer and L. J. Miller, *No Longer a SECRET: Unique Common Sense Strategies for Children with Sensory or Motor Challenges*, Sensory World, Arlington, Tex, USA, 2011.

[18] L. Miller, J. Reisman, D. McIntosh, and J. Simon, "An ecological model of sensory modulation," in *Understanding the Nature of Sensory Integration in Diverse Populations*, S. S. Roley, E. I. Blanche, and R. C. Schaaf, Eds., Therapy Skill Builders, Tuscan, Ariz, USA, 2001.

[19] S. B. Merriam, *Qualitative Research and Case Study Applications in Education*, Jossey-Bass Publishers, San Francisco, Calif, USA, 1998.

[20] IBM Corp., *IBM SPSS Statistics for Windows, Version 22.0*, IBM Corp., Armonk, NY, USA, 2013.

[21] T. A. Creel, "Chat rooms and level II fieldwork," *Occupational Therapy in Health Care*, vol. 14, no. 2, pp. 55–59, 2001.

[22] E. Murphy, "An instrument to support thinking critically about critical thinking in online asynchronous discussions," *Australasian Journal of Educational Technology*, vol. 20, no. 3, pp. 295–318, 2004.

[23] J. N. Scanlan and N. Hancock, "Online discussions develop students' clinical reasoning skills during fieldwork," *Australian Occupational Therapy Journal*, vol. 57, no. 6, pp. 401–408, 2010.

[24] A. Thomas and C. Storr, "WebCT in occupational therapy clinical education: implementing and evaluating a tool for peer learning and interaction," *Occupational Therapy International*, vol. 12, no. 3, pp. 162–179, 2005.

[25] L. Trujillo and J. Painter, "The effectiveness of discussion board usage for occupational therapy fieldwork II students," *Journal of the Research Center for Educational Technology*, vol. 5, pp. 80–88, 2009.

[26] D. Wooster, "An exploratory study of web-based supports for occupational therapy students during level II fieldwork," *Occupational Therapy in Health Care*, vol. 18, no. 1-2, pp. 21–29, 2004.

[27] L. J. Miller, D. A. Fuller, and J. Roetenberg, *Sensational Kids Revised Edition: Hope and Help for Children with Sensory Processing Disorder (SPD)*, Penguin, London, UK, 2014.

18

Validity and Reliability of the Korean Version of the Utrecht Scale for Evaluation of Rehabilitation-Participation

Joo-Hyun Lee,[1] Ji-Hyuk Park,[1] Yeong Jo Kim,[1] Sang Heon Lee,[2] Marcel W. M. Post,[3] and Hae Yean Park[1]

[1] *Department of Occupational Therapy, Yonsei University, Wonju, Republic of Korea*
[2] *Department of Occupational Therapy, Soonchunhyang University, Cheonan, Republic of Korea*
[3] *Brain Center Rudolf Magnus and Center of Excellence in Rehabilitation Medicine, University Medical Center Utrecht and De Hoogstraat Rehabilitation, Utrecht, Netherlands*

Correspondence should be addressed to Ji-Hyuk Park; otscientist@yonsei.ac.kr

Academic Editor: Claudia Hilton

This study investigated the reliability and validity of the Korean version of the Utrecht Scale for Evaluation of Rehabilitation-Participation (K-USER-P) in patients with stroke. Stroke patients participated in this study. The Utrecht Scale for Evaluation of Rehabilitation-Participation was translated from English into Korean. A total of 120 questionnaires involving the K-USER-P were distributed to rehabilitation hospitals and centers by mail. Of those, 100 questionnaires were returned and 67 were included in the final analysis after exclusion of questionnaires with insufficient responses. We analyzed the questionnaires for internal consistency, test-retest reliability, and construct validity. The results indicated that internal consistency coefficients of the frequency, restriction, and satisfaction domains were 0.69, 0.66, and 0.67, respectively. Test-retest reliability was 0.63, 0.45, and 0.71 for the three domains, respectively. Intercorrelations between the SF-12 and the London Handicap Scale were generally moderate to good. The Korean version of the Utrecht Scale for Evaluation of Rehabilitation-Participation can be used as a measure of the participation level of stroke patients in clinical practice and the local community.

1. Introduction

Participation is an important outcome of rehabilitation treatment. Particularly in community-based settings and outpatient clinics, the final goal of rehabilitation is to improve the level of activities of daily life participation rather than the level of function [1]. The participation has been described as involvement in actual life situations by International Classification of Functioning, Disability and Health (ICF) framework [2]. For patients with disabilities, increasing this participation in daily livings not only strengthens the well-being of them, but also helps reduce the long-term costs of treatment and support [3]. Thus, in rehabilitation field, there is a growing interest in participation enhancement in daily activities and meaningful life roles and then improvement of functional ability after becoming disabled [4]. A participation measure is therefore needed as an outcome measure to evaluate the effects of rehabilitation interventions.

It is important for therapists to measure objective and subjective participation for patients because participation can explain objective experience such as frequency and duration and subjective expression of patient's values such as satisfaction and importance [5]. Since the introduction of the ICF in 2001, various tools for participation measurements have been developed [6, 7]. However, there is a lack of measures that include both the subjective and objective aspects of participation [1]. Of tools for participation measurement, most tools are objective and normative tools that were used variables such as frequency, duration, and limitations of activities, but not subjective tools [6, 8].

The Utrecht Scale for the Evaluation of Rehabilitation-Participation (USER-P) was developed to measure both objective and subjective participation [9]. Also, the USER-P is a valid and reliable measurement of participation in rehabilitation [1].

Among all neurological disorders, stroke is the leading cause of death and disability in Korea. Stroke survivors experience motor and cognitive impairment or decline such as paralysis, abnormal muscle tone, attention, and memory loss [10]. These stroke-related disabilities can severely restrict participation in meaningful activities of daily living [11]. In other words, patients with stroke are dependent upon others in some of the basic activities of daily living (BADL) such as dressing, transferring to shower, and walking outside as well as the instrument activities of daily living (IADL) such as household tasks [12]. These results can decrease quality of life with patients. So, nowadays goal of intervention and assessment in rehabilitation area aims to promote independence and reintegration into the community of people with stroke [13]. To do this, it is important to measure participation of activities of daily living with stroke patients.

However, participation limitation is not yet widely used as measurement index in the rehabilitation area of Korea [14]. Thus the USER-P can be used to verify effectiveness of intervention and measure the recovery after stroke in Korea.

Therefore, we translated the USER-P into Korean in order to use the tool in our country. The purpose of this study was to test the validity and reliability of the Korean translation of the USER-P.

2. Methods

2.1. Participants. Study participants were recruited through rehabilitation hospitals and centers in Wonju, Korea. Patients were eligible to participate in the study if (i) they were at least 18 years of age, (ii) they had experienced stroke at least six months prior to the study, (iii) they were able to read Korean, (iv) they had participated in rehabilitation therapy for a period of at least four weeks, and (v) they were enrolled from both inpatient or outpatient settings. Exclusion criteria included patients who (i) have severe aphasia and cognitive impairments confirmed by medical records, (ii) have a fast-progressing medical condition after stroke, and (iii) had not signed an informed consent. Informed consent was obtained from all participants.

2.2. Procedure. This study was performed over a period of three months from November 2013 to January 2014. In the first month, the USER-P was translated from English to Korean, and it was back translated into English and compared to the original English USER-P questionnaire by two experienced occupational therapists (bilingual Korea-English speaker). The USER-P Korean version was subsequently developed through review about understanding of contents by a committee of experts (two occupational therapists and two professors) [15]. In the second month, a total of 120 questionnaires involving the USER-P Korean version were distributed to the head or person in charge of rehabilitation hospitals and centers by mail. The questionnaires then were sent to participants by the head in charge of organization. The stroke patients belonging to each organization were requested to complete the questionnaire with instructions. In addition, to analyze test-retest reliability, we distributed another 30 questionnaires to patients 2 weeks after the first distribution.

2.3. Instruments

2.3.1. USER-P. USER-P was developed as an instrument to objectively and subjectively measure participation in activities of daily living by people with limited physical functions [1]. The tool consisted of a total of 31 items covering three domains: frequency, restriction, and satisfaction. The frequency domain is comprised of both vocational activities and leisure and social activities. The activities related to vocation consist of paid work, unpaid work, volunteer work, and housekeeping and are measured as the number of hours the respondent spends performing these activities in a typical week. For each item, scores range from 0 (not at all) to 5 (36 hours or more). These items also assess the frequency of activities in the previous four weeks. Each item score ranges from 0 (not possible at all) to 5 (19 times or more).

The restriction domain is comprised of 10 items measuring participation restriction in work, leisure, and social activities as a result of health problems. Each item score ranges from 0 (not possible) to 3 (independent without difficulty). Activities that are not relevant to the subject were rated as "not applicable."

The satisfaction domain is comprised of nine items measuring satisfaction with work, leisure, and social activities. Items are rated on a scale of 0 (very dissatisfied) to 4 (very satisfied). The total sum of each frequency, restriction, and satisfaction domain is converted into a score ranging from 0 to 100, with higher scores indicating greater participation. The test-retest intraclass correlation coefficient (ICC) of USER-P was 0.65 (0.45–0.79) for the frequency subscale, 0.85 (0.75–0.92) for the restrictions, and 0.84 (0.73–0.91) for the satisfaction. Cronbach's α was 0.70 for the frequency domain, 0.91 for the restriction domain, and 0.88 for the satisfaction domain. In addition, this tool had good responsiveness among stroke patients [14]. We used the K-USER-P translated into Korea for reliability and validity analysis.

2.3.2. Other Measures. Two criterion measures, which were SF-12 Korean second version and London Handicap Scale Korean version, were used to study the construct validity of the K-USER-P. These measures can be represented with participation concepts that are being measured such as health status, quality of life, and restrictions. The SF-12 Korean second version is an instrument measuring general health status and quality of life related to health [16]. This instrument is a questionnaire with 12 items, including a physical component summary (PCS) and a mental component summary (MCS). The PCS domain is comprised of physical functioning (PF), role physical (RP), bodily pain (BP), and general health (GH). The MCS domain includes mental health (MH), role emotional (RE), social functioning (SF), and vitality (VT). Each item is scored on a 1–6 scale. The total item scores range from 0 to 100, computed by standard score conversion, and higher scores indicate a better health status. This tool has high reliability, with Cronbach's α ranging from 0.81 to 0.84 [17].

The London Handicap Scale (LHS) Korean version is a self-completed questionnaire measuring the effect of chronic disorders on a person's functional ability [16]. It is composed of six items: mobility, physical independence, occupation, social integration, orientation, and the economic self. Each item is scored on a Likert scale of 1 (no disadvantage) to 6 (most severe disadvantage); thus, the total score of the LHS Korean version ranges from 6 to 36, and a higher score indicates greater disability. Cronbach's α was 0.791, and the ICC was 0.983, indicating high reliability [18].

2.3.3. Data Analysis. The psychometric properties of the K-USER-P were examined in two parts. First, we assessed test-retest reliability and internal consistency. Second, we had quantitative comparison of the K-USER-P, SF-12, and LHS. Analyses were performed with SPSS 21.0 (SPSS, Chicago, IL). Internal consistency was assessed with the use of Cronbach's alpha, which should be at least 0.70 [19]. Test-retest reliability was assessed with the use of ICC between the first and second measurement. Construct validity was tested by comparing the K-USER-P with the SF-12 and LHS using Spearman's rank correlation test as a nonparametric approach.

3. Results

3.1. Response and Patient Demographics. A total of 120 questionnaires involving the K-USER-P were distributed to rehabilitation hospitals and centers by mail. We received 100 questionnaires back and included 67 (67%) in the final analysis after excluding questionnaires with insufficient responses. For the test-retest analysis, we also received 20 questionnaires out of a total of 30 and used 13 (65%) for the final analysis. The characteristics for 67 participants were presented in Table 1.

3.2. Internal Consistency. Internal consistency of the K-USER-P was determined using Cronbach's alpha. The alpha values were 0.69 for the frequency scale, 0.66 for the restriction scale, and 0.67 for the satisfaction scale, indicating good internal consistency within the assessment (Table 2).

3.3. Test-Retest Reliability. Table 3 lists the intraclass correlation coefficient (ICC) for the test-retest reliability. The good reliability was found in the K-USER-P satisfaction scale (ICC = 0.71 (95% CI: 0.28~0.90)). However, the reliability of the K-USER-P frequency (ICC = 0.63 (95% CI: 0.15~0.87)) and K-USER-P restriction scale (ICC = 0.45 (95% CI: −0.11~0.79)) was found to be poor.

3.4. Construct Validity. Intercorrelations between the subtests of SF-12 including PCS and MCS and the London Handicap Scale with the K-USER-P scales are listed in Table 4. The K-USER-P scales showed significant, positive correlations with K-SF-12 including PCS and MCS and negative correlations with K-London Handicap. These results indicate that the K-USER-P scales are moderate to good correlated with the K- SF-12 and the K-London Handicap Scales ranging from 0.27 to 0.62.

4. Discussion

This study evaluating the reliability and validity of K-USER-P in stroke patients showed that it is a useful instrument for measuring levels of participation in the local community,

Table 1: Patient characteristics (n = 67).

Gender (n; %)	
Male	46 (68.7)
Female	21 (31.3)
Age in years (mean; SD)	55.3 (13.3)
Education (n; %)	
No education	10 (14.9)
Elementary school	5 (7.5)
Middle school	6 (9.0)
High school	30 (44.8)
College/university	16 (23.8)
Occupation (n; %)	
Yes	11 (16.4)
No	56 (83.6)
Residence (n; %)	
Own house	17 (25.4)
Rehabilitation hospital	43 (64.2)
Care hospital	7 (10.4)
Marital status (n; %)	
Married	36 (53.7)
Unmarried	17 (25.4)
Divorced	3 (4.5)
Widowed	11 (16.4)
Caregiver (n; %)	
None	25 (37.3)
Family	13 (19.4)
Caregiver	29 (43.3)

Table 2: Internal consistency of K-USER-P (N = 67).

K-USER-P frequency	K-USER-P restriction	K-USER-P satisfaction
0.69	0.66	0.67

Note: K-USER-P: Korean version of Utrecht Scale for Evaluation of Rehabilitation-Participation; data represent Cronbach's α.

hospital, and sanatorium settings. The results of this study on internal consistency, test-retest reliability, and construct validity of the K-USER-P were generally moderate to good.

The results of the internal consistency analysis showed moderate reliability in the restriction subscale, frequency, and satisfaction subscale. Our study found that the reliability of the Korean version of the USER-P was not similar to that of the original USER-P, which was studied in multidisciplinary outpatient rehabilitation subject [1]. These results indicated that because the subscales of K-USER-P consisting of activities relate to daily life, social relationship, and work, some subscales such as work, leisure activity, and relationship were not suitable to inpatients among participants of this study. However, the K-USER-P is a useful instrument with moderate reliability. In addition, test-retest reliability was measured as an additional method of assessing reliability. Considering that correlation coefficients in the range of 0.50 to 0.75 generally represent moderate to high reliability and a correlation coefficient of over 0.75 indicates very high

TABLE 3: Test-retest reliability ($N = 13$).

Items	Test M (SD)	Retest M (SD)	Mean difference M (SD)	p	ICC	95% CI
K-USER-P frequency	15.71 (12.10)	12.53 (10.15)	3.19 (9.58)	0.25	0.63	0.15~0.87
K-USER-P restrictions	40.79 (23.66)	42.2 (28.6)	−1.40 (27.54)	0.86	0.45	−0.11~0.79
K-USER-P satisfaction	35.19 (18.91)	35.39 (21.29)	−0.19 (15.36)	0.97	0.71	0.28~0.90

TABLE 4: Construct validity for USER-P ($N = 67$).

K-USER-P	K-SF-12 PCS	K-SF-12 MCS	K-SF-12 Total	K-London Handicap
	Rho	Rho	Rho	Rho
K-USER-P frequency	0.33**	0.35**	0.38**	−0.54**
K-USER-P restriction	0.41**	0.27*	0.35**	−0.58**
K-USER-P satisfaction	0.43**	0.45**	0.50**	−0.62**

Note: K-USER-P: Korean version of Utrecht Scale for Evaluation of Rehabilitation-Participation; K-SF-12: The 12-Item Short-Form Health Survey (SF-12) Korean version; K-London handicap: London Handicap Scale Korean version.
Note: data represent Pearson's correlation.
* p value < 0.05 (bilateral).
** p value < 0.01 (bilateral).

reliability [20], this study found high test-retest reliability in the satisfaction and frequency subscales and moderate reliability in the restriction subscales. Of these three areas, the correlation coefficient of the restriction area was somewhat lower, indicating that changes in participation restriction of patients occurred during the 2 weeks after first test administration.

Correlations between the K-USER-P and subscales of SF-12 or the London Handicap Scale were low. The subscales of SF-12 showed a positive correlation with the K-USER-P, and coefficients of correlation were higher in the satisfaction subscale than frequency and restriction subscales. And there is a good correlation between the London Handicap Scale and K-USER-P. Particularly, a correlation satisfaction subscale of K-USER-P is stronger than for the frequency and restriction subscales. Our results suggest that the SF-12 is not sufficiently sensitive or responsive to changes in participation level because the items of the SF-12 are related to health status, while the K-USER-P and the London Handicap Scale measure participation restriction. In addition, the SF-12 contains a small number of items.

One limitation of this study is that only subjects who had experienced stroke were included. Studies involving subjects with other conditions, such as spinal cord injury or musculoskeletal disease, are also needed. Second, because subjects had certain limitations on participation caused by hospitalization, some items of the K-USER-P did not apply. Third, our study lacked methods for assessing the validity of the K-USER-P because we only calculated construct validity. Finally, the number of participants for test-retest analysis is very small. Also, factor analysis was not conducted because of inadequate sample size. However, the K-USER-P showed high reliability similar to that of the original USER-P instrument, indicating that it is a very important tool for identifying activities of daily living participation in Korea. Therefore, our data suggest that the K-USER-P can be reliably used among stroke patients to evaluate the effects of rehabilitation interventions. This study is significant because the K-USER-P can be used by occupational therapists in hospitals and local communities for measurement of the participation level of people with stroke in Korea.

Competing Interests

The authors report no competing interests.

Acknowledgments

The authors would like to thank Marcel Post and Hae Yean Park for analysis and interpretation of the data and drafting the manuscript or revising it for important intellectual contents.

References

[1] M. W. M. Post, C. H. van der Zee, J. Hennink, C. G. Schafrat, J. M. A. Visser-Meily, and S. B. van Berlekom, "Validity of the utrecht scale for evaluation of rehabilitation-participation," *Disability and Rehabilitation*, vol. 34, no. 6, pp. 478–485, 2012.

[2] World Health Organization, *International Classification of Functioning, Disability and Health: ICF*, World Health Organization, Geneva, Switzerland, 2011.

[3] E.-Y. Park and Y.-I. Choi, "Rasch analysis of the London Handicap Scale in stroke patients: a cross-sectional study," *Journal of NeuroEngineering and Rehabilitation*, vol. 11, no. 1, article no. 114, 2014.

[4] A. A. Timmermans, H. A. Seelen, R. D. Willmann, and H. Kingma, "Technology-assisted training of arm-hand skills in stroke: concepts on reacquisition of motor control and therapist guidelines for rehabilitation technology design," *Journal of NeuroEngineering and Rehabilitation*, vol. 6, article 1, 2009.

[5] J. Hammel, S. Magasi, A. Heinemann, G. Whiteneck, J. Bogner, and E. Rodriguez, "What does participation mean? An insider perspective from people with disabilities," *Disability and Rehabilitation*, vol. 30, no. 19, pp. 1445–1460, 2008.

[6] S. Magasi and M. W. Post, "A comparative review of contemporary participation measures' psychometric properties and content coverage," *Archives of Physical Medicine and Rehabilitation*, vol. 91, no. 9, supplement, pp. S17–S28, 2010.

[7] M. W. M. Post, L. P. de Witte, E. Reichrath, M. M. Verdonschot, G. J. Wijlhuizen, and R. J. M. Perenboom, "Development and validation of IMPACT-S, an ICF-based questionnaire to measure activities and participation," *Journal of Rehabilitation Medicine*, vol. 40, no. 8, pp. 620–627, 2008.

[8] M. Brown, M. P. J. M. Dijkers, W. A. Gordon, T. Ashman, H. Charatz, and Z. Cheng, "Participation objective, participation subjective: a measure of participation combining outsider and insider perspectives," *Journal of Head Trauma Rehabilitation*, vol. 19, no. 6, pp. 459–481, 2004.

[9] C. H. Van Der Zee, A. R. Priesterbach, L. D. Van Dussen et al., "Reproducibility of three self-report participation measures: the ICF measure of participation and activities screener, the participation scale, and the utrecht scale for evaluation of rehabilitation-participation," *Journal of Rehabilitation Medicine*, vol. 42, no. 8, pp. 752–757, 2010.

[10] K.-S. Hong, O. Y. Bang, D.-W. Kang et al., "Stroke statistics in Korea: part I. Epidemiology and risk factors: a report from the Korean stroke society and clinical research center for stroke," *Journal of Stroke*, vol. 15, no. 1, pp. 2–20, 2013.

[11] T. Tse, J. Douglas, P. Lentin, and L. Carey, "Measuring participation after stroke: a review of frequently used tools," *Archives of Physical Medicine and Rehabilitation*, vol. 94, no. 1, pp. 177–192, 2013.

[12] A. Hartman-Maeir, N. Soroker, H. Ring, N. Avni, and N. Katz, "Activities, participation and satisfaction one-year post stroke," *Disability and Rehabilitation*, vol. 29, no. 7, pp. 559–566, 2007.

[13] A. O. Obembe and J. J. Eng, "Rehabilitation interventions for improving social participation after stroke: a systematic review and meta-analysis," *Neurorehabilitation and Neural Repair*, vol. 30, no. 4, pp. 384–392, 2015.

[14] C. H. Van Der Zee, A. Kap, R. R. Mishre, E. J. Schouten, and M. W. M. Post, "Responsiveness of four participation measures to changes during and after outpatient rehabilitation," *Journal of Rehabilitation Medicine*, vol. 43, no. 11, pp. 1003–1009, 2011.

[15] D. L. Streiner and G. R. Norman, *Health Measurement Scales: A Practical Guide to Their Development and Use*, Oxford University Press, Oxford, UK, 4th edition, 2008.

[16] S. H. Yoo, *The Characteristics and Risk Factors of Pain Among Older Adults in Single District of Korea*, Seoul National University, Seoul, Republic of Korea, 2006.

[17] L. L.-Y. Lim and J. D. Fisher, "Use of the 12-item Short-Form (SF-12) Health Survey in an Australian heart and stroke population," *Quality of Life Research*, vol. 8, no. 1-2, pp. 1–8, 1999.

[18] Y. I. Choi, W. H. Kim, and E. Y. Park, "Validity and reliability of the Korean version of the London handicap scale," *Journal of the Korea Academia-Industrial Cooperation Society*, vol. 12, no. 11, pp. 5102–5109, 2011.

[19] C. B. Terwee, S. D. M. Bot, M. R. de Boer et al., "Quality criteria were proposed for measurement properties of health status questionnaires," *Journal of Clinical Epidemiology*, vol. 60, no. 1, pp. 34–42, 2007.

[20] L. G. Portney and M. P. Watkins, *Foundations of Clinical Research: Applications to Practice*, Prentice Hall, New Jersey, NJ, USA, 3rd edition, 2009.

19

The Immediate Effects of Deep Pressure on Young People with Autism and Severe Intellectual Difficulties: Demonstrating Individual Differences

Lana Bestbier[1] **and Tim I. Williams**[1,2]

[1] *Priors Court Foundation, Thatcham, UK*
[2] *Institute of Education, University of Reading, Reading, UK*

Correspondence should be addressed to Tim I. Williams; timothy.williams@reading.ac.uk

Academic Editor: Lynette A. MacKenzie

Background. Deep pressure is widely used by occupational therapists for people with autism spectrum disorders. There is limited research evaluating deep pressure. *Objective.* To evaluate the immediate effects of deep pressure on young people with autism and severe intellectual disabilities. *Methods.* Mood and behaviour were rated for 13 pupils with ASD and severe ID before and after deep pressure sessions. *Results.* Sufficient data was available from 8 participants to be analysed using Tau-U, a nonparametric technique that allows for serial dependence in data. Six showed benefits statistically. Five of these showed benefits across all domains, and one showed benefits on three out of five domains. *Relevance to Clinical Practice.* Deep pressure appears to be of immediate benefit to this population with autism and severe ID, but the heterogeneity of response suggests that careful monitoring of response should be used and deep pressure discontinued when it is no longer of benefit. *Limitations.* This is an open label evaluation study using rating scales. *Recommendations for Future Research.* Future studies of the use of deep pressure should use physiological response measures, in addition to blinded raters for aspects of behaviours such as attitude to learning psychological health not captured physiologically.

1. Introduction

Deep pressure has been defined as the "sensation produced when an individual is hugged, squeezed, stroked, or held" [1]. It is widely used by occupational therapists working with children with autism spectrum disorders (ASD) [2] and is thought to be rewarding, reducing symptoms of stress and anxiety and improving performance in school [3]. Deep pressure is based on sensory integration theory [4] as initially developed by Ayres in the 1960s and 1970s [5]. The use of deep pressure for individuals with autism spectrum disorders has been widely discussed since Temple Grandin described her self-designed machine (hug machine) for giving her the pressure sensations that she craved [6]. Other types of deep pressure therapy include weighted garments, swaddling, holding, stroking, hugging, squeezing, and therapeutic brushing [7].

A number of reviews have concluded that sensory integration has insufficient evidence for therapeutic and educational use unless it is carefully evaluated [2]; however, other reviews have reached different conclusions. Case-Smith et al. [8] helpfully distinguished between sensory integration techniques (SI, "play and sensory-enhanced interactions to elicit the child's adaptive responses") and sensory-based interventions (SBI, "adult-directed sensory modalities that are applied to the child to improve behaviours associated with modulation disorders"). Deep pressure is generally a technique that is administered by caregivers and so falls into the category of SBI rather than being an implementation of sensory integration.

The evidence for SBIs such as deep pressure is less convincing, in part because of the heterogeneity of interventions and in part because the reviews do not examine the same sets of studies. For instance, Case-Smith et al. [8] identified 2 studies of brushing and joint compression as compared with 7 studies using weighted vests, 2 studies using therapy balls, and 4 studies using multiple methods including deep pressure. Losinski et al. [4] reviewed 14 studies of weighted or snug vests and 2 of Wilbarger brushing. Yunus et al. [9] reviewed

4 studies of weighted vests, three of massage, and one each of brushing, horse riding intervention, and therapy ball chairs.

There seems to be agreement between the systematic reviews that weighted vests do not seem to confer any benefit on participants. However, Chen et al. [7] using a within subjects design ($N = 12$) found that weighted blankets reduced signs of dental anxiety in typically developing students when measured physiologically but not behaviourally. Blairs et al. [10] provided a programme of noncontingent deep pressure using bed linen (swaddling) to an adult with autism, severe anxiety, and intellectual disability. They proposed that he might benefit, because he had previously benefitted from being hugged by his mother when upset and because he chose to wear a tightly fitting coat when he was in anxiety provoking situations. As an adult he was observed to be more relaxed when tightly tucked into bed and when being physically restrained. Following the introduction of noncontingent deep pressure, episodes of restraint and as required medication were used less often to control his behaviour. Physiological indicators of stress (blood pressure, heart rate, and respiration rate) also reduced following the introduction of this form of deep pressure.

Other types of SBI have been less well studied. Losinski et al. [4] concluded that Wilbarger brushing had no effect. A previous systematic review of the Wilbarger brushing studies [11] found four studies (only one of which is reviewed by Losinski et al. [4]) from which they concluded that "emerging evidence from these studies warrants future robust research on this topic." Similarly, Yunus et al. [9] concluded that tactile based therapies (such as massage or brushing) offered level 1 evidence of efficacy in managing behaviour problems.

There is some evidence of short term beneficial effects of squeezing which was not analysed by Case-Smith et al. [8], Losinski et al. [4], or Yunus et al. [9]. A "squeeze machine" controlled by participants themselves (cf. Grandin's "hug machine") was found to feel more relaxing than a control treatment, although objective measures showed no difference [1]. Edelson et al. [12] tested deep pressure in the Grandin style squeeze machine using a randomized allocation of 12 young people with autism compared with being placed in the machine but without any pressure. Physiological measures (Galvanic Skin Response, GSR) did not show any difference but a parent rating of anxiety did. A post hoc analysis suggested that those with higher arousal preintervention seemed to benefit more than the lower arousal group, suggesting that there might be individual differences in responses.

McGinnis et al. [13] offer a different perspective on sensory-based interventions. Three children with ASD aged between 2 and 7 years who were receiving ABA therapy in a private clinic were allowed to choose objects (blanket, gym mat, and pillow) which could be used to provide deep pressure. The experimental phase required the young people to choose whether to have free play or deep pressure. Two of the children showed a clear preference for deep pressure over free play. The third's preferences were confounded by ill health during the experimental phase. The authors concluded that deep pressure was rewarding for the children. Unlike previous studies of SBI this study uses a contingent application of SBI dependent on requesting it. They had planned their study to investigate whether deep pressure could be rewarding, since they were concerned that the use of deep pressure to help individuals calm when distressed might inadvertently reward signs of distress.

In summary, the evidence for deep pressure is equivocal [4, 8, 9], but the reviews cited above fail to cite evidence from case studies. Another evidence suggests that there may be idiosyncratic responses as has been highlighted by McGinnis et al. [13] who demonstrated that only some people will find deep pressure rewarding. A further issue is when to provide deep pressure. With the exception of McGinnis et al. [13] all research cited above seems to have used deep pressure as a means of improving mood and adaptability to the environment. As a result it was used noncontingently and regularly. McGinnis et al. [13] provided deep pressure as a form of rewarding stimulation following task completion and point out that the form of deep pressure may be person specific. An alternative would be to use deep pressure at times when the person was distressed or otherwise in a non-optimal state. This study was designed to provide information about the extent of variability of the immediate responses of young people with autism and severe intellectual disability to deep pressure by providing regular access to deep pressure.

2. Methods

2.1. Research Design. A pretest-posttest design was employed to evaluate the effects of deep pressure sessions on young people with autism spectrum disorder and severe intellectual disabilities. The study was approved by the ethics subcommittee of the trustees of Priors Court Foundation (Education & Care Committee 2012-2013: Minute number 650 dated November 8, 2012). The agreed procedure included requesting consent from the parents of each of the participants.

2.2. Participants. The study took place in a residential school for children with autism and severe intellectual disabilities. 13 young people (2 girls) were selected to take part in the study based on behaviours that were deemed by staff to indicate a desire for deep pressure (cf. [10]). The behaviours that were thought to indicate a need for deep pressure included trying to get in very small spaces, placing people's hands upon their heads, head-banging, and stamping feet. The ages of the young people ranged from 7 yrs and 10 mths to 18 yrs and 7 mths. Table 1 shows further details of the young people who were involved in the study and whose data included information from more than 15 sessions of deep pressure.

2.3. Measures. Visual analogue scales [16] are routinely used by the staff in the school to measure mood and activity of the young people. The visual analogue scales are 10 cm lines anchored at each end with the modifiers "not at all" and "very." All staff are trained during induction to use these scales. Each young person is usually rated on individually designed scales, but for the purposes of this study the same five areas of mood and behaviour were rated by the one of the staff working with the young person: calmness, engagement

TABLE 1: It shows the characteristics of the participants. Not all participants had been tested on the psychoeducational profile [14], but all of them had been assessed educationally using the *P* scales as recommended for pupils with special educational needs in England [15].

Participant (number of sessions)	Age (yrs:mths)	Psychoeducational profile [14] Cognitive verbal/preverbal	Expressive language	Receptive language	Fine Motor	Gross Motor	VMI	Academic levels	Communication Skills	Reasons for deep pressure
Alison (130)	07:10	38	26	23	39	29	30	P5	PECS level 3	Banging her head against people
Brian (45)	17:09							P5	PECS level 4	Hitting self, body slamming against walls
Carl (40)	12:10	20	<12	19	23	25	25	P5	PECS level 1	Biting hand
David (17)	13:09	25	21	23	29	27	25	P5	PECS level 4	Dropping to floor
Eric (49)	15:03	26	13	15	23	22	18	P6		Slapping walls
Fenella (17)	14:06	<12	<12	<12	<12	<12	<12	P4	PECS level 4	Dropping to floor
Graham (39)	15:10							P5	PECS level 3	Slapping own head
Herbert (48)	09:05							P4	PECS level 1	Wraps himself in blanket, extremely sensitive to sound

with activities, responsiveness to instructions or other stimuli in the environment, happiness, and communicativeness (e.g., the two anchor points for the calmness visual analogue scale were "not at all calm" and "very calm"). The measures were designed to be simple and quick to complete and yet provide indicators of possible short term responses to deep pressure. The staff were also encouraged to provide further written information on the reactions of the young people to planned sessions, and if the young people seemed distressed by the procedures or attempted to withdraw, they were allowed to.

2.4. Procedure. Three deep pressure techniques were used: brushing, massage, and squeezing. They were delivered in quiet places with minimal distraction by care and education staff who had been trained by an occupational therapist with a sensory integration qualification. Deep pressure sessions between five and fifteen minutes were scheduled to be delivered up to three times per day during school hours. The deep pressure was delivered over a period of three months on weekdays when the young people were in school. Variations in numbers of sessions per child were due to reasons such as the child being absent from school through ill health, school trips, or insufficient trained staff available to carry out sessions. The staff administering the deep pressure rated the young person's behaviour for the half hour before the session and again thirty minutes after the session.

2.5. Analysis. Data will be presented for 8 young people for whom there were more than 15 sessions to evaluate. Additional 5 young people had not completed sufficient sessions for reliable statistical analysis. The statistical analysis uses the Tau-U statistic [17] which measures the difference in data range (nonoverlap) between two phases (A and B), while being able to correct for a moving baseline. It is a nonparametric technique, with statistical power of 91% to 95% of linear regression but when data violates the assumptions of parametric data analysis the power of Tau-U can exceed the parametric techniques to 115% [17]. For the analysis reported here the two phases are before and after deep pressure.

3. Results

Table 2 shows the results as means and standard deviations of the five ratings before and after deep pressure sessions together with associated levels of statistical significance for the changes for each young person aggregated over all of their sessions. Four of the young people showed benefits in all areas measured, two showed no benefits in any area, and further two showed benefits on three and two ratings each. Figure 1 shows radar plots of the mean change for all five scales and eight participants. The radar plot has five "axes" representing each of the ratings. The five sided shapes (pentagons) represent the mean changes for an individual. It can be seen that Fenella shows the least benefit (the pentagon has short sides). On the other hand Alison shows large consistent benefits across all five ratings. Carl's pentagon is quite irregular which suggests that he benefits in some areas more than others.

4. Discussion

Deep pressure appears to be beneficial for most of the young people in this study. The effects were not uniform across all areas of functioning and it is clear that there are individual differences in response to deep pressure that should be taken into account when providing deep pressure interventions. As Figure 1 shows the largest changes across all the participants seem to be in the area of happiness, with possibly the least consistency in calmness. In the course of the study significant numbers of staff rated the behaviour and mood of the young people, which has probably diminished the effect sizes by introducing additional variability in ratings.

The variability of responses to deep pressure may be of importance clinically. Of the eight participants, four (Alison, Brian, Carl, and Eric) showed a wide ranging improvement in rated behaviours. David and Graham's responses to deep pressure were less wide ranging. Both showed improvements in calmness and David was more responsive and engaged. Graham surprisingly showed an increase in communicativeness following sessions of deep pressure suggesting that, for some individuals with autism, communication skills learning may be enabled. Neither Fenella nor Herbert seemed to benefit from deep pressure. It was unclear why this was, but we might note that Fenella differed from the other participants in being a very placid individual who moved around rather slowly. Herbert too was different, in that, left to his own devices, he chose to wrap himself in a blanket suggesting he would prefer a type of swaddling deep pressure rather than the more localized versions being provided in this study. It follows that one question for future research is whether it is possible to predict which individuals will derive benefit from the intervention. There are a number of measures of sensory sensitivity and processing that are believed to predict response to sensory stimulation (cf. [18]) and which could be evaluated.

All but one of the studies so far reported on deep pressure have used the technique noncontingently. For example, Blairs et al. [10] successfully used deep pressure noncontingently as a means to reduce levels of challenging behaviour. However, one of the main claims for the efficacy of deep pressure is that it can be used to improve the mood of the person receiving it when they are already anxious or otherwise upset. Longer term information on the mood and behaviour of people receiving deep pressure could help suggest answers to this question, although it might require further studies using quasi-experimental designs to determine the feasibility of a randomized controlled trial. Consideration should also be given to how deep pressure could be used to improve behaviour, if it is rewarding. If it is rewarding, then people might show more challenging behaviour in order to obtain deep pressure, in a similar way to the participant in Blairs et al. [10] study who was using challenging behaviour as a way of obtaining restraint and therefore deep pressure.

The study would have been improved if the individuals could have been randomized to different start dates (known as a multiple baseline design [19]). For instance, it could have been organised so that participants began to receive the intervention at weekly intervals, so Alison and Brian might have

TABLE 2: Means and standard deviations recorded for the scales before and after deep pressure sessions.

Participant (number of sessions)	Scale	Before session mean (SD)	After session mean (SD)	Z value of Tau-U statistic
Alison (130)	Calmness[a]	7.84 (2.40)	8.99 (1.59)	6.95**
	Engaged[a]	7.73 (2.37)	8.87 (1.54)	7.05**
	Responsivity[a]	8.17 (4.74)	8.88 (1.56)	6.66**
	Happy	7.26 (2.83)	8.78 (1.62)	5.80**
	Communicative[a]	7.94 (2.10)	8.87 (1.59)	7.49**
Brian (45)	Calmness	5.74 (2.51)	7.20 (2.16)	2.96*
	Engaged	4.66 (2.40)	6.59 (2.32)	3.65*
	Responsivity	4.74 (2.43)	6.39 (2.50)	3.28**
	Happy	4.92 (2.68)	6.91 (2.19)	3.66**
	Communicative	5.64 (1.64)	6.78 (1.93)	3.30*
Carl (40)	Calmness	7.35 (2.65)	8.84 (1.12)	3.55*
	Engaged[a]	6.78 (2.58)	8.51 (1.49)	3.55***
	Responsivity[a]	6.93 (2.56)	8.66 (1.35)	3.72***
	Happy[a]	6.85 (2.83)	8.67 (1.31)	3.71***
	Communicative[a]	5.92 (2.87)	8.08 (2.19)	3.54***
David (17)	Calmness	5.89 (2.49)	8.48 (1.08)	3.29**
	Engaged	5.52 (2.58)	8.03 (1.57)	2.81*
	Responsivity	5.87 (2.44)	8.24 (1.20)	2.91*
	Happy	6.15 (2.59)	8.19 (1.53)	2.50
	Communicative	6.22 (2.96)	8.06 (1.78)	1.66
Eric (49)	Calmness	4.68 (2.78)	7.69 (2.04)	4.98**
	Engaged	4.65 (2.61)	7.27 (2.15)	5.94**
	Responsivity	5.29 (2.37)	7.65 (2.08)	5.32**
	Happy[a]	5.69 (2.61)	8.02 (1.86)	3.50**
	Communicative	5.06 (2.35)	7.55 (1.98)	5.01**
Fenella (17)	Calmness	5.71 (2.35)	5.99 (2.40)	0.29
	Engaged	4.49 (2.60)	4.90 (2.60)	−0.03
	Responsivity	4.99 (2.36)	4.99 (2.64)	−0.21
	Happy	5.30 (3.01)	5.19 (2.75)	0.26
	Communicative	4.71 (2.76)	4.85 (2.53)	−0.59
Graham (39)	Calmness	7.51 (1.91)	8.66 (1.10)	3.33**
	Engaged[a]	7.04 (2.41)	8.24 (2.18)	2.20
	Responsivity[a]	7.32 (2.35)	8.31 (1.85)	1.69
	Happy	8.12 (1.86)	9.04 (0.94)	2.56
	Communicative	7.58 (2.14)	8.66 (1.16)	2.85**
Herbert (48)	Calmness	5.83 (1.91)	6.83 (1.92)	0.11
	Engaged	4.61 (2.13)	6.33 (2.08)	0.12
	Responsivity	5.39 (1.97)	6.40 (1.95)	0.12
	Happy	5.84 (2.13)	6.82 (1.89)	0.11
	Communicative	4.89 (2.07)	5.90 (2.20)	0.12

Notes. [a]Corrected baseline Tau-U statistic used; $^{*}p < 0.01$; $^{**}p < 0.001$; $^{***}p < 0.0005$. Significance figures corrected for multiple imputation per participant using the Bonferroni correction, that is, $(0.05/5 = 0.01)$ used as the highest level of significance reported.

started on the first week, Carl and David the second week, and so on through the first few weeks of the term. The shift patterns of the staff did not allow this possibility. We would also recommend more systematic measures to ensure reliability and possibly the use of observational measures such as counts of behaviour to evaluate reactions to different techniques of administering deep pressure. Systematisation of observational measures such as those used in this study could include estimation of the reliability of the rating scales and potentially trained raters so as to ensure consistency of measures across raters and occasions. Recent studies of sensory integration have used Goal Attainment Scaling (e.g., [20]) as a method of measuring progress, but other measures such as the Problem Behaviour Inventory [21] might be more relevant when the goal of sensory integration therapy is improved mood or behaviour. Although it is difficult to envisage how this

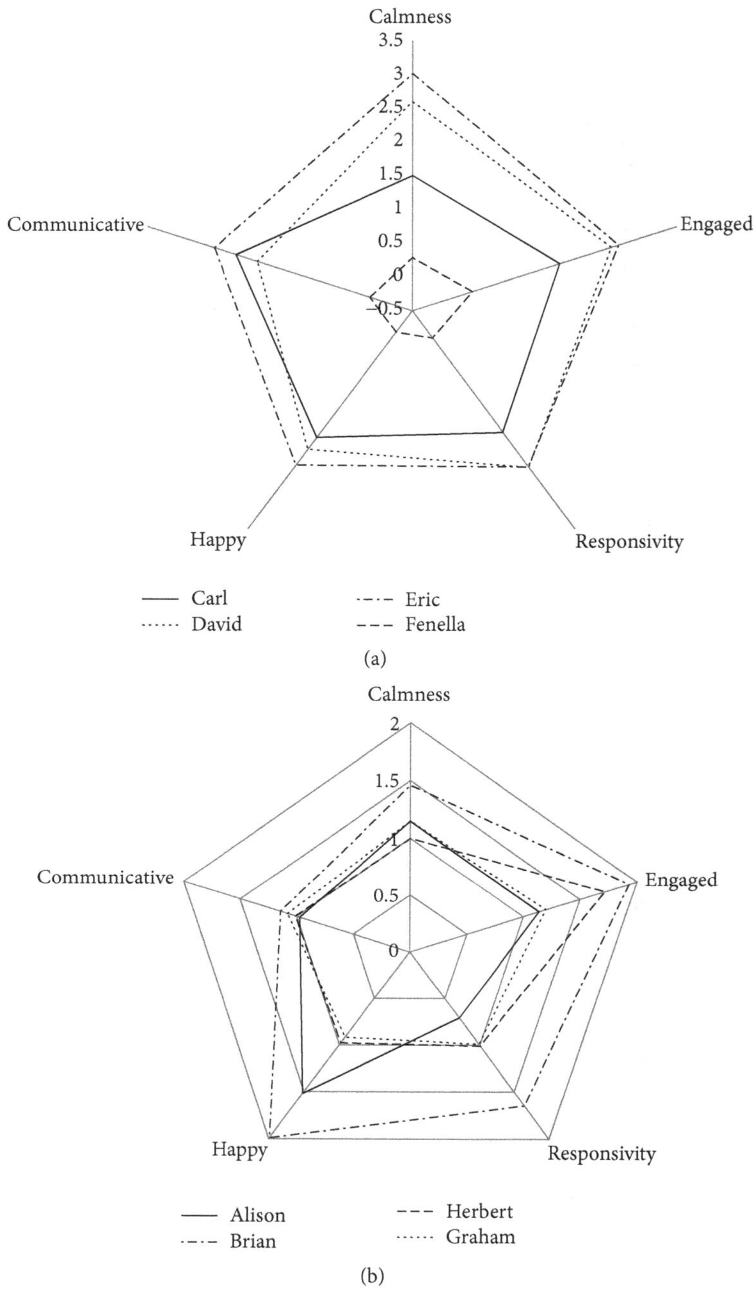

FIGURE 1: Radar plot of mean change in five rating scales (happy, communicative, calmness, engaged(-ness), and responsivity) for each of the eight participants. The radar plot shows the 5 ratings for each participant, such that the distance from the centre (at which point the change in rating scale = −0.5, i.e., a deterioration) indicates the magnitude of the changes. If every participant made an equal improvement the shapes would be regular pentagons. Rating scales are designed to display positive values for improved functioning in that domain.

particular group of participants would have reacted to more intrusive measures of response such as galvanic skin response or heart rate monitoring, the development of small wearable monitors offers the potential for still further refinements.

In summary, our study has demonstrated that stimulating skin pressure sensory systems seems to benefit most of a population of young people with autism and severe intellectual disability on whom it was trialled. Importantly, not all participants benefit to the same extent, which suggests that more research is needed to define the populations who might find it most effective.

Additional Points

Deep pressure benefits most participants to a statistically significant degree. The variability in individual responses indicates that deep pressure should be tailored to the individual needs of the recipient. Deep pressure seems to have benefits in many areas for most people, but individual responses must be considered in the design of future research.

Competing Interests

The authors declare that they have no competing interests.

Acknowledgments

The authors are grateful to the many school staff who recorded information about the young people before and after deep pressure sessions. Ms. Bestbier passed away after a short illness in December 2016. This paper is dedicated to her memory.

References

[1] K. E. Krauss, "The effects of deep pressure touch on anxiety," *The American Journal of Occupational Therapy*, vol. 41, no. 6, pp. 366–373, 1987.

[2] R. Lang, M. O'Reilly, O. Healy et al., "Sensory integration therapy for autism spectrum disorders: a systematic review," *Research in Autism Spectrum Disorders*, vol. 6, no. 3, pp. 1004–1018, 2012.

[3] A. A. Owen-Smith, S. Bent, F. L. Lynch et al., "Prevalence and predictors of complementary and alternative medicine use in a large insured sample of children with Autism Spectrum Disorders," *Research in Autism Spectrum Disorders*, vol. 17, pp. 40–51, 2015.

[4] M. Losinski, S. A. Sanders, and N. M. Wiseman, "Examining the use of deep touch pressure to improve the educational performance of students with disabilities: a meta-analysis," *Research and Practice for Persons with Severe Disabilities*, vol. 41, no. 1, pp. 3–18, 2016.

[5] A. J. Ayres, *Sensory Integration and Learning Disorders*, Western Psychological Services, Los Angeles, Calif, USA, 1972.

[6] T. Grandin and M. Scariano, *Emergence: Labeled Autistic*, Arena Press, Novato, Calif, USA, 1986.

[7] H.-Y. Chen, H. Yang, H.-J. Chi, and H.-M. Chen, "Physiological effects of deep touch pressure on anxiety alleviation: the weighted blanket approach," *Journal of Medical and Biological Engineering*, vol. 33, no. 5, pp. 463–470, 2013.

[8] J. Case-Smith, L. L. Weaver, and M. A. Fristad, "A systematic review of sensory processing interventions for children with autism spectrum disorders," *Autism*, vol. 19, no. 2, pp. 133–148, 2015.

[9] F. W. Yunus, K. P. Y. Liu, M. Bissett, and S. Penkala, "Sensory-based intervention for children with behavioral problems: a systematic review," *Journal of Autism and Developmental Disorders*, vol. 45, no. 11, pp. 3565–3579, 2015.

[10] S. Blairs, S. Slater, and D. J. Hare, "The clinical application of deep touch pressure with a man with autism presenting with severe anxiety and challenging behaviour," *British Journal of Learning Disabilities*, vol. 35, no. 4, pp. 214–220, 2007.

[11] S. Weeks, K. Boshoff, and H. Stewart, "Systematic review of the effectiveness of the Wilbarger protocol with children," *Pediatric Health, Medicine and Therapeutics*, no. 3, pp. 79–89, 2012.

[12] S. M. Edelson, M. G. Edelson, D. C. R. Kerr, and T. Grandin, "Behavioral and physiological effects of deep pressure on children with autism: a pilot study evaluating the efficacy of Grandin's Hug Machine," *American Journal of Occupational Therapy*, vol. 53, no. 2, pp. 145–152, 1999.

[13] A. A. McGinnis, E. Q. Blakely, A. C. Harvey, A. C. Hodges, and J. B. Rickards, "The behavioral effects of a procedure used by pediatric occupational therapists," *Behavioral Interventions*, vol. 28, no. 1, pp. 48–57, 2013.

[14] E. Schopler, *Psychoeducational Profile: PEP-3; TEACCH Individualized Psychoeducational Assessment for Children with Autism Spectrum Disorders*, Pro-Ed, Austin, Tex, USA, 2005.

[15] Department for Education, *Performance—P Scale—Attainment Targets for Pupils with Special Educational Needs*, Department for Education, London, UK, 2014.

[16] R. A. Stern, J. E. Arruda, C. R. Hooper, G. D. Wolfner, and C. E. Morey, "Visual analogue mood scales to measure internal mood state in neurologically impaired patients: Description and initial validity evidence," *Aphasiology*, vol. 11, no. 1, pp. 59–71, 1997.

[17] R. I. Parker, K. J. Vannest, J. L. Davis, and S. B. Sauber, "Combining nonoverlap and trend for single-case research: Tau-U," *Behavior Therapy*, vol. 42, no. 2, pp. 284–299, 2011.

[18] A. E. Lane, R. L. Young, A. E. Z. Baker, and M. T. Angley, "Sensory processing subtypes in autism: association with adaptive behavior," *Journal of Autism and Developmental Disorders*, vol. 40, no. 1, pp. 112–122, 2010.

[19] A. E. Kazdin, *Single-Case Research Designs: Methods for Clinical and Applied Settings*, Oxford University Press, 2011.

[20] R. C. Schaaf, T. W. Benevides, D. Kelly, and Z. Mailloux-Maggio, "Occupational therapy and sensory integration for children with autism: a feasibility, safety, acceptability and fidelity study," *Autism*, vol. 16, no. 3, pp. 321–327, 2012.

[21] J. Rojahn, J. L. Matson, D. Lott, A. J. Esbensen, and Y. Smalls, "The behavior problems inventory: an instrument for the assessment of self-injury, stereotyped behavior, and aggression/destruction in individuals with developmental disabilities," *Journal of Autism and Developmental Disorders*, vol. 31, no. 6, pp. 577–588, 2001.

20

Information Management for the Assistive Technology Provision in Community: Perspectives of Local Policymakers and Health Service Providers

Suchitporn Lersilp,[1] **Supawadee Putthinoi**,[1] **and Sayaka Okahashi**[2]

[1]*Department of Occupational Therapy, Faculty of Associated Medical Sciences, Chiang Mai University, Chiang Mai, Thailand*
[2]*Division of Occupational Therapy, Department of Human Health Sciences, Graduate School of Medicine, Kyoto University, Kyoto, Japan*

Correspondence should be addressed to Suchitporn Lersilp; suchitporn.l@cmu.ac.th

Academic Editor: Wendy B. Stav

Background. Assistive technology (AT) is a way to enhance the performance of daily activities in people with disabilities and help them live more independently. However, an important problem in providing AT lies in the effectiveness of information management. Local policymakers and health service providers have become aware of this problem and their perspectives are the key to solving it. *Methods.* This study explored the types of AT provided for people with disabilities in the community and the perspectives on information management of local policymakers and health service providers. A survey checklist and semistructured in-depth interview were the instruments of this study. The key informants in this study included administrators, nurses, and physical therapists from four community areas in Chiang Mai, Thailand. *Results.* The medical records showed that the types of AT provided were mostly second-hand (57.24%) and borrowed devices (57.73%). All of them were low-tech devices (crutch, cane, walker, wheelchair, and adaptive tricycle). In addition, the results indicated three perspective aspects related to information management: (1) problems in the database recording system, (2) different policies and processes of information management, and (3) improvement of the AT provision system. *Conclusion.* The perspectives of local policymakers and health service providers indicated related problems, impacts of policies, and ways to improve the AT provision system by applying information technology.

1. Introduction

Information management is essential for a successful community and district health system, where the information from local, national, and other available resources is linked. District health systems for primary health care are concerned with health systems management and other sectors such as health care service providers, district health managers, and agencies [1]. Willem and Buelens [2] suggested that information from other units can provide interunit knowledge sharing to enhance a positive organizational outcome. Management of information from one or more sources in community health at the district health level is useful for both community and national policy. Information in the community helps the health service providers and public health officials direct the community in meeting its needs. Village health volunteers (VHVs) in Thailand are key persons in gathering data on community resources for national policy, and community-based resource management requires information from many different related groups such as community hospitals, local governments, and village health volunteers. The information from each group is used for support in qualifying disability rights and making decisions in providing direct and indirect services and disability benefits. Jokandan et al. [3] showed that Information and Communication Technology (ICT) had heavy impact on the formality of municipal and urban management as well as all employees. ICT functions are able to manage the complex information of community health services and provide assistive technology (AT) in community contexts. Thus, this study aimed to explore the information process among the people at the community level.

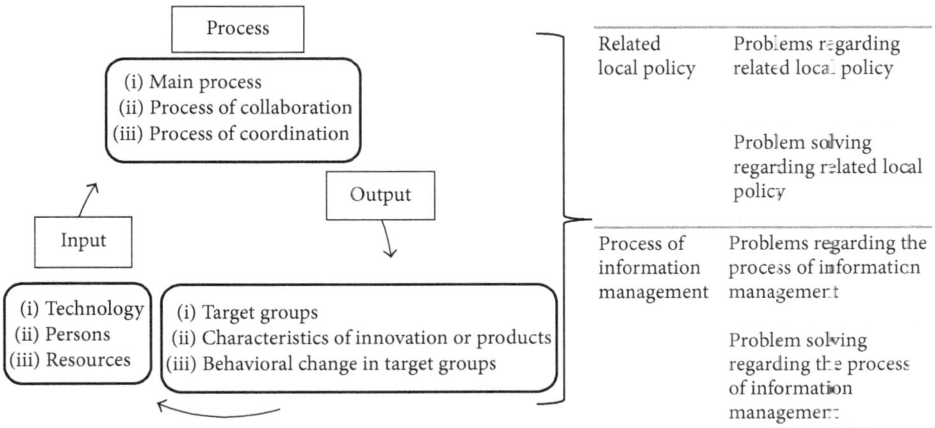

FIGURE 1: The information management system in community health at the district health level.

Assistive technology (AT) includes adaptive and assistive devices that enable improved performance in living independently for people with disabilities. AT not only impacts these people directly, but also could provide caregivers with immediate relief, reduced stress, and help in providing care more easily and safely [4]. Mann et al. [5] found that AT and home modifications can reduce home care costs.

Many countries have laws and legislations regarding AT: for example, Bausch and Hasselbring [6] reported that types of AT and related services were regulated many years ago in the Individuals with Disabilities Act Amendments PL 105-17 (USA). However, many studies reported that people with disabilities could not use the technologies because of the time it takes to learn, train in, and practice their use, and some clients refused to use them. Besides the problem of use, the provision of AT is an important issue for people with disabilities in the community. Indeed, some communities receive a great deal of AT from the government and through donations, while many communities lack some types of the technology. Different situations create various problems; for example, some communities have maintenance and storage problems, while others lack AT. A main cause of this situation is the need for an information management system or an incomplete one. Based on the concept of "access for all," AT could make an important contribution to the care of dependent people, such as those with disabilities, children with special needs, and elderly people in institutions and at home. This could be carried out by video-monitoring, remote health monitoring, electronic sensors, assistive devices, and adaptive equipment [7]. Cooper et al. [8] pointed out that not only modern or high technologies, but also problem trends in developing AT are related to ineffective delivery systems, changes to public policy, and coordination among people with disabilities, policymakers, manufacturers, researchers, and service providers. These concerns highlight the current ineffectiveness of AT. Ocepek et al. [9] reported that using AT improved quality of life in the majority of the participants. AT was recommended to the user mostly by a general practitioner or consultant physician, nurse, specialist, or relatives, as there are no AT specialists in community hospitals or community healthcare centers. As medical teams or a public health team carry out work in the municipality, the information management system providing AT is recorded in medical or informal records that are difficult to locate. For these reasons, this study explored the types of AT and perspectives of local policymakers and health service providers on information management in providing AT for people with disabilities in the community.

2. Materials and Methods

This study used quantitative and qualitative research methods in four community areas in Chiang Mai, Thailand. A survey checklist explored the types of AT provided for people with disability in the community, and a semistructured in-depth interview was used to study the perspectives of local policymakers and health service providers.

A survey method was planned and processed for the objective of exploring types of AT provided for people with disabilities in the community. Information was collected during 2015 and 2016 from secondary sources of data in the medical and informal records of community hospitals and subdistrict municipalities in four community areas of Chiang Mai province, Thailand. In addition, a semistructured in-depth interview was administered for the objective of studying the perspectives of local policymakers and health service providers on information management in providing AT for people with disabilities in the community. This objective applied to the information management system in community health at the district health level [10] in order to create the scope of the interview as shown in Figure 1.

Probing questions comprised four points as follows:

(1) Related local policy of AT provision for people with disabilities in the community

(2) Problems and problem solving regarding related local policy of AT provision for people with disabilities in the community

(3) Process of information management regarding AT provision for people with disabilities in the community

TABLE 1: AT provision information collected from community hospitals (2015, 2016).

Information	Number	Percentage
Type of AT		
Crutch	80	27.59
Cane	80	27.59
Walker	69	23.79
Wheelchair	57	19.66
Adaptive tricycle	4	1.38
Total	*290*	*100.00*
Category of AT		
Second-hand device	166	57.24
New device	124	42.76
Total	*290*	*100.00*
Way of provision		
Borrowed	167	57.59
Disability benefits	123	42.41
Total	*290*	*100.00*

(4) Problems and problem solving regarding the process of information management regarding AT provision for people with disabilities in the community

There were 16 key informants in this study comprising 10 administrators of subdistrict municipalities and 6 health service providers, including nurses, physical therapists, and community-developers of local community hospitals in four community areas in Chiang Mai, Thailand. They were interviewed and recorded individually. Data from interviewing were analyzed by content analysis.

3. Results and Discussion

The results showed that all four community areas did not have a database management system of AT provision, which was recorded in the hospitals' general medical records for 2015 and 2016. It was found that 289 people with disability were provided with AT in the four community areas. The results showed that 55.71% and 44.29% were female and male, respectively. Besides gender, there was no other personal information in the database of these people. In addition, the types of AT provided were mostly second-hand (57.24%) and borrowed devices (57.59%). One person was provided with two AT devices, a walker and cane; therefore, the number of AT devices was greater than that of people with disabilities. All of the devices were low-tech such as a crutch, cane, walker, wheelchair, and an adaptive tricycle, as shown in Table 1.

In addition, the results indicated three perspective aspects related to the information management system that emerged from the local policymakers and health service providers. The first aspect was a problem in database records, including lack of a type of AT system, lack of personal and disability information of clients receiving AT, and an incomplete system of lending and returning AT. The second aspect was the policy and process of different organizations. There are three main related organizations providing AT; the local community hospital, district hospital, and subdistrict municipality. Policies of the local community and district hospital come under the Provincial Health Office. On the other hand, those of the subdistrict municipality come from the mayor. Therefore, there are different policies and processes of information management regarding AT provision. The local community hospital has a system of finding people in the community who need AT, assessing which AT meets their needs, coordinating with district hospitals for receiving AT, and providing AT directly to the people, as well as participating in home visit teams with the district hospital and subdistrict municipality. District hospitals that participate in home visit teams with the subdistrict municipality directly provide evaluation, training, and repair of AT (both new and used) and issue certificates of disabilities. Subdistrict municipalities register people with disabilities in the community in order to provide living allowance, home visits, and coordination with the provincial hospital or disability center that receives AT. The last aspect was improvement of the AT provision system. The local policymakers and health service providers pointed out the importance of a lending system, which is a way to manage and exchange second-hand AT between communities. Furthermore, they indicated that when the lending system is linked between communities, the information management system and resource sharing occur, as well as an increase in the efficiency of services for the people in the community. In addition, they also thought of setting up the AT center in the community, as a hub of sharing information, demonstrating, evaluating, training and repairing AT, and modifying the home for independent living. Moreover, the AT specialists provide services that help to decrease waiting times and transportation or traveling costs (as it is extremely difficult for some clients to get to and from the hospital). Content analysis of these perspectives is shown in Figure 2.

The findings indicated that the types of AT provided in the community were low-tech and used for the purpose of mobility. These findings were related to Putthinoi et al. [11] in that AT homes of the elderly were assistive products and technology for personal use in daily living, indoor-outdoor mobility, and transportation. This was because the legal rights of people with disabilities in Thailand are still limited by government budgets. Low-tech AT devices are inexpensive, simple to make, and easily obtainable for all [12]. This result relates to Lersilp [13], who indicated that although there was a related regulation and an assistive technology provision system in each university, many types of assistive technologies were not used, and some were not even received.

Furthermore, these findings were fundamental to the design of an effective information management system by applying information technology in providing AT for people with disabilities in the community. According to the above results, it was found that the database records on providing AT in community hospitals and subdistrict municipalities were recorded in informal notebooks and did not contain any personal information, except for name and gender. This was because the community hospitals and subdistrict municipalities were not responsible for providing AT directly. Community hospitals have the role of a hybrid health service, including health promotion, disease prevention and control,

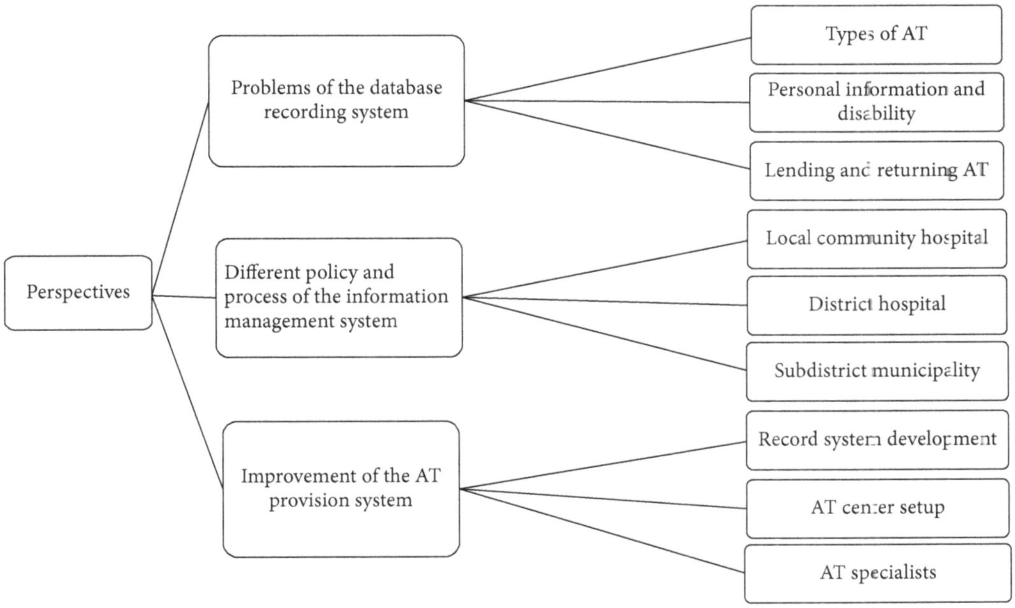

FIGURE 2: Perspectives of local policymakers and health service providers on information management in providing AT in the community.

medical treatment, rehabilitation, and health risk factor management [14]. AT provision is a part of rehabilitation; therefore, no AT specialist or specific AT officer is responsible for the database recording system in community hospitals.

The results above show that communities incur problems of the database recording system and related policy. According to Lersilp et al. [15], this information shows that a major problem in the provision and use of AT was the criteria of educational policy. When developed countries are considered in similar contexts, Japan is a good model of AT provision, as the rental system is an interesting AT provision system in that country. After hospital discharge, people or local residents usually start using AT rental services under Long-Term Care Insurance, which came into force in 2000. Approximately 67% of these people receive advice from a care manager and about 68% select AT rental agencies near their home through the "care manager advisory," usually without comparing prices. People pay only 10% of the rental charge under Long-Term Care Insurance. Although prices are not the same between agencies, they are often within the standard price area [16].

The charge in this system can be determined freely for some products by each AT rental agency. Wholesale AT rental agencies are responsible for profit and general, distribution, and maintenance costs; consecutively, while "in-house" or retail rental agencies are responsible for maintenance cost, profit, and general and distribution costs, consecutively. Sometimes people buy their own AT according to specific needs, while considering the rental charge per month, purchase price, frequency of everyday use, and so on. Unfortunately, there are no good websites such as "comparison shopping websites" providing comprehensive information that shows comparisons of specific AT rental charges or purchases prices [17, 18].

Care managers, who are under Long-Term Care Insurance, play an important role in managing each person's future plan of care/rehabilitation service and AT rental according to the severity of disability. However, it is possible that they only have information on AT depending on their own specialty (e.g., nurse and dentist). Important information includes not only the rental details, but also AT safety, especially physical safety after long-term use. Some cases indicated the need for AT that had been discontinued. The AT business model should be considered in terms of the AT distribution system. Manufacturers of AT mainly contact rental agencies without having information of individual users, thus making it difficult for the former to understand user needs [16–18]. An AT supply system set up by the medical and welfare combination team will be needed to solve these problems.

Regarding Japanese Occupational therapists, there are 47 branches of the Japan Association of Occupational Therapists in all prefectures of Japan. Thirty-four of them have had the "AT advice system" since July 2014 to support occupational therapists who have problems with AT matching/adaptation for their patients. Several occupational therapists, who have specialized in AT, are registered as mentors in each branch, and inexperienced occupational therapists can communicate with them whenever necessary. It is important to set up both a hard and soft AT supply system in the aging community [17, 18].

4. Conclusion

This study explored the types of AT provided for people with disabilities in the community and the perspectives on information management of local policymakers and health service providers. Results showed that 289 people with disabilities were provided with AT in the study areas. The types of AT provided were mostly second-hand and borrowed devices. All of them were low-tech such as a crutch, cane, walker, wheelchair, and an adaptive tricycle. However, it was found that the hospitals' general medical records of information on AT provision were incomplete in the AT database and contained no personal information of people receiving AT. The local policymakers and health service providers reflected three perspective aspects related to the information management system such as problems of the database recording system, different policies and processes of the information management system, and improvement of the AT provision system. These findings were fundamental to the development of an effective information management system providing AT for people with disabilities in the community by applying information technology.

Conflicts of Interest

The authors declare no conflicts of interest regarding the publication of this paper.

Acknowledgments

This research was supported by a grant from the International College of Digital Innovation, Chiang Mai University, under the ASEAN+3 Cross Border Research Project.

References

[1] World Health Organization, *District Health Facilities: Guidelines for Development and Operations*, World Health Organization: the Regional Office for the Western Pacific, Manila, Philippines, 1998.

[2] A. Willem and M. Buelens, "Knowledge sharing in inter-unit cooperative episodes: The impact of organizational structure dimensions," *International Journal of Information Management*, vol. 29, no. 2, pp. 151–160, 2009.

[3] A. D. Jokandan, M. Fattahi, and S. F. Ghane, "Examining the role of information and communication technology in the organizational structure of the QaemShahr municipality," *International Journal on Leadership*, vol. 4, pp. 493–501, 2015.

[4] L. N. Gitlin, W. Mann, M. Tomit, and S. M. Marcus, "Factors associated with home environmental problems among community-living older people," *Disability and Rehabilitation*, vol. 23, no. 17, pp. 777–787, 2001.

[5] W. Mann, K. Ottenbacher, L. Fraas, M. Tomita, and C. Granger, "Effectiveness of assistive technology and environmental interventions in maintaining independence and reducing home care costs for frail elderly: a randomized controlled trial," *Archives of Family Medicine*, vol. 8, no. 3, pp. 210–217, 1999.

[6] M. E. Bausch and T. S. Hasselbring, "Assistive Technology: Are the Necessary Skills and Knowledge Being Developed at the Preservice and Inservice Levels?" *Teacher Education and Special Education*, vol. 27, no. 2, pp. 97–104, 2004.

[7] F. G. Miskelly, "Assistive technology in elderly care," *Age and Ageing*, vol. 30, no. 6, pp. 455–458, 2001.

[8] R. A. Cooper, R. Cooper, and M. L. Boninger, "Trends and issues in wheelchair technologies," *Assistive Technology*, vol. 20, no. 2, pp. 61–72, 2008.

[9] J. Ocepek, Z. Prosič, and G. Vidmar, "Assistive Technology and Its Role among the Elderly – a Survey," *Informatica Medica Slovenica*, vol. 17, no. 2, 2012.

[10] T. Yana and R. Sirapanichkul, *Manual of Community Health System Development*, Sahamitr Printing and Publishing Company, Bangkok, Thailand, 2015.

[11] S. Putthinoi, S. Lersilp, and N. Chakpitak, "Home Features and Assistive Technology for the Home-Bound Elderly in a Thai Suburban Community by Applying the International Classification of Functioning, Disability, and Health," *Journal of Aging Research*, vol. 2017, Article ID 2865960, 2017.

[12] A. M. Cook and S. M. Hussey, *Assistive Technologies: Principles and Practices*, Mosby, Missouri, USA, 2nd edition, 2002.

[13] T. Lersilp, "Access to information for learning by using assistive technology for undergraduate students with disabilities in Northern Thailand," *Information (Switzerland)*, vol. 7, no. 4, article no. 54, 2016.

[14] C. Supawong, S. Chunharat, L. Damrikarnlerd, S. Sriwanichakorn, K. Wechsutranon, and S. Sirilak, *Service Providing Manual of Community Hospital*, TAP co. ltd, Bangkok, Thailand, 2009.

[15] S. Lersilp, S. Putthinoi, and N. Chakpitak, "Model of Providing Assistive Technologies in Special Education Schools," *Global Journal of Health Science*, vol. 8, no. 1, pp. 36–44, 2016.

[16] Ministry of Health, Labour and Welfare. Long-term Care Insurance in Japan. 2002. Available online: http://www.mhlw.go.jp/english/topics/elderly/care/.

[17] T. Fujiwara, "Assistive devices consultation support system," *Journal of the Osaka Occupational Therapy Association*, vol. 28, no. 2, pp. 122–124, 2015.

[18] K. M. Marasinghe, J. M. Lapitan, and A. Ross, "Assistive technologies for ageing populations in six low-income and middle-income countries: A systematic review," *BMJ Innovations*, vol. 1, no. 4, pp. 182–195, 2015.

Sensory Overresponsivity, Loneliness, and Anxiety in Taiwanese Adults with Autism Spectrum Disorder

Ya-Cing Syu[1] and Ling-Yi Lin[1,2]

[1]Department of Occupational Therapy, College of Medicine, National Cheng Kung University, Tainan, Taiwan
[2]Institute of Allied Health Sciences, College of Medicine, National Cheng Kung University, Tainan, Taiwan

Correspondence should be addressed to Ling-Yi Lin; lingyi@mail.ncku.edu.tw

Academic Editor: Erna I. Blanche

Purpose. Sensory overresponsiveness is highly prevalent in individuals with autism spectrum disorders (ASD) and typically persist into adulthood. However, the role of sensory processing difficulties in influencing emotional well-being among adults with ASD remains unclear. Additionally, the associations between sensory overresponsiveness, anxiety, and loneliness are yet to be examined among adults with ASD. Therefore, to address these critical gaps in the literature, we aimed to investigate the relationships among sensory avoiding, anxiety, and loneliness in a sample of adults with ASD. *Participants.* Seventy adults (age, 20–39 years) completed three self-reported measures. All participants had a documented diagnosis of ASD and had normal IQ. *Methods.* Sensory processing, loneliness, and anxiety were assessed with the Adult Sensory Profile, short-form UCLA loneliness scale, and Beck Anxiety Inventory, respectively. *Results.* Autism spectrum traits and sensory avoiding were associated with anxiety and loneliness. Participants who experienced sensory avoiding more frequently reported higher anxiety and feelings of loneliness, with loneliness mediating the relationship between sensory avoiding and anxiety. More anxiety symptoms in participants with greater sensory avoiding were associated with their higher level of loneliness. *Conclusion.* This study demonstrates that the relationships existed between sensory processing difficulties, loneliness, and anxiety among adults with ASD. Interventions regarding sensory processing difficulties and emotional well-being are substantial need for adults with ASD, and our results highlight the importance of sensory overresponsiveness and anxiety in evaluating and improving the psychological well-being of adults with ASD.

1. Introduction

Autism spectrum disorder (ASD) is a developmental disorder characterized by problems with communication and social interaction and repetitive body movements or behaviors [1]. Atypical sensory processing is considered a core feature of ASD, and sensory features (hyperactivity or hypoactivity or unusual interest to sensory input) have been included in the criteria for ASD in the fifth edition of the *Diagnostic and Statistical Manual of Mental Disorders* [1].

People experience and process the sensory stimuli from the environment and the body itself continually. Dunn constructed a model using the relationship between neuroscience and behavior concepts to illustrate the way that people manage, process the stimuli, and elicit responses [2]. Every individual has a unique sensory processing pattern [3]. Individual responses to sensory inputs present as a bell-shaped distribution, with most of the people exhibiting moderate responses to sensory stimuli and few people responding more or less intensively [3]. Not all the stimuli can produce responses; the stimuli have to exceed the neurological threshold to activate the nerve cells or the nervous system [3]. With low neurological thresholds, people frequently sense most of the stimuli and trigger the response; on the contrary, people with high neurological thresholds will often overlook the stimuli that others may notice [3]. Another critical construct is the behavior pattern that people perform after they take in and process the sensory inputs [2]. A person may use a passive or active self-regulatory strategy reacting to the things happening around them [3].

Using the interaction of neurological threshold continuum and behavior response continuum, Dunn introduced the four quadrants of sensory processing patterns, including low registration, sensory seeking, sensory sensitivity, and sensory avoiding [2].

According to Dunn's model [3], low registration refers to a passive behavioral response pattern (unable to detect the stimuli that most other individuals have noticed) that is related to a high neurological threshold (require more intense sensory stimuli inputs to generate a response). Sensory seeking refers to an active behavioral response pattern (actively searching or seeking for sensory stimuli) that is related to a high neurological threshold. Sensory sensitivity refers to a passive behavioral response pattern that is related to a low neurological threshold (requires lower magnitude sensory stimuli inputs to generate a response). Individuals in this category may exhibit unpleasant feelings or negative reactions to certain sensory stimuli. Sensory avoidance refers to an active behavioral response pattern that is related to a low neurological threshold. Individuals in this category may establish their own routines or ritual behaviors to reduce their exposure to stimuli [3].

Additionally, Miller et al. [4] indicated that sensory sensitivity and sensory avoiding are two types of sensory overresponsivity patterns. Brown and Dunn [5] and Pfeiffer et al. [6] hypothesized that individuals who overrespond to sensory stimuli have low neurological thresholds, such that minimal stimuli provoke a strong reaction. Thus, sensory overresponsivity refers to an exaggerated or negative response to sensory stimuli. Individuals may experience unpleasant feelings or pain and may perform avoidance or hypervigilance behaviors [4].

Unusual sensory processing negatively influences the daily lives of people with ASD. For example, sensory overresponsivity was highly correlated with sleep problems in children and adolescents with ASD [7, 8]. Another study that looked at sensory processing patterns in higher education students with ASD reported that auditory sensitivity might affect the student's ability to absorb information in a study environment [9]. Students also described sensory preferences related to their choice of leisure activity and social life, and these were linked to lower levels of social skills and adaptive behavior [9]. Pfeiffer et al. [6] found that hypersensitivity was inversely associated with community use and social skills in children and adolescents with Asperger's disorder.

Sensory overresponsivity is common in children and adolescents with ASD. It has been linked to higher levels of anxiety [6, 10, 11] and together with anxiety predicts an increasing number of gastrointestinal problems [12]. Although ASD is a lifelong condition persisting into adulthood, most studies have focused on the pediatric population. Only few studies that included adults with ASD have shown that sensory overresponsivity persists into adulthood [9, 13]. Sensory overresponsivity is prevalent in adulthood and is present in each sensory modality (vision, hearing, touch, smell, taste, and proprioception) among adults with ASD [13]. Moreover, previous findings suggest that overresponsiveness to sensory stimuli is correlated with psychological well-being in children [6, 7, 12, 14]. However, little is known about this issue in adults with ASD, and, therefore, it warrants further investigation.

Anxiety is one of the most common psychiatric symptoms in adults with ASD. According to a recent report, autistic adults are more likely to have an anxiety disorder and behavioral challenges [15]. There is growing interest in the relationship between sensory overresponsivity and anxiety in this population. It has been observed that sensory overresponsivity emerges before anxiety and positively predicts the subsequent increasing levels of anxiety in toddlers with ASD [14]. Similarly, another study found a strong, positive association between anxiety and sensory overresponsivity in children with ASD, but not adults [12]. Although the underlying mechanism that connects sensory overresponsivity to anxiety is not understood, individuals with low neurological thresholds may be uncomfortable with sensory stimuli from the surroundings, which might induce feelings of unease, worry, or anxiety.

Another problematic condition associated with anxiety in ASD is loneliness. Loneliness is a subjective and negative experience and may affect an individual's self-esteem, social functioning, and mental and physical health. Individuals with ASD may face social isolation because of their difficulties with social skills, leading to deeper feelings of loneliness. Many studies have explored the connection between loneliness and external factors, such as friendship and social support; however, research on the association of loneliness and mental health problems in adults with ASD is limited. Evidence suggests that loneliness correlates with increased depression and anxiety in adults with ASD, even after controlling for the effect of ASD symptoms. This suggests that loneliness may be a consequence of social deficits or negative emotional well-being [16].

Considering the high proportion of sensory overresponsivity and anxiety in individuals with ASD, it is logical to speculate that the relationship between sensory overresponsivity and anxiety also manifests in adults with ASD. Adults with ASD who have sensory avoiding or sensory sensitivity may feel overwhelmed by the sensory stimuli, resulting in aggressive or negative reactions. These extreme sensory-responsive patterns may negatively affect the experience of interacting with others or the environment, further elevating feelings of loneliness [17]. Loneliness as a potential mediator might be related to the higher level of anxiety [18, 19]. Compared to Western countries, individuals in Eastern countries are more likely to feel lonely because they pay more attention to interpersonal bonds and their existing social network [20]. Thus, sensory processing and loneliness may result in negative emotional well-being in this population, but critical gaps exist in the literature about this issue, which the current study seeks to address. The present study is aimed at exploring relationships between sensory processing, loneliness, and anxiety in a sample of adults with ASD.

2. Materials and Methods

2.1. Procedures. The principal investigator has obtained the Institutional Review Board of National Cheng Kung University Hospital approval for the research (A-BR-101-074).

We recruited adults with ASD from the local autism groups and organizations. The principal investigator explained all study procedures to the participants. Written informed consent was gathered from all participants.

2.2. Participants. The sample size for a linear multiple regression was estimated using G*Power (version 3.1.2) [21]. With a medium effect size ($f^2 = 0.15$), an alpha of 0.05, a test power of 0.80, and two predictors, the minimum sample size would be 68 participants to achieve adequate power. The statistical power was 0.81.

The characteristics of study participants are presented in Table 1. Participants were adults with ASD ($n = 70$, 46 men and 24 women; mean age: 27.8 years; range: 20–39 years). All participants had a documented diagnosis of ASD by a registered psychiatrist. Individuals had been diagnosed with pervasive developmental disorders using the DSM-IV-TR criteria [22] of autistic disorder, Asperger's disorder, or pervasive developmental disorder not otherwise specified should be diagnosed with ASD [1]. The principal investigator reviewed the disability certificates issued by Taiwan Department of Social Welfare to confirm diagnosis of ASD. The exclusion criterion was marked intellectual disabilities (IQ < 70). To determine participants' reading and writing skills, we asked them to read a newspaper paragraph and then immediately write five of the words they had read. All participants with ASD could read and write Mandarin Chinese.

Table 1: Demographic characteristics.

Characteristics	Mean ± SD or n (%)	Median	Range
Gender			
Male	46 (65.7%)		
Female	24 (34.3%)		
Age (years), mean ± SD	27.8 ± 5.0	27.0	20–39
Autism spectrum quotient	32.9 ± 6.0	34.0	20–43
Social skills	7.0 ± 2.3	7.0	2–10
Attention switching	6.9 ± 1.7	7.0	3–9
Attention to detail	6.3 ± 1.9	6.0	2–10
Communication	6.5 ± 1.8	6.0	1–10
Imagination	6.3 ± 1.6	6.0	1–9
Educational level			
High school and below	16 (22.9%)		
College and above	54 (77.1%)		
Employed	33 (47.1%)		
Marital status: single	70 (100%)		
Comorbid psychiatric disorders	15 (21.4%)		
Sensation sensitivity	43.2 ± 9.7	43	22–67
Sensation avoidance	45.9 ± 8.2	44	33–69
Sensation seeking	43.6 ± 8.1	44	27–64
Low registration	41.6 ± 8.6	43	23–66
Anxiety	21.2 ± 11.9	20	2–43
Loneliness	21.9 ± 4.9	22	11–31

2.3. Measures

2.3.1. Sensory Profile. The Chinese version of the Adult Sensory Profile, which is reliable and valid, was used to examine patterns of sensory processing [23]. It consists of 60 items, which is divided into four quadrants of sensory processing: sensation seeking (an intensive craving for sensory stimuli), sensory sensitivity (overresponsive reactions to sensory input), sensation avoiding (a tendency to reduce stimulation), and low registration (a tendency to not notice everyday sensory events and to respond slowly to them). The score range for each quadrant is 15–75. Sensory overresponsive individuals are hypersensitive and tend to avoid certain sensations. In contrast, sensory-underresponsive individuals are hyposensitive and often engage in sensation-seeking behaviors. Higher scores indicate that certain sensory patterns occur more frequently than others.

2.3.2. Anxiety. The Beck Anxiety Inventory (BAI) was used for measuring the severity of anxiety [24]. The Chinese version has strong construct validity and an excellent reliability [25]. The BAI consists of 21 items that measure the severity of anxiety symptoms in adults. Participants were asked to answer the question "Did you feel anxious this past week?" using a scale of 0 to 3 (0 = "not at all," 3 = "severely"). The BAI consists of four factors: (1) neurophysiological; (2) subjective; (3) autonomic; and (4) panic. The scores range from 0 to 63, with higher scores indicating more severity of anxiety symptoms. The scores are categorized as follows: minimal level of anxiety (0–7), mild anxiety (8–15), moderate anxiety (16–25), and severe anxiety (26–63). On the Chinese version of the BAI, a cut-off score of 14 was used to discriminate between individuals with and without anxiety [25].

2.3.3. Loneliness. The short-form UCLA loneliness scale (ULS-8) assessed the extent of loneliness and social isolation. A total of 8 items were selected from the revised UCLA loneliness scale [26]. The ULS-8 demonstrates high internal reliability and good validity [27]. Each item was scored on a 4-point Likert scale ranging from 1 (never) to 4 (always). The scale generates loneliness score in the range of 8–32, with higher scores indicating higher degrees of loneliness and greater social isolation.

2.3.4. Autism Spectrum Quotient. The Taiwanese Chinese translation [28] of the autism spectrum quotient (AQ) [29] was used to quantify the autistic traits. The Chinese version demonstrates adequate test-retest reliability and validity [28]. The AQ contains 50 questions divided into five domains: social skills, communication, imagination, attention to detail, and attention switching. The scores range from 0 to 50, with higher scores indicating greater level of autistic traits.

2.3.5. Demographic Information. Participants were asked to report the demographic information including age, sex, comorbid psychiatric disorders, education, employment status, marital status, smoking habits, and drinking habits.

2.4. Data Analysis. SPSS 17.0 for Windows (SPSS Inc., Chicago, IL, USA) was used in the analysis of the demographic

TABLE 2: Intercorrelations of sensory processing, anxiety, and loneliness.

Variables	AQ	Sensation sensitivity	Sensation avoidance	Sensation seeking	Low registration	Anxiety	Loneliness
AQ	–						
Sensation sensitivity	0.221	–					
Sensation avoidance	0.008	0.709***	–				
Sensation seeking	−0.224	0.244*	0.291*	–			
Low registration	0.173	0.636***	0.517***	0.447***	–		
Anxiety	0.248*	0.217	0.302*	0.061	0.232	–	
Loneliness	0.381*	0.221	0.305*	−0.109	0.274*	0.501***	–

*$p < 0.05$, **$p < 0.01$, and ***$p < 0.001$. AQ = autism spectrum quotient.

data and outcome measures for the study variables. Normality was assessed using the Shapiro-Wilk test of normality. We performed Pearson's correlations and multivariate regression analysis to examine relationships between all variables. Statistical significance was set at $p < 0.05$.

3. Results

The mean (standard deviation [SD]) scores for the four sensory quadrants (sensory sensitivity, sensation avoiding, sensation seeking, and low registration) were 43.2 (9.7), 45.9 (8.2), 43.6 (8.1), and 41.6 (8.6), respectively. They scored in more than most people in the quadrants of sensation avoiding (35.7%), sensory sensitivity (27.1%), sensation seeking (22.9%), and low registration (21.4%). The mean (SD) score for anxiety was 21.2 (11.9). Using the cut-off score of 14, we determined that more than 70% of the participants (77.9%) reported moderate or severe level of anxiety. The mean (SD) score for loneliness was 21.9 (4.9) on the ULS-8, with about one-third of the participants (32.9%) having scores over 24. The Shapiro-Wilk normality test suggested that loneliness was normally distributed ($p = 0.083$). The median and the range of the three measures can be found in Table 1.

The correlation matrix for the study variables was used to evaluate relationships between study variables. There were significant correlations among sensory avoiding, anxiety, and loneliness (Table 2). A significant positive correlation was observed between sensory avoiding and anxiety, suggesting that participants reported greater anxiety when sensory avoiding occurred more frequently. Sensory avoiding was positively correlated with loneliness, such that the higher the level of reported sensory avoiding, the greater the severity of loneliness. Moreover, participants reported a greater anxiety severity when they experienced greater loneliness.

Separate multiple regression analysis models were applied to investigate whether the sensory processing and autism spectrum traits were associated with levels of anxiety and loneliness (Table 3). Regression analyses indicated that the autism spectrum traits ($\beta = .268$, $p = 0.039$) and sensory avoiding ($\beta = .362$, $p = 0.035$) were significant predictors of anxiety ($R^2 = 0.16$, $F(5, 64) = 2.50$, $p = 0.039$). Autism spectrum traits ($\beta = .345$, $p = 0.004$) and sensory avoiding ($\beta = .413, p = 0.009$) were significantly associated with loneliness ($R^2 = 0.29$, $F(5, 64) = 5.28$, $p < 0.001$).

TABLE 3: Multiple regressions of autism spectrum traits and sensory processing on anxiety and loneliness (standardized coefficients).

Variables	Anxiety	Loneliness
AQ	0.268*	0.345**
Sensation sensitivity	−0.163	−0.262
Sensation avoidance	0.362*	0.413**
Sensation seeking	0.012	−0.203
Low registration	0.097	0.258
R^2	0.16*	0.29***

*$p < 0.05$, **$p < 0.01$, and ***$p < 0.001$.

The method outlined by Hayes [30] was followed to examine whether loneliness was a mediating variable that accounts for the relationship between sensory avoiding and anxiety. This hypothesis was tested by a series of regression analysis. Sensory avoiding was significantly associated with loneliness and anxiety (Table 2). After controlling the relation between the loneliness and anxiety, the significant relationship between sensory avoiding and anxiety was reduced or became nonsignificant. A mediation effect would be supported. Figure 1 shows that loneliness was a mediator that accounts for the relationship between sensory avoiding and anxiety. Analyses using Sobel's test [31] indicated that the mediation effect was supported. This figure indicates that the higher level of anxiety in participants with greater sensory avoiding was mediating by their higher level of loneliness.

4. Discussion and Conclusion

The purpose of the present study was to investigate the relationship among sensory avoiding, anxiety, and loneliness in adults with ASD. The results indicate that in adults with ASD, more sensory avoiding was associated with higher reported anxiety and feelings of loneliness. In addition, loneliness served as a mediator between sensory avoiding and anxiety, indicating that adults with ASD reported high levels of anxiety if high sensory avoiding was accompanied by greater loneliness.

Consistent with previous research [13], sensory processing difficulties not only affect children with ASD but also persist into adulthood. In our sample, more than 25% of participants scored more than most people in the sensation

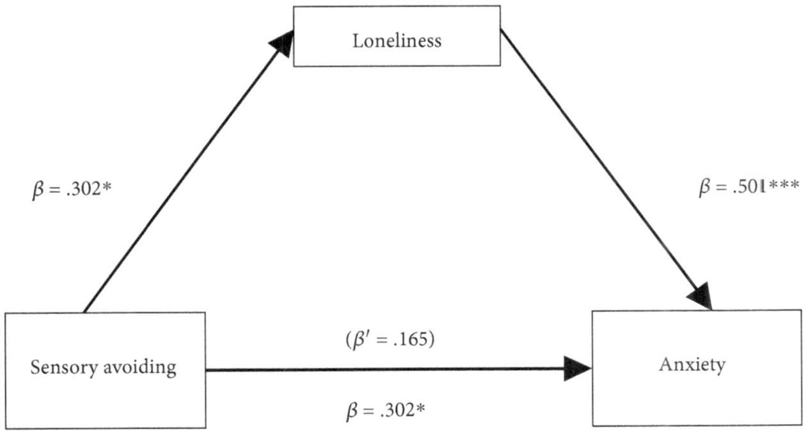

FIGURE 1: Results of testing for mediation by loneliness on relationship between sensory avoiding and anxiety. Note: $^*p < 0.05$, $^{***}p < 0.001$. β' referred to standardized coefficient after controlling for anxiety. Type of mediation = full, Sobel's z value = 2.178, $p = 0.0294$. Standardized coefficient of sensory avoiding on anxiety: direct = 0.165, indirect = 0.137.

avoiding and sensory sensitivity quadrants. This result is partially consistent with that of a study by Clince et al. [9], which revealed that adults with ASD scored higher than most people in the quadrants of sensory avoidance, sensory sensitivity, and low registration. However, contrary to our findings, their participants did not score more than most people in the sensation seeking quadrant. This discrepancy may be attributable to the age difference of the participants; the participants of the previous study were mostly 18–23 years old, whereas the average age of our participants was 28 years. The sensory feature may vary according to age, but this hypothesis warrants further investigation.

Adults with ASD who reported a higher level of sensory avoiding are also experiencing more feeling of loneliness in the present study. Furthermore, loneliness was a significant mediator of the relationship between sensory avoiding and anxiety. To our knowledge, no previous study has demonstrated that loneliness is a mediator of the relationship between sensory processing and anxiety. Our results extend the prior findings in children and adolescents to adults, with a more holistic view of psychological well-being [6, 12, 32]. It is possible that adults with ASD were sensitive to sensory stimuli, which may lead to them avoiding the sensory stimuli encountered in an environmental or social context, resulting in social isolation or loneliness. The negative experience may cause uncomfortable feelings or even anxiety when interacting with the environment or others [33]. Moreover, the lack of strategies for dealing with sensory processing difficulties could also affect their emotional status.

Increased anxiety was significantly associated with loneliness. Cumulative evidence indicates that loneliness has a negative effect on physical health and psychosocial well-being in the general population [34, 35]. The findings from studies of individuals with ASD are highly consistent [16, 32, 36]. Adults with ASD may be more prone to anxiety if they experience more sensory overresponsiveness and perceive greater loneliness. Thus, our results confirm that feelings of loneliness have considerable impacts on the psychosocial well-being of adults with ASD.

The present study does have some limitations. We only included adults with ASD with an IQ above 70, i.e., high-functioning adults with ASD. Due to the inclusion criteria, the percentage of participants with a college education is slightly high. This sample might not be representative of the general adult population with ASD. Additionally, because of the heterogeneity of ASD, the findings of our study may not apply to all adults with ASD. Further research with larger and more diverse sample size from a broader community is required to arrive at conclusions that are more generally applicable. Another limitation is that we only investigated the relationships among anxiety, loneliness, and sensory processing. Recent research reported that adults with ASD were less likely to have friends and more likely to live at home than adults without an ASD diagnosis [15]. Because social networks include family, peers, and friends, future research should consider the influence of external factors on loneliness, such as intimate relationships with others, amount of social support, depression, and living at home vs. living alone. Furthermore, the cross-sectional survey may exhibit bias. Future research should focus on the longitudinal effects of the sensory processing difficulties and emotional well-being of adults with ASD. Despite the limitation, the present findings have important implications for the evaluation of sensory issues and subsequent therapeutic interventions in adults with ASD.

To the best of our knowledge, this study is the first to investigate the relationships among sensory processing, loneliness, and anxiety in Taiwanese adults diagnosed with ASD. It is clinically important to consider the sensory components and emotional status of adults with ASD in their daily lives to effectively evaluate and improve their psychological well-being. Appropriate therapeutic interventions targeting sensory processing issues may have beneficial effects on loneliness and further reduce or prevent anxiety in adults with ASD. Further research should prospectively examine changes in sensory processing and emotional well-being by performing a longitudinal survey and also investigate the relationships among the sensory response and social and emotional functioning in greater detail.

Conflicts of Interest

The authors report no conflicts of interest.

Acknowledgments

Support for this research was provided by grant MSOT 102-2314-B-006-068 from the Taiwan Ministry of Science and Technology. We thank the individuals who participated in this research and the autism associations in Taiwan.

References

[1] American Psychiatric Association, *Diagnostic and Statistical Manual of Mental Disorders*, American Psychiatric Association, Washington, DC, USA, 5th edition, 2013.

[2] W. Dunn, "The impact of sensory processing abilities on the daily lives of young children and their families: a conceptual model," *Infants & Young Children*, vol. 9, no. 4, pp. 23–35, 1997.

[3] W. Dunn, "Supporting children to participate successfully in everyday life by using sensory processing knowledge," *Infants & Young Children*, vol. 20, no. 2, pp. 84–101, 2007.

[4] L. J. Miller, M. E. Anzalone, S. J. Lane, S. A. Cermak, and E. T. Osten, "Concept evolution in sensory integration: a proposed nosology for diagnosis," *American Journal of Occupational Therapy*, vol. 61, no. 2, pp. 135–140, 2007.

[5] C. Brown and W. Dunn, *Adolescent-Adult Sensory Profile: User's Manual*, Therapy Skill Builders, Tucson, AZ, USA, 2002.

[6] B. Pfeiffer, M. Kinnealey, C. Reed, and G. Herzberg, "Sensory modulation and affective disorders in children and adolescents with Asperger's disorder," *American Journal of Occupational Therapy*, vol. 59, no. 3, pp. 335–345, 2005.

[7] M. O. Mazurek and G. F. Petroski, "Sleep problems in children with autism spectrum disorder: examining the contributions of sensory over-responsivity and anxiety," *Sleep Medicine*, vol. 16, no. 2, pp. 270–279, 2015.

[8] S. Reynolds, S. J. Lane, and L. Thacker, "Sensory processing, physiological stress, and sleep behaviors in children with and without autism spectrum disorders," *OTJR: Occupation, Participation and Health*, vol. 32, no. 1, pp. 246–257, 2012.

[9] M. Clince, L. Connolly, and C. Nolan, "Comparing and exploring the sensory processing patterns of higher education students with attention deficit hyperactivity disorder and autism spectrum disorder," *American Journal of Occupational Therapy*, vol. 70, no. 2, pp. 7002250010p1–7002250010p9, 2015.

[10] M. Kinnealey and M. Fuiek, "The relationship between sensory defensiveness, anxiety, depression and perception of pain in adults," *Occupational Therapy International*, vol. 6, no. 3, 206 pages, 1999.

[11] J. Lidstone, M. Uljarević, J. Sullivan et al., "Relations among restricted and repetitive behaviors, anxiety and sensory features in children with autism spectrum disorders," *Research in Autism Spectrum Disorders*, vol. 8, no. 2, pp. 82–92, 2014.

[12] M. O. Mazurek, R. A. Vasa, L. G. Kalb et al., "Anxiety, sensory over-responsivity, and gastrointestinal problems in children with autism spectrum disorders," *Journal of Abnormal Child Psychology*, vol. 41, no. 1, pp. 165–176, 2013.

[13] T. Tavassoli, L. J. Miller, S. A. Schoen, D. M. Nielsen, and S. Baron-Cohen, "Sensory over-responsivity in adults with autism spectrum conditions," *Autism*, vol. 18, no. 4, pp. 428–432, 2013.

[14] S. A. Green, A. Ben-Sasson, T. W. Soto, and A. S. Carter, "Anxiety and sensory over-responsivity in toddlers with autism spectrum disorders: bidirectional effects across time," *Journal of Autism and Developmental Disorders*, vol. 42, no. 6, pp. 1112–1119, 2012.

[15] D. Hiersteiner, V. Bradley, A. Ne'eman, J. Bershadsky, and A. Bonardi, "Putting the research in context: the life experience and outcomes of adults on the autism spectrum receiving services in 29 states," *Inclusion*, vol. 5, no. 1, pp. 45–59, 2017.

[16] M. O. Mazurek, "Loneliness, friendship, and well-being in adults with autism spectrum disorders," *Autism*, vol. 18, no. 3, pp. 223–232, 2014.

[17] R. S. Smith and J. Sharp, "Fascination and isolation: a grounded theory exploration of unusual sensory experiences in adults with Asperger syndrome," *Journal of Autism and Developmental Disorders*, vol. 43, no. 4, pp. 891–910, 2013.

[18] M. E. Beutel, E. M. Klein, E. Brähler et al., "Loneliness in the general population: prevalence, determinants and relations to mental health," *BMC Psychiatry*, vol. 17, no. 1, p. 97, 2017.

[19] M. Muyan, E. C. Chang, Z. Jilani, T. Yu, J. Lin, and J. K. Hirsch, "Loneliness and negative affective conditions in adults: is there any room for hope in predicting anxiety and depressive symptoms?," *The Journal of Psychology*, vol. 150, no. 3, pp. 333–341, 2015.

[20] V. A. Lykes and M. Kemmelmeier, "What predicts loneliness? Cultural difference between individualistic and collectivistic societies in Europe," *Journal of Cross-Cultural Psychology*, vol. 45, no. 3, pp. 468–490, 2013.

[21] F. Faul, E. Erdfelder, A. Buchner, and A.-G. Lang, *G*Power Version 3.1.2*, Computer Software, 2008, Retrieved from http://www.psycho.uni-duesseldorf.de/abteilungen/aap/gpower3/download-and-register.

[22] American Psychiatric Association, *Diagnostic and Statistical Manual of Mental Disorders*, American Psychiatric Association, Washington, DC, USA, 4th, Text Revision edition, 2000.

[23] M. H. Tseng and W. S. Chen, *Chinese Version of Adolescent-Adult Sensory Profile: User's Manual*, Chinese Behavioral Science Corporation, Taipei, Taiwan, 2009.

[24] A. T. Beck and R. A. Steer, *Manual for the Beck Anxiety Inventory*, Psychological Corporation, San Antonio, TX, USA, 1990.

[25] H. H. Che, M. L. Lu, H. C. Chen, S. W. Chang, and Y. J. Lee, "Validation of the Chinese version of the Beck anxiety inventory," *Formosan Journal of Medicine*, vol. 10, pp. 447–454, 2006.

[26] R. Hays and M. R. DiMatteo, "A short-form measure of loneliness," *Journal of Personality Assessment*, vol. 51, no. 1, pp. 69–81, 1987.

[27] C. H. Wu and G. Yao, "Psychometric analysis of the short-form UCLA loneliness scale (ULS-8) in Taiwanese undergraduate students," *Personality and Individual Differences*, vol. 44, no. 8, pp. 1762–1771, 2008.

[28] M. J. Liu, "Screening adults for Asperger syndrome and high-functioning autism by using the autism-spectrum quotient (AQ) (Mandarin version)," *Bulletin of Special Education*, vol. 33, no. 1, pp. 73–92, 2008.

[29] S. Baron-Cohen, S. Wheelwright, R. Skinner, J. Martin, and E. Clubley, "The autism-spectrum quotient (AQ): evidence

from Asperger syndrome/high-functioning autism, males and females, scientists and mathematicians," *Journal of Autism and Developmental Disorders*, vol. 31, no. 1, pp. 5–17, 2001.

[30] A. F. Hayes, *PROCESS: A Versatile Computational Tool for Observed Variable Mediation, Moderation, and Conditional Process Modeling*, Guilford Press, 2012, Retrieved from http://www.afhayes.com/public/process2012.pdf.

[31] K. J. Preacher and A. F. Hayes, "SPSS and SAS procedures for estimating indirect effects in simple mediation models," *Behavior Research Methods, Instruments, & Computers*, vol. 36, no. 4, pp. 717–731, 2004.

[32] S. W. White and R. Roberson-Nay, "Anxiety, social deficits, and loneliness in youth with autism spectrum disorders," *Journal of Autism and Developmental Disorders*, vol. 39, no. 7, pp. 1006–1013, 2009.

[33] J. Landon, D. Shepherd, and V. Lodhia, "A qualitative study of noise sensitivity in adults with autism spectrum disorder," *Research in Autism Spectrum Disorders*, vol. 32, pp. 43–52, 2016.

[34] D. W. Nangle, C. A. Erdley, J. E. Newman, C. A. Mason, and E. M. Carpenter, "Popularity, friendship quantity, and friendship quality: interactive influences on children's loneliness and depression," *Journal of Clinical Child and Adolescent Psychology*, vol. 32, no. 4, pp. 546–555, 2003.

[35] J. G. Parker and S. R. Asher, "Friendship and friendship quality in middle childhood: links with peer group acceptance and feelings of loneliness and social dissatisfaction," *Developmental Psychology*, vol. 29, no. 4, pp. 611–621, 1993.

[36] N. Bauminger, C. Shulman, and G. Agam, "The link between perceptions of self and of social relationships in high-functioning children with autism," *Journal of Developmental and Physical Disabilities*, vol. 16, no. 2, pp. 193–214, 2004.

22

Effect of Community-Based Occupational Therapy on Health-Related Quality of Life and Engagement in Meaningful Activities of Women with Breast Cancer

Daiva Petruseviciene,[1] **Deive Surmaitiene**,[2] **Daiva Baltaduoniene**,[1] **and Egle Lendraitiene**[1]

[1]*Department of Rehabilitation, Medical Academy, Lithuanian University of Health Sciences, Kaunas, Lithuania*
[2]*Kulautuva Hospital of Rehabilitation, Hospital of Lithuanian University of Health Sciences Kauno Klinikos, Kaunas, Lithuania*

Correspondence should be addressed to Daiva Petruseviciene; daiva.petruseviciene@lsmuni.lt

Academic Editor: Mélanie Levasseur

We aimed to evaluate the short-term effects of community-based occupational therapy on health-related quality of life and engagement in meaningful activities among women with breast cancer. An open label randomized controlled trial study design was applied. The participants were members of various societies of women with cancer. In total, 22 women have participated in the study. Participants of the experimental group ($n = 11$) participated in a 6-week community-based occupational therapy program and the usual activities of various societies, whereas the control group ($n = 11$) women participated in the usual activities of the societies only. 1 of the participants withdrew during the course; therefore 21 completed the study successfully. Participants of both groups were assessed for health-related quality of life and the participants of the experimental group were assessed for engagement in meaningful activities. The evaluation was carried out during the nonacute period of the disease—at the beginning of the study and after 6 weeks. Women of the experimental group demonstrated statistically significantly better scores in the global quality of life, role functions, physical, emotional, cognitive, and social functions, fatigue, insomnia, financial impact, systemic therapy side effects, and breast symptoms scales compared to the control group participants ($p < 0.05$) after the 6 weeks, as measured by the *EORTC QLQ-C30* questionnaire and its breast cancer module *QLQ-BR23*. Furthermore, women of the experimental group demonstrated significant greater engagement in meaningful activities when applying community-based occupational therapy ($p < 0.05$), as measured by using the Engagement in Meaningful Activities Survey (EMAS). The evaluation of the associations between the women's engagement in meaningful activities and changes in health-related quality of life showed that greater engagement in meaningful activities was associated with better emotional functions and a lower level of insomnia ($p < 0.05$). Based on the results of our study, we recommend applying occupational therapy in the field of community healthcare in order to maintain or improve breast cancer patients' health-related quality of life and suggest involving women into meaningful activities during community-based occupational therapy after clarifying which activities are important to them.

1. Introduction

On the global scale, cancer causes one-seventh of all deaths. According to the most recent estimates, there have been over 14 million new cases of cancer and over 8 million deaths from cancer registered worldwide, and it is expected that, due to the increasing numbers and aging of the population, these numbers will increase to, accordingly, 21.7 million and 13 million by the year 2030 [1].

Breast cancer, defined by the National Cancer Institute as cancer forming in breast tissues, is the most common malignant tumor among women and in as many as 19 out of 21 regions it is the leading cause of death among women in both the developed and the developing countries [2–4].

Over 1.5 million new cases of invasive breast cancer are registered globally every year, and this is the single most common form of cancer among women that is prevalent in absolutely all regions of the world [2, 5]. In European countries, breast cancer is also the most frequently diagnosed malignant tumor in women, and the prevalence of this disease has been increasing in most countries over the last decades [3, 6]. Despite the continuous improvement in the diagnostic and treatment techniques, breast cancer remains one of the most common cancers among women in Lithuania as well as in the rest of the world (in Lithuania, breast cancer is currently the second most common cancer after skin cancer (melanoma) and is undoubtedly their most urgent health problem). Even though survival rates in Lithuania are among the lowest, the overall situation is improving: breast cancer is detected at increasingly earlier stages, and women's survival is improving [7].

Unfortunately, the completion of breast cancer treatment does not mean the end of the disease [8]. Healthcare institutions with all the necessary services and specialists ensure integrated assistance to breast cancer patients. However, after discharge, women frequently experience emotional stress because of short-term or long-term adverse effects of the therapy, the risk of recurrence, difficulty getting information about their health status and its possible changes, financial problems, difficulty getting back to work, impaired sexual life, and so forth. Improving survival rates and the risk of late-onset adverse reactions increase the need for healthcare and rehabilitation services on the community level [3, 9, 10]. Consequently, quality of life questions related to the financial impact of the disease, concern about the future of the family, fear of disease recurrence, insufficient preparation for possible late-onset adverse reactions to the treatment, and possible changes in social support become increasingly relevant [11].

Today, it is the field of health-related quality of life that is being most actively developed in Lithuania as well as abroad [12]. Over the last several decades, breast cancer treatment has become more effective, which resulted in a significant increase in patients' long-term survival. Schoormans et al. (2015) stated that because of this, researchers had to focus increasingly on long-term consequences of the disease or the treatment, which they related to the quality of life, thus developing the concept of breast cancer patients' health-related quality of life [13].

The impact of the diagnosis and treatment of breast cancer differs depending on the patient, resulting in varying numbers and degrees of physical and psychological sequelae. The consequences may significantly impair a woman's ability to participate in meaningful activities, including housework, return to work, and adequate performance of the main social roles and responsibilities. This, in turn, may negatively affect the economic status and disrupt interpersonal relations, thus further impairing the woman's engagement in meaningful activities as well as her psychoemotional status and the quality of life. Despite the fact that the combined effect of breast cancer and its treatment may manifest themselves at any moment and last for a very long time, it is essential for the patients to resume their daily roles as soon as possible after the completion of the treatment and this is where the role of the occupational therapist is especially important [14]. According to Pergolotti et al. (2016), the economic effectiveness of occupational therapy and its usefulness in reducing disease consequences have already been proven, and yet occupational therapy is still rarely applied in the rehabilitation of cancer patients [15].

The theory of occupational therapy states that human subsistence is a social process, and people need meaningful activity; its absence is a major threat to human health, and thus occupational therapists in their professional practice strive to achieve their patients' maximum capacity to increase their ability to engage in activities that they see as important and meaningful [16, 17]. According to Cook and Thompson (2015), the meaningfulness of life significantly affects a person's physical, mental, and social wellbeing. Engagement in purposeful activities contributes to the satisfaction of the need for the meaningfulness of life, but only if this activity motivates the person, is interesting, can be successfully completed, and helps to achieve other significant aims. Engagement in purposeful activities directly affects a person's emotional condition, self-esteem, and self-confidence. Purposeful activities have been recognized as directly affecting the quality of life, and thus an important task when working with a patient is to clarify which activities are important for him or her. When purposeful activity is selected in accordance with the person's interests and priorities, it becomes meaningful [18]. Occupational therapists strive to and can help cancer patients live a meaningful life, be self-sufficient, participate in activities, be able to manage themselves and others, engage in work, leisure, and health promotion activities, and be a part of social groups and the family [16]. Occupational therapists' holistic approach and creative decisions may improve breast cancer patients' cognitive and physical capacity, mental health, and the quality of life [15].

When working in communities, occupational therapists have to be familiar with the characteristics of community-based activity in order to be able to pursue meaningful activities based on the community members' priorities. Active participation in community activities, social support, and engagement in meaningful activities positively affect community members' health and the quality of life [19]. Based on this theory, we wanted to determine the influence of community-based occupational therapy on breast cancer patients' health-related quality of life and engagement in meaningful activities.

No similar research was found and we were the first in Lithuania who made a study analyzing changes in health-related quality of life, engagement in meaningful activities, and its associations among breast cancer patients when applying occupational therapy in the field of community healthcare. We hope that the results of our study will be useful for occupational therapists working with breast cancer patients' communities.

Consequently, all these reasons have affected the following aim of the study: to evaluate the short-term effects of community-based occupational therapy on health-related quality of life and engagement in meaningful activities among women with breast cancer.

2. Methods

This randomized controlled trial was conducted with the permission of the Bioethics Center of the Lithuanian University of Health Sciences (number BEC-SR(M)-186), the permission of the European Organization for Research and Treatment of Cancer (EORTC) Quality of Life Group to use the quality of life questionnaire EORTC QLQ-C30 and its module EORTC QLQ-BR23 in the study, and the permission of the Associate Professor A. M. Eakman from Colorado State University to use the Engagement in Meaningful Activities Survey (EMAS) in the study. The study was performed during May–June 2016 in Kaunas city, with the mediation of the chairwomen of two societies of women who either had overcome their breast cancer or were still fighting it on the community level.

Eligible women were adult (≥18 years of age) and Lithuanian-speaking, with diagnosed breast cancer and functional status being ≤2b according to the ECOG *(Eastern Cooperative Oncology Group)* scale of performance status, were able to understand the essence of the study and simple instructions, were familiarized with the aim of the study, and volunteered to participate. Exclusion criteria were the following: refusal to participate in the study, women with severe decompensated comorbidities and mental diseases, and being incapable of independently filling out the questionnaires, and whose functional status was >2b according to the ECOG scale of performance status.

All the participants who met the inclusion criteria were in advance familiarized with the study, its aims, objectives, and methods, the confidentiality of the data, and the possibility of withdrawing from the study at any time and provided a written consent to participate in the study.

In total, 22 members of breast cancer patients' societies met the inclusion criteria. All participants had been diagnosed with breast cancer (code C50 according to the ICD-10-AM). The participants were randomly distributed into two groups: the experimental group and the control group, following simple randomization procedure (computerized random numbers). The distribution of the participants was equal in both groups. The participants were also distributed into two groups based on the analyzed characteristics: age, employment status, the duration of the disease, the stage of the disease, the location of the tumor, metastases, and functional status according to the ECOG. Detailed characteristics of the participants are presented in Table 1.

There were no significant differences in the participants' distribution between the groups concerning their age ($\chi^2(1) = 0$, $p = 1$), employment status ($p = 1$), the duration of the disease ($\chi^2(1) = 0$, $p = 1$), the stage of the disease ($p = 0.311$), the location of the tumor ($\chi^2(1) = 0$, $p = 1$), metastases ($p = 1$), or functional status according to the ECOG ($p = 1$), $p > 0.05$.

During the study, we evaluated changes in women health-related quality of life and experimental group participants' engagement in meaningful activities during the nonacute period of the disease. The methods used in the study were the following: a survey using a questionnaire designed by the author, testing, experiment, and statistical data analysis. During the survey, we evaluated the participants' sociodemographic data (age and employment status) and clinical factors: the duration of the disease, the stage of the disease, the location of the tumor, metastases, and functional status according to the ECOG. Testing was conducted twice: at the beginning of the study and after 6 weeks. In order to evaluate changes in the participants' health-related quality of life, we used the EORTC QLQ-C30 questionnaire and its module QLQ-BR23. The principal questionnaire, EORTC QLQ-C30, consists of 30 questions forming the global health status and quality of life scale, five functional scales, three symptom scales, and six separately evaluated components. The EORTC module QLQ-BR23 is a more specific questionnaire designed for breast cancer patients and consisting of 23 questions forming four functional scales and four symptom scales. After the calculation of the results according to the formulas presented by the authors, the score intervals in all scales and separately evaluated components ranged from 0 to 100 points. The questionnaires have been translated and adapted in many languages including Lithuanian and are suitable for the evaluation of cancer patients' health-related quality of life. In Lithuania, Banienė and Šinkariova (2015) evaluated the internal consistency of the scales of those questionnaires ($0.6 \leq \alpha \leq 0.9$) and, based on the obtained results, stated that the questionnaires are suitable for studies of breast cancer patients [20].

The testing of the experimental group participants' engagement in meaningful activities was also conducted at baseline and at the end of the study, using the Engagement in Meaningful Activities Survey. This survey has not been translated into Lithuanian and has not been adapted in Lithuania. For this reason, studies for the evaluation of the reliability and validity of the survey should be conducted. The results of the survey on engagement in meaningful activities reflect the level of the subjects' engagement in meaningful activities. The survey consists of 12 statements, each of which has the minimal value of 1 point and the maximal value of 4 points, where 1 point means "rarely"; 2 points, sometimes; 3 points, often; and 4 points, always. Engagement in meaningful activities was evaluated by a sum score. There is a growing body of scientific literature validating the psychometric properties of this test. The association of the results of this test with those of the evaluation of satisfaction with life and health-related quality of life has already been proven. Eakman with coauthors (2010) have proven the test-retest reliability of this instrument ($r = 0.56$) and evaluated the internal consistency of the scale ($\alpha = 0.89$), using the English version of this test in adult population [21]. All study participants filled out the questionnaires independently.

During the course of the study, the women participated in a 6-week community-based occupational therapy program and the usual activities of various societies, whereas the control group women participated in the usual activities of the societies only.

The community-based occupational therapy program was designed taking into account the most common sequelae of breast cancer and its treatment identified in literature: arm swelling, reduced range of motion of the arm, fatigue,

TABLE 1: Participants' characteristics.

Characteristic	Total n (%)	Experimental group n (%)	p value ⟷	Control group n (%)
Age				
Young or middle-aged (18–59 years)	11 (50)	6 (54.5)	1*	5 (45.5)
Elderly or old (60–80 years)	11 (50)	5 (45.5)		6 (54.5)
Employment status				
Employed or a student	9 (40.9)	4 (36.4)	1**	5 (45.5)
Unemployed, housewife, retired, or not working because of disability	13 (59.1)	7 (63.6)		6 (54.5)
Duration of disease				
<5 years	11 (50)	5 (45.5)	1*	6 (54.5)
≥5 years	11 (50)	6 (54.5)		5 (45.5)
Stage of the disease				
0, I, or II	17 (77.3)	10 (90.9)	0.311**	7 (63.6)
III or IV	5 (22.7)	1 (9.1)		4 (36.4)
Location of the tumor				
Left	12 (54.5)	6 (54.5)	1*	6 (54.5)
Right	10 (45.5)	5 (45.5)		5 (45.5)
Metastases				
Present	3 (13.6)	1 (9.1)	1**	2 (18.2)
Absent	19 (86.4)	10 (90.9)		9 (81.8)
Functional status according to ECOG				
0 or 1 b.	17 (77.3)	8 (72.7)	1**	9 (81.8)
2 b.	5 (22.7)	(27.3)		2 (18.2)

*Statistical significance was determined according to the χ^2 criterion with Yates correction, no significant differences between the groups, $p \geq 0.05$. **Statistical significance was determined according to Fisher's exact criterion, no significant differences between the groups, $p > 0.05$.

and impaired quality of life. According to Scaffa and Reitz (2014), active participation in community activities, social support, and engagement in meaningful activities have a positive effect on community members' health and quality of life [19]. Cook and Thompson (2015) supported this opinion stating that meaningful activities improve the quality of life [18]. For this reason, by applying this program, we strived to improve not only the experimental group participants' health-related quality of life, but also their engagement in meaningful activities.

During the study, we applied occupational therapy in groups. During each session, purposeful activities were combined with creative techniques, and the sessions were made meaningful through voluntary assistance to others, that is, emotional help when communicating with other women who had the same problems and so forth. The experimental group participants also received individual consultations by an occupational therapist if needed.

Duration of the program consisted of six meetings. The description of the program is provided in Table 2.

Occupational therapy sessions in groups were organized four times: once weekly at an arranged time in the evening (after work), up to 1.5 hours/day.

Note that the sessions in occupational therapy groups took place in a cozy and comfortable environment, and all the tools and materials required for the activities were supplied and were of good quality. Prior to the sessions, the participants received all the necessary information, and the focus during the sessions was on the process rather than on the results.

Statistical data analysis was conducted using the *IBM SPSS Statistics 22* software. The data were described by using the standard numeral characteristics (min and max values, median, and mean). The distributions were compared by applying the nonparametric criteria. Two dependent samples before and after the intervention were compared by applying the nonparametric Wilcoxon criterion and two independent samples by using the Mann–Whitney-Wilcoxon criterion. In order to determine the presence of a relationship between engagement in meaningful activities and health-related quality of life, we calculated Spearman's correlation coefficient. The difference or the relationship between the indices were considered to be statistically significant when $p < 0.05$.

3. Results

After six weeks, of 22 women randomized into the study, 21 completed the trial. The experimental group consisted of 10 participants and the control group consisted of 11. One woman withdrew from the study because of breast cancer recurrence. During the study, when applying occupational

Table 2: Description of the application of the occupational therapy program in the community of women with breast cancer.

	Topic	Aims	Activities
Session I	The beginning of the study	Familiarization, presentation of the study and the planned program, and initiation of the study.	Self-introduction and presentation of the study, a report on the topic of the study, initial filing out of the questionnaires, questions, and answers.
Session *II*	*"Plant and Give"*	Socializing, cooperation, increasing the hand movement amplitude or prevention, development of positive emotions, and sharing positive experience and emotions with those facing the same or similar problems.	Sapling replanting (gardening therapy), advice and discussions about the hand movement amplitude, and donation of saplings to hospitalized women with breast cancer.
Session *III*	*"Origami Crane – the Gift of Hope"*	Experiencing relaxation and calmness, expression of emotions, socialization, prevention or reduction of lymphedema, and sharing positive experience and emotions with those facing the same or similar problems.	Folding paper cranes (art therapy) + a lecture, exercises, and discussions on lymphedema treatment and prevention, as well as on an occupational therapist's assistance.
Session *IV*	*"Sharing the Strength"*	Experiencing relaxation and calmness, expression of emotions, socialization, presentation of the energy conservation principles and their practical application, and sharing positive experience and emotions with those facing the same or similar problems.	Making an original picture postcard (art therapy) while listening to specially selected calm music (music therapy) + a lecture and discussions on fatigue and energy conservation techniques (planning, adjustment of the environment, biomechanics of the body, etc.).
Session *V*	*"Knitting for Preterm Newborns"*	Gratuitous assistance.	Knitting socks + a lecture on the need for socks and donation of socks to preterm newborns.
Session VI	The end of the study	Discussion on the work done, sharing impressions and results, and conclusion of the study.	Summing-up of the program, repeated filling out of the questionnaires, feedback, discussions, questions/answers, etc.

therapy in the community, we strove to improve the participants' engagement in meaningful activities and thus their health-related quality of life. For this reason, the women's active participation in the assignments was highly important for us, and thus, to determine the actual impact of the applied program on the aforementioned indices, we only calculated the results for women who were involved in the study.

The health-related quality of life of women with breast cancer was evaluated during the nonacute period of the disease by calculating the scores in separate scales of the EORTC QLQ-C30 questionnaire and its module QLQ-BR23. The score could range from 0 to 100 points. A higher score in the global quality of life scale indicated better quality of life, a higher score in the functional scales better functioning, and a higher score in the symptom scales a greater degree of the manifestation of the symptom.

The evaluation of the participants' health-related quality of life at baseline using the EORTC QLQ-C30 questionnaire and its module QLQ-BR23 showed that the groups were homogeneous, $p > 0.05$ (Table 3).

Prior to the application of the community-based occupational therapy, the poorest evaluations in the EORTC QLQ-C30 questionnaire among the experimental group participants were on the global quality of life (50 (33.33–83.33; 50.75)), emotional functions (50 (8.33–100; 52.27)), cognitive functions (50 (0–83.33; 54.55)), and social functions (50 (16.67–83.33; 48.49)). The participants were also found to demonstrate the highest degrees of the manifestation of insomnia (66.67 (0–100; 66.67)) and the financial difficulties (66.67 (33.33–100; 69.7)). The results of the EORTC QLQ-BR23 questionnaire showed that the participants gave the poorest evaluations of the future perspective (33.33 (0–66.67; 33.33)) and demonstrated the highest degrees of the manifestation of breast symptoms (41.67 (8.33–75; 38.64)) such as pain, edema, tenderness, or skin problems.

Among the control group participants, the poorest evaluations in the EORTC QLQ-C30 questionnaire at baseline

Table 3: Distribution of evaluation scores in health-related quality of life questionnaire scales in the groups at baseline.

Scales of the quality of life questionnaires	Experimental group n (11)	Experimental group $x_{me}(x_{min}-x_{max}; \bar{x})$	$U; p$ $\longleftrightarrow$	Control group n (11)	Control group $x_{me}(x_{min}-x_{max}; \bar{x})$
		EORTC QLQ C-30			
Global health status/QoL	11	50 (33.33–83.33; 50.75)	41.5; 0.217	11	58.33 (33.33–91.67; 59.85)
Functional scales					
Physical functioning	11	60 (40–86.67; 63.64)	50; 0.519	11	73.33 (46.67–86.67; 67.88)
Role functioning	11	66.67 (16.67–100; 68.18)	60; 1	11	66.67 (33.33–100; 69.7)
Emotional functioning	11	50 (8.33–100; 52.27)	36.5; 0.116	11	66.67 (8.33–100; 65.91)
Cognitive functioning	11	50 (0–83.33; 54.55)	35.5; 0.101	11	83.33 (50–100; 72.73)
Social functioning	11	50 (16.67–83.33; 48.49)	32; 0.065	11	66.67 (50–100; 69.7)
Symptom scales					
Fatigue	11	55.56 (33.33–77.78; 54.55)	54.5; 0.699	11	44.44 (11.11–88.89; 50.5)
Nausea and vomiting	11	0 (0–50; 7.58)	54.5; 0.699	11	0 (0–66.67; 12.12)
Pain	11	33.33 (0–83.33; 34.85)	56; 0.797	11	33.33 (0–83.33; 28.79)
Dyspnoea	11	0 (0–33.33; 15.15)	50; 0.519	11	33.33 (0–66.67; 24.24)
Insomnia	11	66.67 (0–100; 66.67)	39; 0.171	11	66.67 (0–66.67; 48.49)
Appetite loss	11	0 (0–33.33; 9.09)	44; 0.3	11	33.33 (0–33.33; 18.18)
Constipation	11	33.33 (0–100; 42.42)	48; 0.438	11	0 (0–100; 24.24)
Diarrhoea	11	0 (0–66.67; 9.09)	60; 1	11	0 (0–100; 12.12)
Financial difficulties	11	66.67 (33.33–100; 69.7)	42; 0.243	11	66.67 (0–100; 51.52)
		EORTC QLQ BR-23			
Functional scales					
Body image	11	58.33 (0–83.33; 51.51)	28.5; 0.562	11	41.57 (25–91.67; 48.48)
Sexual functioning	11	100 (0–100; 81.82)	60; 1	11	100 (33.33–100; 81.82)
Sexual enjoyment	5	66.67 (33.33–100; 73.33)	9; 0.548	5	66.67 (33.33–100; 60)
Future perspective	11	33.33 (0–66.67; 33.33)	51.5; 0.562	11	33.33 (0–66.67; 27.27)
Symptom scales					
Systemic therapy side effects	11	23.81 (4.76–61.90; 31.6)	58; 0.898	11	28.57 (4.76–57.14; 29)
Breast symptoms	11	41.67 (8.33–75; 38.64)	41; 0.217	11	25 (0–66.67; 28.79)
Arm symptoms	11	33.33 (0–77.78; 37.37)	63; 0.898	11	44.44 (0–88.89; 38.38)
Upset by hair loss	6	16.67 (0–33.33; 16.67)	28.5; 0.573	8	33.33 (0–100; 29.17)

Statistical significance was determined according to the nonparametric Mann–Whitney-Wilcoxon criterion, no significant differences between the groups, $p \geq 0.05$.

were on the global quality of life (58.33 (33.33–91.67; 59.85)), and the participants were found to demonstrate the highest degrees of the manifestation of insomnia (66.67 (0–66.67; 48.49)) and financial impact (66.67 (0–100; 51.52)). The results of the EORTC QLQ-BR23 questionnaire showed that the participants gave the poorest evaluations of the future perspective (33.33 (0–66.67; 27.27)) and demonstrated the highest degrees of the manifestation of arm symptoms (44.44 (0–88.89; 38.38)) such as pain and edema.

The evaluation of changes in the overall scores of the quality of life questionnaire EORTC QLQ-C30 scales between the groups showed that, compared to baseline data, after six weeks (at the end of the study), the experimental group demonstrated statistically significantly better results in the global quality of life ($U = 0$; $p = 0.001$; $r = 0.85$), physical functions ($U = 20$, $p = 0.013$; $r = 0.54$), role functions ($U = 25.5$; $p = 0.036$; $r = 0.46$), emotional functions ($U = 8.5$; $p = 0.001$; $r = 0.72$), cognitive functions ($U = 10$; $p = 0.001$; $r = 0.72$), social functions ($U = 13$; $p = 0.002$; $r = 0.66$), fatigue ($U = 5$; $p = 0.001$; $r = 0.78$), insomnia ($U = 19$; $p = 0.01$; $r = 0.59$), and financial impact ($U = 23.5$; $p = 0.024$; $r = 0.52$) scales, $p < 0.05$. The scores in other functional or symptom scales of the quality of life did not differ statistically significantly between the groups, $p \geq 0.05$ (Table 4).

The evaluation of changes in the overall scores in the scales of the quality of life questionnaire module EORTC QLQ-BR23 between the groups showed that, compared to baseline data, after six weeks (at the end of the study), the experimental group demonstrated statistically significantly better results in the systemic therapy side effects ($U = 11$; $p = 0.001$; $r = 0.68$) and breast symptoms ($U = 24.5$; $p = 0.029$; $r = 0.48$) scales, $p < 0.05$. The scores in other functional or symptom scales did not differ statistically significantly between the groups, $p \geq 0.05$ (Table 5).

Considering the calculated strength of the effect, when a moderate effect was ≥0.5 and a strong effect was ≥0.8, we found not only statistically, but also clinically significant changes ($p < 0.05$) in the scores of the global quality of life (0.85), physical (0.54), emotional (0.72), cognitive (0.72), and social (0.66) functions, fatigue (0.78), insomnia (0.59), financial impact (0.52), and systemic therapy side effects (0.68) scales.

Among the experimental group women with breast cancer, engagement in meaningful activities was evaluated during the nonacute period of the disease. The evaluation was performed based on the results of the Engagement in Meaningful Activities Survey (EMAS)—the sum score that could range from 12 to 48 points, where <29 points indicated insufficient engagement; 29–41 points, moderate engagement; and >41 points, good engagement.

During the evaluation of the participants' engagement in meaningful activities at baseline, the median score in the experimental group was 29 points, the lowest score being 24 points (insufficient engagement) and the highest score being 35 points (moderate engagement). At the end of the study, after the application of the 6-week community-based occupational therapy program, the evaluation scores of the participants' engagement in meaningful activities changed statistically significantly ($Z = -2.829$; $p = 0.005$): the median score was 36 points, the lowest score being 31 points (moderate engagement) and the highest score being 42 points (good engagement), $p < 0.05$ (Figure 1).

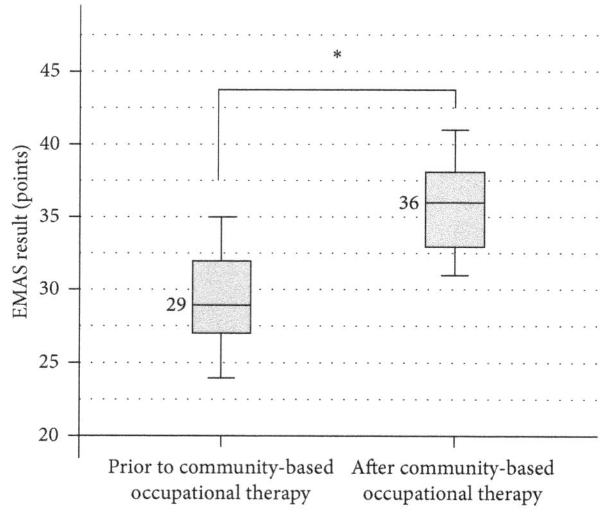

FIGURE 1: Changes in the engagement in meaningful activities in the experimental group participants, $^*p = 0.005$.

We also analyzed the relationship between breast cancer patients' engagement in meaningful activities and changes in their health-related quality of life. The results of the analysis showed that when evaluating the health-related quality of life on the EORTC QLQ-C30 questionnaire, the evaluation scores showed a statistically significant direct moderate relationship ($r(10) = 0.663$; $p = 0.037$) between engagement in meaningful activities and the score in the emotional functions scale: better results of the evaluation of the engagement in meaningful activities (i.e., a greater engagement in meaningful activities) were associated with higher evaluation scores of emotional functions, that is, better emotional functions, $p < 0.05$.

We also found a statistically significant inverse moderate relationship ($r(10) = -0.658$; $p = 0.039$) between engagement in meaningful activities and the evaluation scores in the insomnia scale: better results of the evaluation of the engagement in meaningful activities (i.e., a greater engagement in meaningful activities) were associated with lower evaluation scores of the insomnia scale, that is, a lesser degree of the manifestation of insomnia, $p < 0.05$.

We found a statistically significant inverse moderate relationship ($r(10) = -0.681$; $p = 0.030$) between engagement in meaningful activities and the evaluation scores in the constipation scale: better results of the evaluation of the engagement in meaningful activities (i.e., a greater engagement in meaningful activities) were associated with lower evaluation scores of the constipation scale, that is, a lesser degree of the manifestation of constipation, $p < 0.05$.

We did not find any statistically significant relationship for the evaluation scores of other functional or symptom scales of the quality of life questionnaire EORTC QLQ-C30 or any scale of the module EORTC QLQ-BR23, $p \geq 0.05$ (Tables 6 and 7).

TABLE 4: Characteristics of changes in the evaluation scores of the scales of the global quality of life questionnaire EORTC QLQ-C30 in the experimental and the control group women.

Scales of the quality of life questionnaire	EGr Before x_{me}	EGr After x_{me}	EGr change $Z; p$	CGr Before x_{me}	CGr After x_{me}	CGr change $Z; p$	Difference between the groups at the end $U; p; r$
			EORTC QLQ C-30				
Global health status/QoL	50	66.67	−2.829; 0.005*	58.33	50	−1.956; 0.05	0; 0.001**; 0.85
Functional scales							
Physical functioning	60	70	−2.384; 0.017*	73.33	60	−1.012; 0.311	20; 0.013**; 0.54
Role functioning	66.67	75	−1.023; 0.306	66.67	66.67	−1.409; 0.159	25.5; 0.036**; 0.46
Emotional functioning	50	62.5	−2.670; 0.008*	66.67	58.33	−1.480; 0.139	8.5; 0.001**; 0.72
Cognitive functioning	50	66.67	−2.060; 0.039*	83.33	50	−2.388; 0.017*	10; 0.001**; 0.72
Social functioning	50	66.67	−1.951; 0.051	66.67	50	−2.410; 0.016*	13; 0.002**; 0.66
Symptom scales							
Fatigue	55.56	44.44	−2.555; 0.011*	44.44	66.67	−2.568; 0.010*	5; 0.001**; 0.78
Nausea and vomiting	0	0	−1.089; 0.276	0	0	−1.289; 0.197	51; 0.809
Pain	33.33	16.67	−0.933; 0.351	33.33	33.33	−0.213; 0.832	41.5; 0.349
Dyspnoea	0	0	−1; 0.317	33.33	33.33	−1.382; 0.167	32.5; 0.114
Insomnia	66.67	33.33	−2.280; 0.023*	66.67	66.67	−1.890; 0.059	19; 0.01**; 0.59
Appetite loss	0	0	−0.707; 0.480	33.33	33.33	−1.633; 0.102	48; 0.654;
Constipation	33.33	16.67	−1.890; 0.059	0	0	−0.730; 0.465	48; 0.654;
Diarrhoea	0	0	−1; 0.317	0	0	−0.816; 0.414	40.5; 0.314;
Financial difficulties	66.67	66.67	−1.236; 0.216	66.67	66.67	−2.041; 0.041*	23.5; 0.024**; 0.52

*Statistical significance was determined according to the nonparametric Wilcoxon criterion; the differences between the groups were significant when $p < 0.05$. **Statistical significance was determined according to the nonparametric Mann–Whitney-Wilcoxon criterion; the differences between the groups were significant when $p < 0.05$. *Note.* EGr: experimental group; CGr: control group.

Table 5: Characteristics of changes in the evaluation scores of the scales of the global quality of life questionnaire module EORTC QLQ-BR23 in the experimental and the control group women.

Scales of the quality of life questionnaire	EGr		EGr change	CGr		CGr change	Difference between the groups at the end
	Before x_{me}	After x_{me}	$Z; p$	Before x_{me}	After x_{me}	$Z; p$	$U; p; r$
			EORTC QLQ BR-23				
Functional scales							
Body image	58.33	58.33	−0.512; 0.609	41.67	41.67	−1.2; 0.23	53; 0.918
Sexual functioning	100	66.67	−2.041; 0.041*	100	83.33	0; 1	32.5; 0.114
Sexual enjoyment	66.67	50	−1.604; 0.109	66.67	66.67	−0.816; 0.414	4.5; 0.095
Future perspective	33.33	33.33	−0.184; 0.854	33.33	33.33	−0.184; 0.854	55; 1
Symptom scales							
Systemic therapy side effects	23.81	23.81	−2.092; 0.036	28.57	38.1	−2.371; 0.018*	11; 0.001**; 0.68
Breast symptoms	41.67	25	−2.352; 0.019*	25	33.33	−0.511; 0.61	24.5; 0.029**; 0.48
Arm symptoms	33.33	23.61	−0.986; 0.324	44.44	44.44	−0.106; 0.915	48; 0.654
Upset by hair loss	16.67	33.33	−1.633; 0.102	33.33	33.33	−1.841; 0.066	22.5; 0.852

*Statistical significance was determined according to the nonparametric Wilcoxon criterion; the differences between the groups were significant when $p < 0.05$. **Statistical significance was determined according to the nonparametric Mann–Whitney-Wilcoxon criterion; the differences between the groups were significant when $p < 0.05$.

TABLE 6: Relationship between engagement in meaningful activities and evaluations scores of health-related quality of life (EORTC QLQ-C30) in women with breast cancer.

Scales of the quality of life questionnaire	Relationship with changes in the engagement in meaningful activities $r(n)$; p
	EORTC QLQ-C30
Global health status/QoL	$r(10) = -0.046$; $p = 0.899$
Functional scales	
Physical functioning	$r(10) = 0.26$; $p = 0.469$
Role functioning	$r(10) = 0.21$; $p = 0.561$
Emotional functioning	$r(10) = 0.663$; $p = 0.037^*$
Cognitive functioning	$r(10) = 0.041$; $p = 0.91$
Social functioning	$r(10) = -0.051$; $p = 0.888$
Symptom scales	
Fatigue	$r(10) = -0.316$; $p = 0.374$
Nausea and vomiting	$r(10) = 0.239$; $p = 0.506$
Pain	$r(10) = -0.039$; $p = 0.916$
Dyspnoea	$r(10) = 0.425$; $p = 0.221$
Insomnia	$r(10) = -0.658$; $p = 0.039^*$
Appetite loss	$r(10) = -0.619$; $p = 0.056$
Constipation	$r(10) = -0.681$; $p = 0.03^*$
Diarrhoea	$r(10) = -0.121$; $p = 0.739$
Financial difficulties	$r(10) = -0.326$; $p = 0.359$

*Statistical significance was determined according to Spearman's correlation coefficient; the association was statistically significant when $p < 0.05$.

TABLE 7: Relationship between engagement in meaningful activities and evaluations scores of health-related quality of life (EORTC QLQ-BR23) in women with breast cancer.

Scales of the quality of life questionnaire	Relationship with changes in the engagement in meaningful activities $r(n)$; p
	EORTC QLQ-BR23
Functional scales	
Body image	$r(10) = -0.048$; $p = 0.895$
Sexual functioning	$r(10) = -0.289$; $p = 0.418$
Sexual enjoyment	$r(10) = -0.079$; $p = 0.9$
Future perspective	$r(10) = -0.353$; $p = 0.317$
Symptom scales	
Systemic therapy side effects	$r(10) = 0.177$; $p = 0.624$
Breast symptoms	$r(10) = -0.423$; $p = 0.223$
Arm symptoms	$r(10) = -0.083$; $p = 0.819$
Upset by hair loss	$r(6) = 0.141$; $p = 0.79$

Statistical significance was determined according to Spearman's correlation coefficient; the association was statistically significant when $p < 0.05$.

4. Discussion

A review of both Lithuanian and foreign literature revealed a lack of research or any kind of projects in the context of applying community-based occupational therapy for women with breast cancer, which encouraged us to conduct this study where objectives were set: to evaluate the short-term effects of community-based occupational therapy on changes in health-related quality of life among women with breast cancer and on changes in the experimental group women's engagement in meaningful activities and to analyze the associations between engagement in meaningful activities and changes in health-related quality of life.

In Lithuania, over 1.5 thousand new cases of breast cancer are diagnosed annually [7]. Improving screening programs and modern therapeutic techniques as well as increasing life expectancy of cancer patients result in an increasing relevance of the quality of life questions related to late consequences of the disease and its treatment and this is where the holistic approach and creative decisions of occupational therapists may be of assistance [11, 15, 22]. Based on this idea, in our study we analyzed aforementioned indices among women with breast cancer during the nonacute period of the disease.

In total, 21 women participated in and successfully completed the study. Of these, 10 women participated in a 6-week community-based occupational therapy program consisting of 4 group sessions (once a week, ~1.5 hours/day). The program was designed according to the guidelines provided in the only source of literature describing a study similar to ours—a project by Robinson (2015). The basis for those guidelines was a community-based occupational therapy program for women with breast cancer, aimed at maximizing their capacity for daily activities after the completion of the treatment [23].

We evaluated health-related quality of life by using the questionnaires of the European Organization for Research and Treatment of Cancer (EORTC) Quality of Life Group—the global EORTC QLQ-C30 questionnaire and its module designed specifically for breast cancer, EORTC QLQ-BR23. These questionnaires have been translated into and adapted in many languages, including Lithuanian, and are suitable for the evaluation of health-related quality of life in individuals with breast cancer [24]. In our participants, we evaluated health-related quality of life twice—at baseline and after 6 weeks. The results of our study showed that, at the beginning of the study, the women's quality of life and emotional, cognitive, and social functions were impaired; they experienced stronger manifestations of insomnia and breast and arm symptoms and were concerned about their future perspectives and the financial impact of the disease. Meanwhile, upon completion of the 6-week community-based occupational therapy program, the evaluation results of these and other aspects of health-related quality of life—such as physical functions, role functions, and fatigue—improved statistically significantly, compared to the respective results in the control group participants who did not participate in the program.

EORTC questionnaires have been recommended by a number of foreign researchers [13, 22, 25–28]. The results of a systematic survey conducted by Ghislain et al. (2016) showed that a large proportion (44%) of their analyzed studies on health-related quality of life in women with breast cancer employed EORTC questionnaires. The aforementioned survey showed that the second most frequently used (39%) instrument for the evaluation of health-related quality of life was the FACT-B *(Functional Assessment of Cancer Therapy-Breast)* questionnaire [29]. Apart from those two questionnaires, other researchers applied FACT-G *(Functional Assessment of Cancer Therapy-General)*, FACT-BSC *(Functional Assessment of Cancer Therapy-Breast Cancer Specific Subscale)*, QLACS *(Quality of Life in Adult Cancer Survivors)*, SF-36 *(Medical Outcomes Short-Form Health Survey)*, and other instruments [11, 30, 31].

According to literature data, active engagement in meaningful activities positively affects the quality of life, and thus, in order to improve breast cancer patients' health-related quality of life, the women were involved in meaningful activities during the occupational therapy sessions [18, 19]. To evaluate changes in the study participants' engagement in meaningful activities and its relationship with health-related quality of life, we used the engagement in meaningful activities questionnaire during community-based occupational therapy. The women filled out this questionnaire at the beginning and at the end of the study. A survey of literature failed to identify any Lithuanian or foreign studies on the evaluation of breast cancer patients' engagement in meaningful activities. For this reason, we cannot compare our results, which showed that in the experimental group women who participated in the 6-week community-based occupational therapy program, engagement in meaningful activities improved significantly and that greater result was associated with a significant improvement in emotional functions and a reduction in the level of insomnia. We found only one study conducted by foreign researchers Pergolotti et al. (2015), where, based on the idea of participation in personally important activities for the improvement of the quality of life, the researchers analyzed participation in meaningful activities among older patients with cancer. Of the study subjects, 40% were breast cancer patients, whose participation in meaningful activities was evaluated by applying the MAPA *(The Meaningful Activity Participation Assessment)* test [32].

In this study, we strived to reveal the essence of occupational therapy in the community of women with breast cancer and the influence of this therapy on those women's health-related quality of life. The results of the study showed that occupational therapy significantly improves breast cancer patients' health-related quality of life and engagement in meaningful activities on the community level during the nonacute period of the disease.

One of the limitations of this study is a small number of participants in the groups, and thus in the future, this or a similar study should be performed with a larger sample. We also think that, in further studies, it would be expedient to evaluate whether a longer period of program application or a greater number of sessions would affect the results and improve the effectiveness of the program. In addition, future studies could be expanded by involving specialists of other areas (psychologists, art therapists, marketing specialists, etc.) because a successful implementation of the program requires not only the general competence of an occupational therapist, but also organizational skills, knowledge in marketing, and so forth in order to induce interest, attract, and invite the maximal possible numbers of women. The strong side of the study is that this was a new study in our country and that it provided positive emotions not only for the participants of the study, but also for hospitalized women who did not participate in the study, as voluntary assistance to others added meaningfulness to the sessions.

Conflicts of Interest

The authors declare that there are no conflicts of interest or financial support regarding the publication of this paper.

Authors' Contributions

All the authors have reviewed and approved the manuscript before submission.

Acknowledgments

The study was conducted with the permission of the Bioethics Center of the Lithuanian University of Health Sciences (no. BEC-SR (M)-186), the permission of the European Organization for Research and Treatment of Cancer (EORTC) Quality of Life Group to use the quality of life questionnaire EORTC QLQ-C30 and its module EORTC QLQ-BR23 in the study, and the permission of the Associate Professor A. M. Eakman from Colorado State University to use the Engagement in Meaningful Activities Survey (EMAS) in the study. The manuscript does not concern any commercial product.

References

[1] American Cancer Society, *Global Cancer Facts & Figures*, American Cancer Society, Atlanta, 3rd edition, 2015.

[2] National Cancer Institute, *NCI Dictionary of Cancer Terms*, https://www.cancer.gov/publications/dictionaries/cancer-terms?cdrid=444971.

[3] V. Ostapenko, A. Jackevičius, J. Didžiapetrienė, and V. Atkočius, *Lithuanian Breast Cancer: Scientific and Clinical Aspects. Scientific educational monograph*, National Cancer Institute, Vilnius, Lithuania, 2016.

[4] International Agency for Research on Cancer / World Health Organization, *Cancer Fact Sheet: Breast Cancer*, 2016, http://gco.iarc.fr/today/data/pdf/fact-sheets/cancers/cancer-fact-sheets-15.pdf.

[5] C. Conley, B. Bishop, and B. Andersen, "Emotions and Emotion Regulation in Breast Cancer Survivorship," *Healthcare*, vol. 4, no. 4, p. 56, 2016.

[6] European Network of Cancer Registries Factsheets, *Breast Cancer Factsheet*, European Union/ENCR, 2014, http://www.encr.eu/images/docs/factsheets/ENCR_Factsheet_Breast_2014.pdf.

[7] D. Gudavičienė, L. Steponavičienė, and N. Lachej, "Krūties vėžys Lietuvoje," *Acta Medica Lituanica*, vol. 22, no. 3, pp. 150–160, 2015.

[8] American Cancer Society, *Breast Cancer Facts & Figures 2015-2016*, American Cancer Society, Atlanta, 2015.

[9] E. Juozaitytė, A. Naudžiūnas, L. Valius, D. Krančiukaitytė-Butylkinienė, and et al., "Fundamentals of Family Medicine," in *Practical Skills. Tutorial*, pp. 13–70, UAB Vitae Litera, Kaunas, Lithuania, 2016.

[10] V. T. Devita, T. S. Lawrence, and S. A. Rosenberg, *Cancer: Principles & Practice of Oncology*, Lippincott Williams Wilkins, Wolters Kluwer, Philadelphia, USA, 8th edition, 2008.

[11] S. J. Sohl, B. Levine, and N. E. Avis, "Evaluation of the Quality of Life in Adult Cancer Survivors (QLACS) scale for early post-treatment breast cancer survivors," *Quality of Life Research*, vol. 24, no. 1, pp. 205–212, 2015.

[12] B. Gruževskis and U. L. Orlova, "Sąvokos Gyvenimo kokybė raidos tendencijos," *Socialinis darbas*, vol. 11, no. 1, pp. 7–18, 2012.

[13] D. Schoormans, K. Czene, P. Hall, and Y. Brandberg, "The impact of co-morbidity on health-related quality of life in breast cancer survivors and controls," *Acta Oncologica*, vol. 54, no. 5, pp. 727–734, 2015.

[14] Deluliis E. D. and Hughes J. K., *Occupational Therapy's Role in Breast Cancer Rehabilitation*, The American Occupational Therapy Association Fact Sheet, 2012.

[15] M. Pergolotti, G. R. Williams, C. Campbell, L. A. Munoz, and H. B. Muss, "Occupational therapy for adults with cancer: Why it matters," *The Oncologist*, vol. 21, no. 3, pp. 314–319, 2016.

[16] V. Repšaitė, *The effect of differential training on functional movements and autonomy of persons suffering from stroke*, Lithuanian University of Health Sciences, Medical Academy, 2015.

[17] American Occupational Therapy Association Fact Sheet, *The Role of Occupational Therapy With Health Promotion*, American Occupational Therapy Association, 2015.

[18] G. Cook and J. Thompson, "Purposeful activity," in *Nursing Case Studies on Improving Health-Related Quality of Life in Older Adults*, M. W. Kazer and K. Murphy, Eds., Gasch Printing, USA, 2015.

[19] M. E. Scaffa and S. M. Reitz, *Occupational Therapy in Community-Based Practice Settings*, F. A. Davis Company, Philadelphia, USA, 2th edition, 2014.

[20] I. Banienė and L. Šinkariova, "Relationship between the personality traits of women with breast cancer and the stress-related illness-related strategies for health-related quality of life," *Health Sciences*, vol. 25, no. 3, pp. 11–16, 2015.

[21] A. M. Eakman, M. E. Carlson, and F. A. Clark, "Factor Structure, Reliability, and Convergent Validity of the Engagement in Meaningful Activities Survey for Older Adults," *OTJR: Occupation, Participation, Health*, vol. 30, no. 3, pp. 111–121, 2010.

[22] P. O. Dialla, W.-O. Chu, P. Roignot et al., "Impact of age-related socio-economic and clinical determinants of quality of life among long-term breast cancer survivors," *Maturitas*, vol. 81, no. 3, pp. 362–370, 2015.

[23] H. Robinson, *A community-based occupational therapy program for women afer breast cancer [Master, thesis]*, Afer Cancer Experience, 2015, http://utdr.utoledo.edu/cgi/viewcontent.cgi?article=1601&context=graduate-projects.

[24] N. K. Aaronson, S. Ahinedzai, B. Bergman et al., "The European Organization for Research and Treatment of Cancer QLQ-C30: a quality-of-life instrument for use in international clinical trials in oncology," *Journal of the National Cancer Institute*, vol. 85, no. 5, pp. 365–376, 1993.

[25] M. J. Yuste Sánchez, M. T. Lacomba, B. S. Sánchez et al., "Health related quality of life improvement in breast cancer patients: Secondary outcome from a simple blinded, randomised clinical trial," *The Breast Journal*, vol. 24, no. 1, pp. 75–81, 2015.

[26] K. Almutairi, E. Mansour, and J. Vinluan, "A cross-sectional assessment of quality of life of breast cancer patients in Saudi Arabia," *Public Health*, vol. 136, pp. 117–125, 2016.

[27] D. Moro-Valdezate, E. Buch-Villa, S. Peiró et al., "Factors associated with health-related quality of life in a cohort of Spanish breast cancer patients," *Breast Cancer*, vol. 21, no. 4, pp. 442–452, 2014.

[28] C. Rohani, H.-A. Abedi, R. Omranipour, and A. Langius-Eklöf, "Health-related quality of life and the predictive role of sense of coherence, spirituality and religious coping in a sample of Iranian women with breast cancer: a prospective study with comparative design," *Health and Quality of Life Outcomes*, vol. 13, article 40, 2015.

[29] I. Ghislain, E. Zikos, C. Coens et al., "Health-related quality of life in locally advanced and metastatic breast cancer: methodological and clinical issues in randomised controlled trials," *The Lancet Oncology*, vol. 17, no. 7, pp. e294–e304, 2016.

23

Evaluating Hand Function in Clients with Trigger Finger

Danit Langer,[1] Adina Maeir,[1] Michael Michailevich,[2] and Shai Luria[3]

[1]*School of Occupational Therapy, Hadassah and Hebrew University, Jerusalem, Israel*
[2]*Department of Orthopaedics, Sherutay Briut Clalit, Jerusalem, Israel*
[3]*Department of Orthopedic Surgery, Hadassah-Hebrew University Medical Center, Jerusalem, Israel*

Correspondence should be addressed to Danit Langer; dlanger10@gmail.com

Academic Editor: Claudia Hilton

Background. Trigger finger (TF) is a common hand pathology frequently encountered in hand clinics. Occupational therapists predominantly assess TF symptoms as opposed to using standardized hand functioning assessments. The purpose of this study was to assess the construct validity of dexterity and grip strength assessments for clients with TF. *Method.* Sixty-three participants with TF and 66 healthy controls were administered the Functional Dexterity Test (FDT), Purdue Pegboard Test (PPT), and Jamar® Hydraulic Hand Dynamometer (JD) and completed the Disabilities of Arm Shoulder and Hand questionnaire (DASH). TF symptoms were graded using the Quinnell classification. *Results.* Statistically significant differences were found between the groups in dexterity and grip strength. A statistically significant difference between the three TF grades was found on the PPT. All three test scores were moderately correlated with the DASH scores. *Conclusion.* This study provides innovative evidence for the validity of common hand function assessments for individuals with TF and recommends incorporating these tools in clinical practice. Further research is needed with larger samples and better representation of each TF clinical grade.

1. Introduction

Hand functionis a broad term that incorporates several components, including strength, sensation, range of motion, and dexterity. Normal function of the hand is an important factor in a person's ability to independently engage in daily activities and occupations [1]. Damage to one or more of these components can lead to dysfunction of the hand and limit participation in everyday life [2]. According to the International Classification of Function (ICF), there is an interaction between the elements of *body systems* and *structures* (such as dexterity and strength), *activity* and *participation* in life roles, and *contextual factors* (environmental factors and personal factors) [3].

Trigger Finger (TF), also termed Stenosing Flexor Tenosynovitis, is one of the most common pathologies seen in hand surgery clinics and is the fourth leading cause of referral to these clinics [4]. Triggering of the finger commonly occurs at the fibroosseous tunnel formed by the metacarpal neck and the first annular pulley. The initial complaints associated with TF are pain over the A1 pulley or clicking and may worsen to severe pain and locking of the digit in flexion [5]. The incidence of TF is 28 : 100,000 per year or a lifetime risk of 2.6% in the general population, but it increases to 10% in the diabetic population [6]. The mean age of onset for TF is 58 years and it is diagnosed in women two to six times more frequently than men [5]. The diagnosis of TF is based on symptoms and physical examination, yet in recently published consensus guidelines for managing TF no uniform grading system has been recommended [7]. There are a variety of methods to treat TF; interventions include both nonsurgical and surgical treatment options [8]. In recently published guidelines, experts agreed on the following methods for the management of TF: orthotics, corticosteroid injections, and surgical treatment. When planning a treatment regimen, they recommend considering the severity and duration of the pathology as well as previous treatment [7].

The majority of the intervention studies regarding TF utilized symptom resolution as the outcome measure, as opposed to utilizing hand function outcomes, such as dexterity and strength [9–12]. A similar trend was found among a cohort of 61 occupational therapists from Israel and the

United States, who reported on their assessment practices for clients with TF. These therapists predominantly evaluate TF symptoms, as opposed to the use of standardized hand functioning assessments in clients with other hand conditions [13]. This trend could be attributed to the fact that assessments for hand function have not been validated for individuals with TF. In addition, the lack of validated measures may impede documenting and establishing evidence based occupational therapy for treating individuals with TF [14]. Therefore, the aim of the present study was to assess the construct validity of tools for measuring several components of hand function in clients with TF.

The focus of this study is on hand function measures of dexterity and strength. Dexterity is the ability to use your hands skillfully and is defined as fine, voluntary movement used to manipulate small objects during a specific task [15]. Dexterity can be subcategorized into gross manual dexterity, which is the ability to handle objects with the hand and into fine motor dexterity, which refers to in-hand manipulations using the thumb and second or third digit (McPhee in [16, 17]). Grip strength is defined as the force applied by the hand and fingers or the measurable ability to exert pressure on objects. In the consensus guidelines for the assessment of clients with hand conditions it was agreed that the Jamar Hydraulic Hand Dynamometer (JD) and the Pinch Gauge device should be used to assess strength, yet no consensus was reached regarding the assessment of dexterity [18]. The evaluation of dexterity can provide information about the neuromotor function of the hand, since sensation and intrinsic hand strength are essential for performing manipulative movements [15].

There are many methods available to assess dexterity and the selection of an appropriate tool is often based on a variety of factors, including availability, familiarity, and applicability to a given population and psychometric soundness. For the assessment of dexterity in the present study we used the Functional Dexterity Test (FDT) and the Purdue Pegboard Test (PPT) whose psychometric properties have been well established in other targeted health populations [1, 15] and have been reported to be commonly used by occupational therapists in hand clinics [13].

Study Objectives. The objectives of the study were to assess the construct validity of the FDT, PPT, and the JD for people with TF, specifically to (a) evaluate the ability of these measures to distinguish amongst grades of TF severity; (b) to distinguish between groups with and without TF; (c) to assess whether the side of the involved hand (radial or ulnar) effects grip strength and dexterity; and (d) finally to evaluate the correlation between measures of hand function and self-reported disability. Accordingly the research questions were as follows: (a) Will statistically significant differences be found between the three TF grades in the scores of the FDT, PPT, and JD? (b) Will statistically significant differences be found between the TF and control groups in the scores of the FDT, PPT, and JD? (c) Will statistically significant differences be found between participants with TF on the radial side and the ulnar side in the scores of the FDT, PPT, and JD? (d) Will statistically significant correlation be found between the DASH score and the FDT, PPT, and JD scores of the TF group?

2. Method

2.1. Study Design. The study was a cross-sectional study.

2.2. Participants. The study protocol was approved by the Institutional Helsinki Committee. One hundred and fifty consecutive clients with TF that presented to a central orthopedic clinic of a major health maintenance organization (HMO) and an outpatient clinic in a major hospital between March 1st 2012 and April 30th 2013 were invited to participate in the study. Inclusion criteria were adult clients (age 18 years or above) with a diagnosis of one or more digits with TF of a Quinnell grade one or higher. According to the Quinnell grading system, TF fingers are rated as follows: 0, normal movement of the digit; 1, uneven movement; 2, actively correctable locking of the digit; 3, passively correctable locking; and 4, fixed deformity [19]. The exclusion criteria were upper extremity trauma in the preceding year, known neurological deficits, known cognitive deficits, and pregnant women. Written informed consent was obtained from all participants in the study. The demographic and clinical data of the participants were recorded. Participants were classified as having additional medical conditions if they reported one or more medical condition besides TF. The severity of the TF was recorded by the hand surgeon using the Quinnell grading system. Consenting TF participants were administered the FDT, PPT, JD, numeric pain scale, and the Disabilities of the Arm Shoulder and Hand (DASH) questionnaire immediately after their visit with the doctor. A control group of 66 healthy participants was recruited using a convenience sample and matched for age and gender to the research group. The TF and control groups data was previously analyzed and published [20, 21]. The results of these two studies demonstrated (a) the effect of TF severity on functioning and quality of life as measured by the DASH and the World Health Organization Quality of Life Brief questionnaire (WHOQ-BRIEF) [21] and (b) the wide impact of TF on hand functioning, activities of daily living, and quality of life [20].

2.3. Measures

2.3.1. Functional Dexterity Test (FDT). The FDT tool is suitable for the adult population, 20–70 years old, with various injuries to the upper limb. The FDT gives information regarding the clients' ability to use their hands for functional tasks requiring a dynamic 3-jaw chuck grasp pattern. It is made of a square wooden pegboard with 16 pegs. The examiner documents the time required to turn over all the pegs. Execution time is measured on each hand separately. A five-second penalty is added every time the participant supinates or touches the board and a 10-second penalty is added if the participant drops a peg. Two scores are obtained for each hand: the net time in seconds and the total score (net time plus penalties). The net time score was used in the present study. The FDT was found to have good interrater and good test retest reliability [16, 22].

2.3.2. Purdue Pegboard Test (PPT). The PPT was developed in 1948, in order to assess manual dexterity and precision of applicants for industrial work [23]. Since then, the PPT has been used in rehabilitation and in research [24]. The PPT includes four subtests; in the first three subtests participants are asked within 30 seconds to place the maximum number of metal pins, one at a time, into a row of pegboard holes, first with their dominant hand and then with their nondominant hand followed by placing pairs of pins with both hands simultaneously. In the fourth and final subtest, the participant uses alternate hands to form the maximum number of assemblies consisting of a pin, washer, collar, and second washer within 60 seconds. The PPT tests the quality and speed of performance of the hand as the person accomplishes the four subtests [23].

2.3.3. Jamar Hydraulic Hand Dynamometer (JD). The JD was designed to measure gross power fist grip and is considered to be the most accurate test for this skill. The American Society of Hand Therapists (ASHT) recommended the use of this tool for the assessment of grip strength [25]. The test was administered with the guidelines of the ASHT. Psychometric testing found good interrater reliability and high test retest reliability [26].

2.3.4. Disabilities of the Arm Shoulder and Hand (DASH). The DASH was developed in order to describe the disability experienced by people with upper-limb disorders and also to monitor changes in symptoms and function over time. The questionnaire consists of 30 questions related to physical function, social function, and different symptoms. Each item has five response options. The scores for all items are then used to calculate a scale score ranging from 0 (no disability) to 100 (most severe disability). There are two additional parts with four questions that are relevant for people that engage in sports, music, and work [27]. These parts were not included in the present study.

2.3.5. The Quinnell Grading System. The Quinnell grading system is used to assess clinical severity of TF. According to this classification, TF fingers are rated as follows: 0, normal movement of the digit; 1, uneven movement; 2, actively correctable locking of the digit; 3, passively correctible locking; and 4, fixed deformity [19].

2.3.6. Numerical Pain Rating Scale (NRS). The NRS is a scale with 11 degrees, reflecting the subjective intensity of pain experienced by a person during the preceding day or the previous week (see Figure 2). The pain scale can be administered verbally or by using a visual scale [28].

2.4. Data Analysis. The distribution of variables in the study (FDT, PPT, JD, pain, and age) met the criteria for normality based on the Shapiro-Wilk test of normality ($p > 0.05$). Prior to main hypotheses testing, between groups comparisons of demographics and background clinical data were performed in order to rule out extraneous factors (demographics and background clinical data) that might influence the results. Analysis of variance (ANOVA) was used to compare age and pain intensity between the TF subgroups (TF grades 1–3). A Chi-Square analysis was used to compare gender, hand dominance, affected hand, and presence of additional medical conditions between study and control group and between TF subgroups.

For the hypotheses testing, one-way ANOVA was used in order to compare the mean scores (FDT, PPT, and JD) obtained by the different TF grades and post hoc Tukey HSD test comparisons between groups were conducted. The TF group was divided according to affected finger. If the affected finger was the thumb index or middle finger the participant was assigned to the radial side affected group and if affected finger was the ring or small finger the participant was assigned to the ulnar side affected group. An independent sample t-test was used to compare FDT, PPT, and JD between radial and ulnar affected side groups. The correlations between the FDT, PPT, JD, and DASH were calculated using Pearson's correlations. Effects sizes were calculated according to the statistical test, partial eta squared for ANOVA [29], and Cohen's d for t-test and correlation [30].

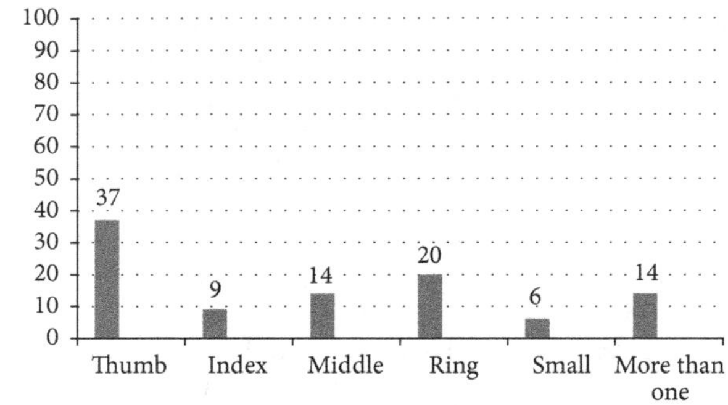

FIGURE 1: Distribution of Trigger finger digits.

2.5. Procedure. Informed consent was obtained by hand surgeons. The hand functioning assessments and questionnaires were administered by experienced occupational therapists to participants immediately after their visit with the doctor. The occupational therapists were trained in the administration of the assessments and were tested for correct administration by the head researcher. Healthy participants were administered the same assessment protocol.

3. Results

Of 150 clients presenting with TF during the study period, a total of 63 met the inclusion criteria, agreed to participate in the study, and completed all assessments. The study group included participants with TF grades 1–3. Demographic and clinical data of participants are presented in Table 1 and distribution of affected digits in Figure 1. No statistically significant differences in demographic and background clinical data were found between subgroups of TF grades, between healthy and control groups, and between radial affected side and ulnar affected side groups ($p > 0.05$).

3.1. Differences in Hand Function between TF Grades. A statistically significant large effect of TF grade was found for PPT subtests demonstrating a decrease in PPT scores with

Table 1: Demographic and clinical data: comparison of TF subgroups.

	TF (n = 63)	TF 1 (n = 11)	TF 2 (n = 43)	TF 3 (n = 9)	Control (n = 66)
	Mean (SD)	Mean (SD)	Mean (SD)	Mean (SD)	Mean (SD)
Age	60.48 (11.34)	57.08 (16.8)	60.53 (9.87)	63.44 (10.87)	58.60 (11.55)
Pain	5.52 (2.45)	5.82 (1.53)	5.48 (2.78)	5.33 (1.58)	
	n (%)	n (%)	n (%)	n (%)	n (%)
Gender					
Male	20 (32)	5 (45)	13 (30)	2 (22)	23 (35)
Female	43 (68)	6 (55)	30 (70)	7 (78)	43 (65)
Dominance					
Right	56 (89)	10 (91)	40 (93)	6 (67)	57 (86)
Left	7 (11)	1 (9)	3 (7)	3 (33)	9 (14)
Affected Hand					
Dominant	36 (57)	9 (82)	21 (49)	6 (67)	
Nondominant	17 (27)	1 (9)	14 (33)	2 (22)	
Both	10 (16)	1 (9)	8 (18)	1 (11)	
Additional conditions					
Yes	34 (54)	5 (45)	24 (56)	4 (44)	27 (41)
No	29 (46)	6 (55)	19 (44)	5 (56)	39 (59)

TF = trigger finger.

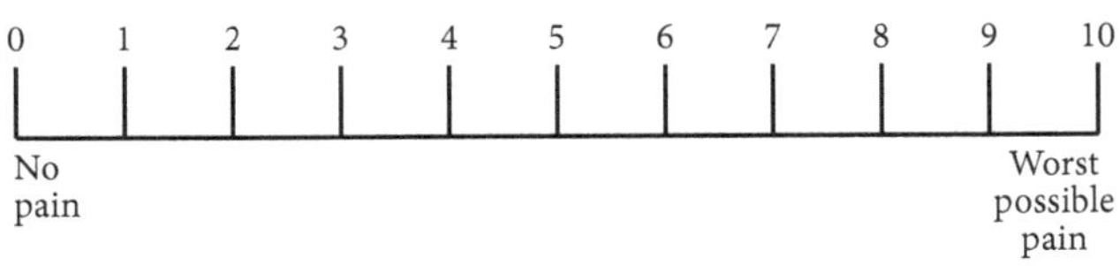

Figure 2: Numerical Pain Rating Scale.

increasing severity of TF ($p < 0.05$) (see Table 2). Post hoc comparisons revealed statistically significant differences between grades 1 and 3 TF subgroups on the affected hand, both hands, and assembly subtests. For both hands subtest a statistically significant difference was also found between grades 2 and 3. As for the FDT, a nonstatistically significant trend was found of increased scores (a higher score reflects reduced dexterity) with higher grade of pathology severity. As for grip strength no group effect was found (see Table 2).

3.2. Decreased Hand Function in TF Group versus Control Group. A statistically significant difference was found between the TF group and controls in all tests scores. The control group achieved superior scores in all the tests (see Table 3).

3.3. Differences in Hand Function between TF Participants with Radial versus Ulnar Side Affected. There were 44 participants with TF on the radial side of the hand and 19 with TF on the ulnar side. No statistically significant differences were found between these two groups in all the measures (see Table 4).

3.4. Dexterity and Grip Strength Test Scores Correlate with Disability Score. Statistically significant moderate correlations were found between the DASH and all the test scores of the affected hand in the TF group except for the PPT affected hand subtest (see Table 5).

4. Discussion

The purpose of the study was to evaluate the construct validity of the FDT, PPT, and JD for participants with TF. The results of the present study demonstrated that all three tools discriminated between people with and without TF. However, only the PPT had a statistically significant group effect on the clinical grades. Statistically significant differences were found between clinical grades 1 and 3 for all subtests of the PPT. No statistically significant differences were found between participants who had TF on the radial or ulnar side. Furthermore, all the tools (excluding one PPT subtest) were statistically significantly correlated with the DASH.

The results of the present study demonstrated the impairment in dexterity among individuals with TF in comparison to controls and that this impairment increased with the severity of TF. The FDT and PPT are both commonly used in clinical settings [13] yet there is a paucity of studies that examined the degree to which these tools are valid for assessing populations with specific hand conditions [24]. The current findings support the validity of the PPT in the TF population and are in line with studies of dexterity in individuals with other hand conditions. A study that examined the validity and reliability of the PPT for people with Carpal Tunnel Syndrome (CTS) found an association between disease severity and all the subtests of the PPT in patients aged 60 and older and statistically significant differences between the CTS group and controls [31]. An earlier study conducted by Ben Shahar et al., in 1998, also found that the PPT differentiated between a group of clients with a variety of hand conditions and controls. In addition to the evidence obtained regarding construct validity, the findings of this study also support

Table 2: Mean difference in FDT, PPT, and JD scores amongst different groups TF grades.

	TF grades											
	TF 1 ($n = 11$)		TF 2 ($n = 42$)		TF 3 ($n = 9$)		ANOVA			I versus II	I versus III	II versus III
	Mean (SD)	95% CI	Mean (SD)	95% CI	Mean (SD)	95% CI	F	p	η_{p2}	p	p	p
FDT affected hand	28.34 (4.98)	13.22–43.45	37.41 (28.74)	29.67–45.14	47.39 (21.43)	30.68–64.11	1.453	0.246	0.046	0.568	0.247	0.558
PPT affected hand	13.18 (2.04)	11.83–14.53	11.55 (2.13)	10.86–12.24	10 (2.87)	10.86–12.24	5.083	0.009*	0.147	0.106	0.010*	0.177
PPT both hands	10.64 (1.21)	9.55–11.73	9.38 (1.89)	8.82–9.94	7.67 (1.94)	8.82–9.94	6.705	0.002*	0.185	0.131	0.002*	0.042*
PPT assembly	28.36 (7.55)	25.12–31.61	23.88 (4.68)	22.22–25.54	19.22 (5.4)	15.64–22.81	7.191	0.002*	0.196	0.056	0.002**	0.070
JD affected hand	21.4 (5.29)	15.72–27.01	16.25 (9.87)	13.34–19.16	16.61 (9.48)	10.33–22.9	1.324	0.274	0.043	0.280	0.531	0.995

TF = trigger finger; FDT = Functional Dexterity Test; PPT = Purdue Pegboard Test; JD = Jamar Hydraulic Hand Dynamometer.
* $p \le 0.05$; ** $p \le 0.001$.

TABLE 3: Mean difference in in FDT, PPT, and JD among TF and control groups.

	TF group mean (SD)	Control group mean (SD)	$t_{(df)}$	p	Effect size	95% CI of the difference
FDT DH ($n = 44$)	36.5 (28.3)	27.7 (8.5)	$2.0_{(108)}$	0.05	0.421	16.1–1.4
FDT NDH ($n = 19$)	38.8 (15.8)	29.2 (7.7)	$2.6_{(83)}$	0.017	0.772	17.5–1.9
PPT DH ($n = 44$)	11.9 (2.5)	13.5 (2.5)	$3.3_{(108)}$	0.001	0.639	0.6–2.5
PPT NDH ($n = 19$)	10.6 (1.9)	13.0 (2.4)	$4.1_{(83)}$	0.001	1.108	1.3–3.6
PPT BH ($n = 63$)	9.3 (2)	10.5 (2.1)	$3.3_{(127)}$	0.002	0.585	0.5–1.9
PPT assembly ($n = 62$)	24 (5.9)	27.5 (8.23)	$2.8_{(126)}$	0.006	0.489	1.1–6.01
JD DH ($n = 44$)	19.2 (8.8)	28.5 (10.2)	$4.9_{(108)}$	0.001	0.976	5.6–13.1
JD NDH ($n = 19$)	11.1 (8.5)	26.4 (10.1)	$6.1_{(83)}$	0.001	1.639	10.3–20.4

TF = trigger finger; FDT = Functional Dexterity Test; PPT = Purdue Pegboard Test; JD = Jamar Hydraulic Hand Dynamometer; DH = dominant hand; NDH = nondominant Hand; BH = both hands.

TABLE 4: Mean difference in FDT, PPT, and JD scores between TF participants with radial versus ulnar side affected.

	Radial affected side group $n = 44$ Mean (SD)	Ulnar affected side group $n = 19$ Mean (SD)	p
FDT affected hand	40.7 (18.5)	45.5 (39.4)	NS
PPT affected hand	11.6 (2.7)	11.4 (1.7)	NS
PPT both hands	9.3 (2.1)	9.3 (1.8)	NS
PPT assembly	23.7 (6.1)	24.7 (5.3)	NS
JD affected hand	16.6 (8.6)	19.4 (11.6)	NS

FDT = Functional Dexterity Test; PPT = Purdue Pegboard Test; JD = Jamar Hydraulic Hand Dynamometer.

TABLE 5: Correlations between FDT, PPT, and JD scores and DASH scores in TF group.

	FDT affected hand	PPT affected hand	PPT both hands	PPT assembly	JD affected hand
DASH	0.301^{*}	−0.214	-0.418^{**}	-0.350^{**}	-0.472^{**}

$^{*}p < 0.05$; $^{**}p < 0.01$.
FDT = Functional Dexterity Test; PPT = Purdue Pegboard Test; DJ = Jamar Hydraulic Hand Dynamometer; DASH = Disabilities of the Arm Shoulder and Hand.

the ecological validity of the PPT for individuals with TF as demonstrated by moderate correlations between PPT subtests and the DASH. These findings are in line with previous studies that demonstrated moderate correlations between the PPT and Activities of Daily Living (ADL) [24, 32]. However, a recent study by Gonzalez et al. [33] demonstrated that the grasping patterns of the fingers while preforming the PPT differed from the patterns observed while performing ADL. The authors suggest that traditional hand function assessments may not capture the complex hand performance that is essential for completing ADL. These findings are in line with the results of the present study that demonstrated only a moderate correlation between the PPT and the DASH. These findings stress the importance of conducting a broad assessment that includes all parts of the ICF model when treating clients with hand conditions.

The findings regarding grip strength differed from dexterity, as no group effect of the clinical grades was demonstrated on the JD. However, TF participants had statistically significant weaker grip strength than the control group. Furthermore, a moderate statistically significant correlation was found between the JD and the DASH, supporting its ecological validity for the TF population. We were unable to find similar studies which used the JD with TF participants. However, several studies have demonstrated a similar trend of decreased grip strength among people with upper extremity musculoskeletal disorders in comparison to healthy controls [34]. Regarding correlation between grip strength and ADL, similar correlations were demonstrated in studies of elderly and individuals after distal radial fracture [35, 36].

5. Conclusions

The current findings suggest that the PPT and FDT are valid tools for measuring dexterity and the JD is a valid measure of strength in clients with TF. According to the results of the current study the PPT was more sensitive to the clinical grades of TF than the other measures. The PPT, FDT, and JD were moderately correlated with a measure of disability (DASH). These findings are important in light of recent findings whereby a very low percentage of occupational therapists use these assessments in their practice with clients with TF, despite the fact that they commonly use these tools with other clients [13]. Based on the findings of the present study therapists may consider incorporating these measures into their assessment protocol for clients with TF.

Additional Points

Study Limitations and Recommendations. The distribution of participants among the TF grades was not equal. Therefore, the findings of this study should be interpreted with caution. Further studies with larger representation of TF grades are recommended.

Competing Interests

The authors declare that they have no competing interests.

References

[1] K. Schoneveld, H. Wittink, and T. Takken, "Clinimetric evaluation of measurement tools used in hand therapy to assess activity and participation," *Journal of Hand Therapy*, vol. 22, no. 3, pp. 221–236, 2009.

[2] M. C. Kasch and J. M. Walsh, "Hand and upper extremity injuries," in *Pedretti's Occupational Therapy: Practice Skills for Physical Dysfunction*, H. M. Pendleton and W. Schultz-Krohn, Eds., pp. 1037–1073, Mosby, St. Louis, Mo, USA, 2013.

[3] World Health Organization, *Towards a Common Language for Functioning, Disability and Health: ICF*, World Health Organization, Geneva, Switzerland, 2001.

[4] C. L. Kerrigan and M. G. Stanwix, "Using evidence to minimize the cost of trigger finger care," *The Journal of Hand Surgery*, vol. 34, no. 6, pp. 997–1005, 2009.

[5] A. H. Makkouk, M. E. Oetgen, C. R. Swigart, and S. D. Dodds, "Trigger finger: etiology, evaluation, and treatment," *Current Reviews in Musculoskeletal Medicine*, vol. 1, no. 2, pp. 92–96, 2008.

[6] W.-L. Tung, L.-C. Kuo, K.-Y. Lai, I.-M. Jou, Y.-N. Sun, and F.-C. Su, "Quantitative evidence of kinematics and functional differences in different graded trigger fingers," *Clinical Biomechanics*, vol. 25, no. 6, pp. 535–540, 2010.

[7] B. M. A. Huisstede, P. Hoogvliet, J. Henk Coert, and J. Fridén, "Multidisciplinary consensus guideline for managing trigger finger: results from the European HANDGUIDE study," *Physical Therapy*, vol. 94, no. 10, pp. 1421–1433, 2014.

[8] M. P. Lee, S. J. Biafora, and D. S. Zelouf, "Management of hand and wrist tendinopathies," in *Rehabilitation of the Hand and Upper Extremity*, T. M. Skirven, A. L. Fedorczy, and P. Amadio, Eds., pp. 569–588, Mosby, Philadelphia, Pa, USA, 2011.

[9] J. Castellanos, E. Muñoz-Mahamud, E. Domínguez, P. Del Amo, O. Izquierdo, and P. Fillat, "Long-term effectiveness of corticosteroid injections for trigger finger and thumb," *The Journal of Hand Surgery*, vol. 40, no. 1, pp. 121–126, 2015.

[10] K. Tarbhai, S. Hannah, and H. P. Von Schroeder, "Trigger finger treatment: a comparison of 2 splint designs," *The Journal of Hand Surgery*, vol. 37, no. 2, pp. 243–249, 2012.

[11] K. Valdes, "A retrospective review to determine the long-term efficacy of orthotic devices for trigger finger," *Journal of Hand Therapy*, vol. 25, no. 1, pp. 89–96, 2012.

[12] R. D. Wojahn, N. C. Foeger, R. H. Gelberman, and R. P. Calfee, "Long-term outcomes following a single corticosteroid injection for trigger finger," *Journal of Bone & Joint Surgery*, vol. 96, no. 22, pp. 1849–1854, 2014.

[13] D. Langer, S. Luria, A. Maeir, and A. Erez, "Occupation-based assessments and treatments of trigger finger: a survey of occupational therapists from Israel and the United States," *Occupational Therapy International*, vol. 21, no. 4, pp. 143–155, 2014.

[14] S. A. Gutman, M. H. Mortera, J. Hinojosa, and P. Kramer, "Revision of the occupational therapy practice framework," *American Journal of Occupational Therapy*, vol. 61, no. 1, pp. 119–126, 2007.

[15] K. E. Yancosek and D. Howell, "A narrative review of dexterity assessments," *Journal of Hand Therapy*, vol. 22, no. 3, pp. 258–270, 2009.

[16] F. Sartorio, E. Bravini, S. Vercelli et al., "The Functional Dexterity Test: test-retest reliability analysis and up-to date reference norms," *Journal of Hand Therapy*, vol. 26, no. 1, pp. 62–68, 2013.

[17] N. Weintraub, N. Gilmour-Grill, and P. L. T. Weiss, "Relationship between handwriting and keyboarding performance among fast and slow adult keyboarders," *American Journal of Occupational Therapy*, vol. 64, no. 1, pp. 123–132, 2010.

[18] L. A. W. Van De Ven-Stevens, M. J. L. Graff, R. W. Selles et al., "Instruments for assessment of impairments and activity limitations in patients with hand conditions: a European Delphi study," *Journal of Rehabilitation Medicine*, vol. 47, no. 10, pp. 948–956, 2015.

[19] R. C. Quinnell, "Conservative management of trigger finger," *The Practitioner*, vol. 224, no. 1340, pp. 187–190, 1980.

[20] D. Langer, A. Maeir, M. Michailevich, Y. Applebaum, and S. Luria, "Using the international classification of functioning to examine the impact of trigger finger," *Disability and Rehabilitation*, vol. 38, no. 26, pp. 2530–2537, 2016.

[21] D. Langer, S. Luria, A. Bar-Haim Erez, M. Michailevich, N. Rogev, and A. Maeir, "Stenosing flexor tenosynovitis: validity of standard assessment tools of daily functioning and quality of life," *Journal of Hand Therapy*, vol. 28, no. 4, pp. 384–388, 2015.

[22] D. H. Aaron and C. W. S. Jansen, "Development of the Functional Dexterity Test (FDT): construction, validity, reliability, and normative data," *Journal of Hand Therapy*, vol. 16, no. 1, pp. 12–21, 2003.

[23] J. Tiffin, *Purdue Pegboard Test*, Science Research, Chicago, Ill, USA, 1948.

[24] R. Ben Shahar, R. Kizony, and A. Nota, "Validity of the Purdue Pegboard Test in assessing patients after traumatic hand injury," *Work*, vol. 11, no. 3, pp. 315–320, 1998.

[25] E. E. Fess, "Grip strength," in *Clinical Assessment Recommendations*, J. S. Casanova, Ed., pp. 41–45, American Society of Hand Therapists, Chicago, Ill, USA, 2nd edition, 1992.

[26] V. Mathiowetz, "Effects of three trials on grip and pinch strength measurements," *Journal of Hand Therapy*, vol. 3, no. 4, pp. 195–198, 1990.

[27] S. Solway, D. E. Beaton, S. McConnell, and C. Bombardier, *The DASH Outcome Measure User's Manual*, Institute for Work and Health, Toronto, Canada, 2nd edition, 2002.

[28] H. Breivik, P. C. Borchgrevink, S. M. Allen et al., "Assessment of pain," *British Journal of Anaesthesia*, vol. 101, no. 1, pp. 17–24, 2008.

[29] G. Keppel, *Design and Analysis: A Researcher's Handbook*, Prentice-Hall, Englewood Cliffs, NJ, USA, 1991.

[30] J. Cohen, *Statistical Power Analysis for the Behavioral Sciences*, Academic Press, 2013.

[31] N. Amirjani, N. L. Ashworth, J. L. Olson, M. Morhart, and K. M. Chan, "Validity and reliability of the purdue pegboard test in carpal tunnel syndrome," *Muscle & Nerve*, vol. 43, no. 2, pp. 171–177, 2011.

[32] G. Sandqvist, M. Eklund, A. Åkesson, and U. Nordenskiöld, "Daily activities and hand function in women with scleroderma," *Scandinavian Journal of Rheumatology*, vol. 33, no. 2, pp. 102–107, 2004.

[33] V. Gonzalez, J. Rowson, and A. Yoxall, "Analyzing finger interdependencies during the Purdue Pegboard Test and comparative activities of daily living," *Journal of Hand Therapy*, 2016.

[34] I. Kjeken, H. Dagfinrud, B. Slatkowsky-Christensen et al., "Activity limitations and participation restrictions in women with hand osteoarthritis: patients' descriptions and associations between dimensions of functioning," *Annals of the Rheumatic Diseases*, vol. 64, no. 11, pp. 1633–1638, 2005.

Role Participation: A Comparison across Age Groups in a Norwegian General Population Sample

Tore Bonsaksen[1,2]

[1]Department of Occupational Therapy, Prosthetics and Orthotics, Faculty of Health Sciences, OsloMet - Oslo Metropolitan University, Oslo, Norway
[2]Faculty of Health Studies, VID Specialized University, Sandnes, Norway

Correspondence should be addressed to Tore Bonsaksen; tore.bonsaksen@hioa.no

Academic Editor: Kathleen M. Matuska

Background. Life events, illness, and disability may alter a person's role participation, in which case occupational therapy may be an appropriate intervention. However, role participation data derived from the general population, which is required for meaningful comparison, is largely missing. This study is aimed at describing past, present, and anticipated role participation in a general population sample from Norway and at examining differences in current role participation between age groups. *Methods.* In 2015, a sample of 140 persons (age range 19–94 years, 65% females) from the Norwegian general population completed the Role Checklist at one occasion. The data were analyzed descriptively and with chi-square tests and one-way analysis of variance. *Results.* The most frequent role was a home maintainer (93.6%), and the least frequent was a religious participant (7.1%). Participants aged 65 years and above had fewer roles compared with their younger counterparts and had to a larger extent experienced role loss over the course of their lives. *Conclusions.* Role continuity was the most prevalent role pattern in the total sample, whereas role loss appeared to be the most prevalent role pattern among those in the oldest age group. Rehabilitation services in general and participation-focused occupational therapy in particular may profit from assessing role participation in clients and potentially target roles through intervention.

1. Introduction

A core aim for occupational therapy services is to promote participation in society by enabling the performance of meaningful, everyday-life occupation [1, 2]. Recently, researchers have suggested that participation may be understood primarily as participation within social roles [3–5]. This idea links the participation concept of the International Classification of Functioning, Disability and Health (ICF) [6] directly with the Model of Human Occupation (MOHO) theory [1], in which social roles are viewed as the main organizing principle of the person's occupational behavior. By performing the tasks and chores associated with social roles, one participates in society. Acting within social roles is *inter*acting—acting in relationship with others, directly or indirectly. The role content is constituted from the ongoing interaction between the person holding the role and their social environment. In other words, acting according to role expectations within the social context constitutes the theoretical definition of role participation [1].

Roles are partly prescribed—for example, one is born as someone's son or daughter. Over the life course, other social roles are acquired, as one takes on various social positions in relationship to others, for example, the role of a student or a teacher. The roles we enact at a given point in time influence what we do and how we do it. With practice, the person gradually identifies with their roles such that their role behaviors come naturally and without much consideration. At this point, the role is internalized within the person—it has become a part of the person's identity [1]. However, when reflecting on the value of roles, a study of Norwegian occupational therapy students showed that most of the performed roles, as reported on the employed Role Checklist, were also highly valued [7]. Subjective well-being among university students in Jordan was associated with having more roles and perceiving roles as more valuable [8], and similarly, participating in more valued roles was associated with higher quality of life among persons who had undergone liver transplantation [9].

Adverse life events, illness, and disability may limit the person's performance in social roles and may consequently change or restrict their social participation [1]. Several studies have been in support of this reasoning. For example, one study found more problems in academic, leisure, and work roles in adolescents with mental illness compared to healthy peers [10]. One year after the landfall of Hurricane Ike at the coast of Texas in September 2008, students in the area experienced that some previous roles were retained whereas others had been disrupted [11]. Scott's [9] study of liver transplant recipients also showed a pattern of disengagement with previously enacted roles, whereas Dickerson and Oakley's [12] study found a consistent pattern of more current roles among nondisabled community-living individuals compared with individuals who had physical or psychosocial disabilities.

However, not only do roles change as an effect of specific events but they also change over the natural life course, and occupational therapy may be relevant for remediating problematic role transitions [13]. In the words of Lee and Kielhofner [14], "Society expects and structures role transitions at various life stages such as entering and exiting the student role, beginning work, and retiring. People also choose to enter and leave roles" (p. 67). One perspective of role patterns across time, encompassing change as well as stability, was provided in a Canadian study of adults with severe mental health problems [15]. Using the Role Checklist [16] to examine roles in a time perspective, the researchers conceptualized role stability in terms of continuity (having the role in the past, present, and foreseen future) and absence (not having the role in the past, nor in the present or foreseen future). Role loss was conceptualized as having the role in the past, but not at present. Conversely, role gain was conceptualized as not having the role in the past, but having it at present. The concept "role change" was used to describe a situation where a role was not enacted at present but was expected in the future.

Conceptually, though, the above example of role change is more precisely one of the "expected role gains," which is merely one of several ways roles can change over time. Adding to this idea, we may therefore differentiate between two aspects of role change: expected role gain and expected role loss. A person heading towards retirement from work could exemplify how role change may involve both aspects. Retirement implies losing the role of a worker (role loss) but may also open up the possibility of taking up, for example, the role of a choir member or a volunteer for a charity organization (role gains).

Two contrasting theories of "successful aging" have traditionally been put forward: the activity theory and the disengagement theory [17, 18]. The latter view emphasizes accepting losses (e.g., of functional ability, activities, roles, and friends) and disengagement from active life, while the former emphasizes holding on—as far as possible—to the roles and activities of middle age. While both views seem valid, recent research evidence seems to favor the activity theory, essentially stating that having a good life in older years is not about giving in, but holding on. For example, Menec's [19] six-year longitudinal study of elderly persons demonstrated that in general, social and productive activities were positively related to higher levels of happiness, better functioning, and lower mortality. As activities are thought to be organized mainly according to roles [1], one could also suggest that having more roles might indicate greater satisfaction with life. Research has shown that currently held roles were often valued roles among students [7] and that participation in more valued roles was related to greater quality of life among liver transplant recipients [9]. However, the notion that having more roles is associated with greater life satisfaction, regardless of the person's valuation of these roles, is an assumption in need of further inquiry.

In summary, the available literature suggests that participating in more valued roles is a source of contentment and satisfaction with life. Moreover, it suggests that adverse life events, illness, and disability can potentially disrupt the individual's social roles. However, role participation is also affected by the normal progression through life. Thus, aging may often imply a need for adapting to new circumstances. Such adaptation may be a difficult process, and occupational therapy may be appropriate as a means to remediate disrupted participation in roles. However, existing studies have largely employed samples with highly specific characteristics, frequently related to a specific illness or disability (see, e.g., [9, 20, 21]). The one study providing comparisons with a general population sample [12] is both dated and concerned with the US context only. To be able to interpret role participation data from different clinical groups, one should preferably be able to compare with current data derived from the general population living in the relevant cultural context.

The present study is aimed at describing past, present, and anticipated role participation in a general population sample from Norway. Second, differences in current role participation between individuals in different age groups were examined. Lastly, building on the procedure described by Hachey and coworkers [15], we described the participants' role patterns.

2. Methods

The study employed a cross-sectional design, utilizing data from an assessment at one point in time. It serves as a Norway-specific substudy associated with a larger cross-cultural study of roles and their links with MOHO as a theoretical framework [3]. The data for the study was collected early in 2015.

2.1. Sample and Recruitment. The sample was a convenience sample of persons from the general population, recruited by personal contact made by nine occupational therapy students and occupational therapist colleagues in Oslo and in the surrounding metropolitan area. Age under 18 years was the only exclusion criterion. The participants were recruited with the aim of making the sample as diverse as possible, representing a blend of men and women and people in different age groups. The participants knew the recruiter in person, or they knew someone known to the researcher, for example, in cases where they were that person's friend or spouse ("snowballing recruitment"). To ensure a diverse sample composition, the recruiters were asked to include both men and women and to continue to include participants until the sample consisted of at least 20 persons in each of the predefined age groups. The age groups represented young persons (aged 18–24), adults (aged 25–44), middle-aged persons (aged 45–64), and elderly persons (aged 65 years and above). Unfortunately, however, the recruitment of participants to the oldest age group was not fully completed due to time restrictions on the part of the recruiters. On the other hand, more than 20 participants were recruited in the other age groups, increasing the statistical power of the analyses.

2.2. Measurement. Role participation was assessed with the Role Checklist [16]. The instrument is widely used—it is available in 13 languages and remains one of the most commonly used assessments in American occupational therapy practice [22]. It is a short self-report assessment that captures a person's perception of their participation in 10 defined roles. The roles are student, worker, volunteer, home maintainer, caregiver, friend, family member, hobbyist/amateur, religious participant, and participant in organizations. Part one of the Role Checklist, which was the only part employed in this substudy, instructs the person to indicate participation in any of the ten roles in the past (up until one week ago), present (today and the preceding week), and anticipated future (tomorrow and any time after tomorrow). The participant's responses to the part one of the Role Checklist are applied to determine the person's participation (or nonparticipation) in each of the listed roles in the past, present, and anticipated future. Scores pertaining to present role participation can also be summed, such that higher sum scores indicate participation in more roles. The roles assessed with the Role Checklist has been found to be consistent with the ICF framework [4], to be linked with the MOHO levels of both performance and participation [3], and to demonstrate concurrent validity with the more extensive Occupational Circumstances Assessment Interview and Rating Scale [5].

Previous translations of the Role Checklist into French [23] and Brazilian Portuguese [24] have both demonstrated good validity and reliability when used in their respective cultures. In addition, measurement properties have been shown to be equivalent when used in paper and electronic version [25], and later modifications of the checklist have similarly been tested with good results [26]. For this study, two independent Norwegian translations of the original instrument were produced and subsequently compared with one another. The comparisons are aimed at ensuring the clarity of concepts as well as the appropriate Norwegian phrasing and sentence structure. After reaching consensus on the forward translation, the instrument was translated back into English, and the back-translated version was checked against the original. Only small modifications were made after this process. Formal guidelines for the translation and adaptation of the Role Checklist have been provided at a later stage in the research process [27]. In addition to completing part one of the Role Checklist, the participants were asked about their age (in years) and gender.

2.3. Data Analysis. Descriptive statistics were used to examine the sample characteristics and their participation in roles. Differences between age groups with a view to the proportions currently participating in each role were examined by the χ^2 test. Differences between age groups with regard to the number of currently enacted roles were examined with one-way analysis of variance (ANOVA). In the ANOVA pairwise comparisons, Tukey's honest significant difference was used to adjust for inflating error levels.

Role patterns were described according to Hachey and coworkers [15]. Role loss was defined as having a role in the past, but not in the present. Role gain was defined as having a role at present, but not in the past. Continuous role was defined as having a role in the past, present, and expected future. Role absence was defined as not having the role in the past, not at present, and not in the expected future. By extending Hachey and coworkers' [15] procedure, expected role loss was defined as having a role at present, while expecting not to have the role in the future. Expected role gain was defined as not having a role at present, while expecting to have the role in the future. All analyses were performed with the software IBM SPSS for Windows [28], and the statistical significance was set at $p < 0.05$.

2.4. Ethics. All participants were verbally informed about the study by the recruitment collaborator. Written information about the study procedures was provided on the front page of the employed checklist. All participants volunteered to take part in the study, and informed consent was implied when we received the completed forms. As neither health-related information nor any person-identifying information was collected for the study, formal ethical approval was not required.

3. Results

3.1. Participants. One hundred and forty persons, 49 (35%) men and 91 (65%) women, opted to participate in the study. The age distribution showed that 45 (32.1%) of the participants were aged 18–24 years, 47 (33.6%) were aged 25–44 years, 31 (22.1%) were aged 45–64 years, and 17 (12.1%) were aged 65 years or older. The sample mean age was 40.2 years (SD = 18.8 years). The gender proportions did not differ significantly between the four age groups ($\chi^2 = 1.26$, $p = 0.74$).

3.2. Role Participation. Role participation in the past, present, and anticipated future is displayed in Figure 1. In the total sample, the most frequently endorsed role was home maintainer at present (93.6%), while the least frequently endorsed role was religious participant at present (7.1%). In the youngest age group (18–24 years), the most frequently endorsed role was home maintainer at present ($n = 45$, 100% within the age group), while the least frequently endorsed role was religious participant at present ($n = 3$, 6.7%). In the adult age group (25–44 years), the most frequently endorsed role was home maintainer at present ($n = 45$, 97.9%), while the least frequently endorsed role was religious participant at

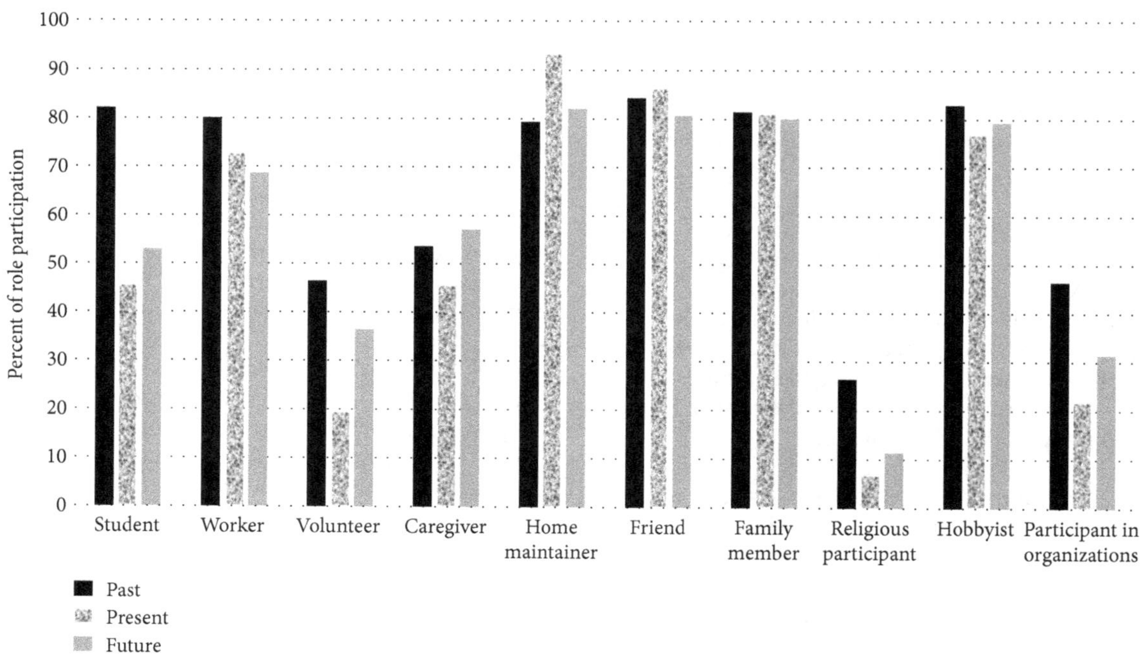

FIGURE 1: Role participation for past, present, and anticipated future roles in the sample ($n = 140$).

present ($n = 0$, 0%). Among the middle-aged participants (45–64 years), the most frequently endorsed role was home maintainer at present ($n = 31$, 100%), while the least frequently endorsed role was student at present ($n = 4$, 12.9%). Among the oldest participants (65 years and over), the most frequently endorsed roles were worker in the past and family member at present (both $n = 31$, 100%), while the least frequently endorsed roles were student at present ($n = 1$, 5.9%), student in the future ($n = 1$, 5.9%), and worker in the future ($n = 1$, 5.9%).

3.3. Current Role Participation according to Age Groups. Table 1 displays the age group comparisons related to currently enacted roles. Statistically significant differences between the age groups were found for the following roles: student, worker, volunteer, caregiver, home maintainer, friend, and religious participant. In addition, the mean number of currently enacted roles was different between participants in the four age groups. The pairwise comparisons revealed that those in the oldest age group participated in fewer roles compared to participants in all other age groups (all $p < 0.001$). Otherwise, no significant differences occurred.

3.4. Continuity and Change in Roles. Table 2 displays the participants' role patterns—that is, the continuity and change in roles across time—as interpreted from the participants' combinations of self-reported past, present, and anticipated future role participation. The roles most frequently lost were student and volunteer, whereas the roles most frequently gained were worker and home maintainer. Home maintainer and friend were the most frequent continuous roles, whereas religious participant and participant in organizations were the roles that most often showed an absent pattern. The roles most frequently expected to be lost were worker and home maintainer. Conversely, the roles most frequently expected to be gained were volunteer and caregiver. Of the predefined role patterns, most of the demonstrated patterns were examples of continuous roles (38.4%).

Considering that the participants in the oldest age group had significantly fewer roles compared to their younger counterparts (see Table 1), there was reason also to examine whether their role patterns across time deviated from the patterns shown for the total sample. The results from this additional analysis of continuity and change in roles for the participants in the oldest age group are displayed in Table 3. In comparison with the total sample, participants in the oldest age group had a higher proportion of the detected role patterns related to role loss and a smaller proportion of the role patterns related to continuous roles and expected role gains.

4. Discussion

The current study is aimed at examining participation in roles and patterns of role participation across time, in a general population sample from Norway. Several of the roles listed on the Role Checklist were currently held among a majority of the sample participants. In the high end of the scale, more than 90% of the sample participated in the role home maintainer. In the low end, fewer than 10% of the sample participated in the role religious participant. Participants over the age of 65 had fewer roles compared to their younger counterparts and showed a somewhat different pattern of continuity and change in role participation across time.

The roles listed in the Role Checklist [16] comprise different levels of necessity—some can be viewed as an integral and inescapable aspect of independent living, such as the most

TABLE 1: Frequency and proportion of individuals currently participating in roles according to age groups.

Current roles	Age groups 18–24 years n (%)	25–44 years n (%)	45–64 years n (%)	≥65 years n (%)	p
Student	43 (95.6)	16 (34.0)	4 (12.9)	1 (5.9)	<0.001
Worker	31 (68.9)	38 (80.9)	30 (96.8)	3 (17.6)	<0.001
Volunteer	8 (17.8)	8 (17.0)	11 (35.5)	0 (0.0)	0.02
Caregiver	9 (20.0)	30 (63.8)	19 (61.3)	6 (35.3)	<0.001
Home maintainer	43 (95.6)	46 (97.9)	31 (100.0)	11 (64.7)	<0.001
Friend	45 (100.0)	41 (87.2)	23 (74.2)	12 (70.6)	<0.01
Family member	33 (73.3)	39 (83.0)	26 (83.9)	18 (94.1)	0.27
Religious participant	3 (6.7)	0 (0.0)	5 (16.1)	2 (11.8)	<0.05
Hobbyist	34 (75.6)	37 (78.8)	24 (77.4)	13 (76.5)	0.99
Participant in organizations	7 (15.6)	11 (23.4)	9 (29.0)	4 (23.5)	0.56
	M (SD)	M (SD)	M (SD)	M (SD)	
Number of current roles	5.69 (1.56)	5.66 (1.20)	5.87 (1.65)	4.0 (1.37)	<0.001

Note. Differences by χ^2 tests for separate roles and by one-way ANOVA F-test for the number of current roles.

TABLE 2: Continuity and change in role participation across time in the total sample ($n = 140$).

Role	Loss n (%)	Gain n (%)	Continuous n (%)	Absence n (%)	Expected loss n (%)	Expected gain n (%)
Student	61 (43.6)	10 (7.1)	49 (35.0)	8 (5.7)	11 (7.9)	21 (15.0)
Worker	34 (24.3)	24 (17.1)	75 (53.6)	2 (1.4)	23 (16.4)	17 (12.1)
Volunteer	48 (34.3)	10 (7.1)	15 (10.7)	51 (36.4)	10 (7.1)	34 (24.3)
Caregiver	24 (17.1)	13 (9.3)	50 (35.7)	34 (24.3)	8 (5.7)	24 (17.1)
Home maintainer	3 (2.1)	23 (16.4)	107 (76.4)	3 (2.1)	19 (13.6)	3 (2.1)
Friend	15 (10.7)	18 (12.9)	103 (73.6)	3 (2.1)	17 (12.1)	9 (6.4)
Family member	18 (12.9)	18 (12.9)	94 (67.1)	4 (2.9)	18 (12.9)	16 (11.4)
Religious participant	27 (19.3)	0 (0.0)	10 (7.1)	100 (71.4)	0 (0.0)	6 (4.3)
Hobbyist	22 (15.7)	14 (10.0)	92 (65.7)	7 (5.0)	14 (10.0)	17 (12.1)
Participant in organizations	40 (28.6)	6 (4.3)	24 (17.1)	63 (45.0)	6 (4.3)	19 (13.6)
Total	292	136	619	275	126	166
Role patterns	18.1%	8.4%	38.4%	17.0%	7.8%	10.3%

Note. Role loss was defined as having a role in the past, but not in the present. Role gain was defined as having a role at present, but not in the past. Continuous role was defined as having a role in the past, present, and expected future. Role absence was defined as not having the role in the past, not at present, and not in the expected future. Expected role loss was defined as having a role at present, while expecting not to have the role in the future. Expected role gain was defined as not having a role at present, while expecting to have the role in the future.

frequently endorsed roles of worker and in particular home maintainer (see Figure 1). Other roles, such as the hobbyist and religious participant roles, are not connected to independent living. It is fully possible to lead both independent and fulfilling lives without these roles, and therefore, adopting these roles needs other sources of motivation. Empirical studies have shown that differently composed samples will have each own unique composition of the roles in which participants engage more and less frequently (compare, e.g., [7, 9, 12, 20, 29]). On the other hand, one should be able to assume that role participation in general has a relationship to basic human needs. As suggested by Deci and Ryan [30], such "human motivational universals" are comprised from basic needs for mastery, affiliation, and autonomy. In line with such a view, one may see the worker and home maintainer roles as linked with the need for autonomy, while roles like family member and religious participant link more strongly with the need for affiliation. However, affiliation needs may be expressed and met in different ways. People who live without a family may, for example, rely more on friends, neighbors, and interest groups as sources of companionship and support. This line of reasoning mirrors the recently introduced Model of Occupational Wholeness [31–33], suggesting that personal satisfaction with what we do is based on our tacit judgment of how our doing contributes to our satisfaction of needs. Taken together, this suggests that a majority of participants in any given sample will be expected to participate in some roles (worker, home maintainer, and friend), whereas the level of participation in other roles (e.g., hobbyist, religious participant, and

TABLE 3: Continuity and change in role participation across time among the participants in the oldest age group ($n = 17$).

Role	Loss n (%)	Gain n (%)	Continuous n (%)	Absence n (%)	Expected loss n (%)	Expected gain n (%)
Student	14 (82.4)	0 (0.0)	1 (5.9)	2 (11.8)	0 (0.0)	0 (0.0)
Worker	14 (82.4)	1 (5.9)	1 (5.9)	0 (0.0)	2 (11.8)	0 (0.0)
Volunteer	11 (64.7)	0 (0.0)	0 (0.0)	5 (29.4)	0 (0.0)	2 (11.8)
Caregiver	9 (52.9)	2 (11.8)	4 (23.5)	2 (11.8)	0 (0.0)	1 (5.9)
Home maintainer	3 (17.6)	3 (17.6)	7 (41.2)	3 (17.6)	3 (17.7)	0 (0.0)
Friend	3 (17.6)	2 (11.8)	10 (58.8)	2 (11.8)	2 (11.8)	0 (0.0)
Family member	1 (5.9)	3 (17.6)	13 (76.5)	0 (0.0)	2 (11.8)	0 (0.0)
Religious participant	3 (17.6)	0 (0.0)	2 (11.8)	12 (70.6)	0 (0.0)	0 (0.0)
Hobbyist	4 (23.5)	4 (23.5)	8 (47.1)	0 (0.0)	4 (23.5)	1 (5.9)
Participant in organizations	8 (47.1)	0 (0.0)	4 (23.5)	5 (29.4)	0 (0.0)	0 (0.0)
Total	70	15	50	31	13	4
Role patterns	38.3%	8.2%	27.3%	16.9%	7.1%	2.2%

Note. Role loss was defined as having a role in the past, but not in the present. Role gain was defined as having a role at present, but not in the past. Continuous role was defined as having a role in the past, present, and expected future. Role absence was defined as not having the role in the past, not at present, and not in the expected future. Expected role loss was defined as having a role at present, while expecting not to have the role in the future. Expected role gain was defined as not having a role at present, while expecting to have the role in the future.

participant in organizations) will depend more on the specific sample characteristics and the given cultural and environmental context [1, 34].

In line with the theoretical assumptions [1, 13, 17, 18], participants in the age group of 65 years and over participated in fewer roles than their counterparts of younger age (see Table 1). The participants in the oldest age group also experienced role loss more frequently compared to the younger participants (see Tables 2 and 3). Reduced role participation may be associated with reduced physical capacity and the onset of illness and functional limitations, which is more often the case in older years. In addition, reaching the normal retirement age (which in Norway is 67 years) directly implies loss of the worker role. Indirectly, it opens up the possibility that friends and family members of similar age may fall ill and eventually die. Consequently, roles like friend, family member, and caregiver may also be lost in the natural progression through life. Nonetheless, occupational therapists should be aware of the potential threats related to role loss. According to the MOHO [1], people organize their everyday lives according to roles. We do what we do much because we enact our roles as researchers, rock band guitarists, amateur kitchen chefs, and a multitude of others. Losing roles as an organizing principle for our everyday lives may further lead to a loss of meaning and purpose.

In most cases, people value the roles they have. In a previous Norwegian study, occupational therapy students demonstrated positive and statistically significant associations between currently enacted roles and their valuation of the same roles [7]. Further, participating in more valued roles appears to lead to more satisfaction, compared to having fewer roles. In support of this, researchers have demonstrated significant associations between participation in more valued roles and having higher quality of life [9] and more life satisfaction [35]. Thus, occupational therapists should pay attention to role loss. Such loss may indicate that the client may be at risk of experiencing reduced quality of life, and he or she may need help to remediate his or her role composition to restore life satisfaction.

In a study conducted in the midnineties, Dickerson and Oakley [12] compared an American nondisabled community sample with a matched sample of persons with physical or mental disabilities. They found that participants in the disabled sample not only had significantly fewer roles compared with the nondisabled sample but also had anticipated fewer future roles and tended to place lower value on several roles, compared to their nondisabled counterparts. The present study augments these previous results by indicating that role loss may not only be an effect of illness and disability but can also be an effect of the aging process itself, regardless of illness or disability (see Tables 2 and 3). At the same time, however, participants in the oldest age group did experience substantial role continuity across the past, present, and anticipated future. Moreover, building on Hachey and coworkers' [15] concept of "role change," we found that the possibility of *gaining* a role in the future was in fact expected by some of the older participants (Table 3). Two participants expected to gain the role of volunteer, one expected to become a caregiver, and one expected to enter the hobbyist role. Thus, in spite of reaching older age, role participation does not have to be all about losing roles, although this should also be expected.

4.1. Study Strengths and Limitations. The sample size, in particular for the oldest age group, was small. Thus, the reliability of the results for this age group is uncertain—there may not have been sufficient variability within the group, and this may have caused biased results. Further studies using larger sample subgroups are needed to shed light on the potential age differences in role participation. Participants were also recruited by convenience, such that we are unable to speak about how well they represent the Norwegian general population. The cross-sectional study design precludes us from establishing cause-effect relationships between the study variables. A trusted group of students and occupational therapist colleagues were used as collaborators in recruiting the participants and informing them about the study procedures. In addition, the employed Role Checklist is relatively straightforward to use, so there is good reason to trust the validity of the collected data. It provides, however, one particular set of roles with a particular set of definitions. Other ways of conceptualizing and measuring role participation may lead to different results. Thus, a limitation of the study is the use of a single measure to look at a complex phenomenon. Moreover, a weakness is the focus on role participation only, not taking into account the participants' valuation of the roles. In addition, potentially associated outcomes, like measures of health or quality of life, were not included. Thus, although previously demonstrated in a clinical sample [9], the study renders the question of whether role participation is related to significant outcomes in a general population sample. If indeed related to such outcomes, we should also ask whether role participation is important in and of itself or whether role participation only matters when the roles in question are personally valued. Future research may also include the Role Checklist in a variety of longitudinal rehabilitation studies to examine whether role participation outcomes are affected as a result of intervention, be they interprofessional or occupational therapy specific.

5. Conclusion

The most frequently endorsed current role in the sample was home maintainer, while the least frequently endorsed current role was religious participant. Compared with the total sample, the participants in the oldest age group participated less frequently in most listed roles, and they had a lower total number of current roles. The role patterns for the total sample indicated for the most part a continuity of roles, while the most frequent role pattern for the oldest group of participants was role loss. More health-related problems, but also the reaching retirement age itself, may lead to role loss as one moves towards older age. Rehabilitation services in general and participation-focused occupational therapy in particular may profit from assessing role participation in clients and potentially target roles through intervention.

Conflicts of Interest

There are no conflicts of interest related to this article.

References

[1] R. R. Taylor, *Kielhofner's Model of Human Occupation*, Lippincott Williams & Wilkins, Philadelphia, 5th edition, 2017.

[2] E. A. Townsend and H. J. Polatajko, *Enabling Occupation II: Advancing an Occupational Therapy Vision for Health, Well-Being, & Justice through Occupation*, Canadian Association of Occupational Therapists, Ottawa, 2007.

[3] T. Bonsaksen, U. Meidert, D. Schuman et al., "Does the Role Checklist measure occupational participation?," *The Open Journal of Occupational Therapy*, vol. 3, no. 3, p. 2, 2015.

[4] P. J. Scott, "Measuring participation outcomes following life-saving medical interventions: the Role Checklist version 2: quality of performance," *Disability and Rehabilitation*, vol. 36, no. 13, pp. 1108–1112, 2014.

[5] P. J. Scott, D. Cacich, M. Fulk, K. Michel, and K. Whiffen, "Establishing concurrent validity of the Role Checklist version 2 with the OCAIRS in measurement of participation: a pilot study," *Occupational Therapy International*, vol. 2017, Article ID 6493472, 6 pages, 2017.

[6] World Health Organization, *International Classification of Functioning, Disability and Health (ICF)*, WHO, Geneva, 2001.

[7] T. Bonsaksen and H. Kvarsnes, "Role performance and role valuation among occupational therapy students in Norway," *The Open Journal of Occupational Therapy*, vol. 4, no. 1, p. 7, 2016.

[8] F. Yazdani, M. Jibril, and G. Kielhofner, "A study of the relationship between variables from the Model of Human Occupation and subjective well-being among university students in Jordan," *Occupational Therapy In Health Care*, vol. 22, no. 2-3, pp. 125–138, 2008.

[9] P. J. Scott, "Participation in valued roles post-liver transplant," *British Journal of Occupational Therapy*, vol. 73, no. 11, pp. 517–523, 2010.

[10] R. Barris, G. Kielhofner, R. M. B. Martin, I. Gelinas, M. Klement, and B. Schultz, "Occupational function and dysfunction in three groups of adolescents," *The Occupational Therapy Journal of Research*, vol. 6, no. 5, pp. 301–317, 1986.

[11] T. M. Smith, A. Drefus, and G. Hersch, "Habits, routines, and roles of graduate students: effects of Hurricane Ike," *Occupational Therapy In Health Care*, vol. 25, no. 4, pp. 283–297, 2011.

[12] A. E. Dickerson and F. Oakley, "Comparing the roles of community-living persons and patient populations," *American Journal of Occupational Therapy*, vol. 49, no. 3, pp. 221–228, 1995.

[13] R. Wright and L. Sugarman, *Occupational Therapy and Life Course Development*, Wiley-Blackwell, Chichester, UK, 2009.

[14] S. W. Lee and G. Kielhofner, "Habituation: patterns of daily occupations," in *Kielhofner's Model of Human Occupation*, R. R. Taylor, Ed., pp. 57–73, Wolters Kluwer, Philadelphia, 2017.

[15] R. Hachey, G. Boyer, and C. Mercier, "Perceived and valued roles of adults with severe mental health problems," *Canadian Journal of Occupational Therapy*, vol. 68, no. 2, pp. 112–120, 2001.

[16] F. Oakley, G. Kielhofner, R. Barris, and R. K. Reichler, "The Role Checklist: development and empirical assessment of reliability," *The Occupational Therapy Journal of Research*, vol. 6, no. 3, pp. 157–170, 1986.

[17] R. J. Havighurst, "Successful aging," *The Gerontologist*, vol. 1, no. 1, pp. 8–13, 1961.

[18] R. Havighurst, "Successful aging," in *Processes of Aging*, R. Williams, C. Tibbitts, and W. Donahue, Eds., vol. 1, pp. 299–320, Atherton, New York, NY, USA, 1963.

[19] V. H. Menec, "The relation between everyday activities and successful aging: a 6-year longitudinal study," *The Journals of Gerontology Series B: Psychological Sciences and Social Sciences*, vol. 58, no. 2, pp. S74–S82, 2003.

[20] S. Corr and S. Wilmer, "Returning to work after a stroke: an important but neglected area," *British Journal of Occupational Therapy*, vol. 66, no. 5, pp. 186–192, 2003.

[21] J. M. Sepiol and J. Froehlich, "Use of the Role Checklist with the patient with multiple personality disorder," *American Journal of Occupational Therapy*, vol. 44, no. 11, pp. 1008–1012, 1990.

[22] S. W. Lee, R. Taylor, G. Kielhofner, and G. Fisher, "Theory use in practice: a national survey of therapists who use the Model of Human Occupation," *American Journal of Occupational Therapy*, vol. 62, no. 1, pp. 106–117, 2008.

[23] R. Hachey, J. Jumoorty, and C. Mercier, "Methodology for validating the translation of test measurements applied to occupational therapy," *Occupational Therapy International*, vol. 2, no. 3, 203 pages, 1995.

[24] J. R. Cordeiro, A. Camelier, F. Oakley, and J. R. Jardim, "Cross-cultural reproducibility of the Brazilian Portuguese version of the Role Checklist for persons with chronic obstructive pulmonary disease," *American Journal of Occupational Therapy*, vol. 61, no. 1, pp. 33–40, 2007.

[25] P. J. Scott, R. McFadden, K. Yates, S. Baker, and S. McSoley, "The Role Checklist v2: QP: establishment of reliability and validation of electronic administration," *British Journal of Occupational Therapy*, vol. 77, no. 2, pp. 96–102, 2014.

[26] M. Avrech Bar, V. Rubin, G. Gavrieal-Tyjchman, and T. Jarus, "The validity and reliability of the modified version of the Role Checklist (M-RCL)," *Scandinavian Journal of Occupational Therapy*, vol. 20, no. 6, pp. 454–462, 2013.

[27] L. R. Van Antwerp, L. Haglund, K. Fenger, and P. Scott, *Translation Guidelines: The Role Checklist*, Indiana University, Indianapolis, 2016.

[28] IBM Corporation, *SPSS for Windows, Version 24*, IBM Corporation, Armonk, NY, 2016.

[29] M. A. Watson and C. L. Ager, "The impact of role valuation and performance on life satisfaction in old age," *Physical & Occupational Therapy In Geriatrics*, vol. 10, no. 1, pp. 27–62, 1991.

[30] E. L. Deci, R. M. Ryan, P. J. Corr, and G. Matthews, Eds., "Self-determination theory: a consideration of human motivational universals," in *The Cambridge Handbook of Personality Psychology*, pp. 441–456, Cambridge University Press, Cambridge, 2009.

[31] F. Yazdani and T. Bonsaksen, "Introduction to the Model of Occupational Wholeness," *ErgoScience*, vol. 12, no. 1, pp. 32–36, 2017.

[32] T. Bonsaksen and F. Yazdani, "The Norwegian occupational wholeness questionnaire (N-OWQ): scale development and psychometric properties," *Scandinavian Journal of Occupational Therapy*, pp. 1–10, 2018.

[33] T. Bonsaksen and F. Yazdani, "Sociodemographic factors associated with the Norwegian occupational wholeness questionnaire scales," *ErgoScience*, vol. 13, no. 1, pp. 14–20, 2018.

[34] M. K. Duellman, R. Barris, and G. Kielhofner, "Organized activity and the adaptive status of nursing home residents," *American Journal of Occupational Therapy*, vol. 40, no. 9, pp. 618–622, 1986.

[35] M. S. Elliott and R. Barris, "Occupational role performance and life satisfaction in elderly persons," *The Occupational Therapy Journal of Research*, vol. 7, no. 4, pp. 215–224, 1987.

25

Occupational Therapy Students' Perceptions of the Role of Robots in the Care for Older People Living in the Community

Sławomir Tobis,[1] Mirosława Cylkowska-Nowak,[1] Katarzyna Wieczorowska-Tobis,[2] Mariola Pawlaczyk,[3] and Aleksandra Suwalska[4]

[1] *Laboratory of Occupational Therapy, Department of Geriatric Medicine and Gerontology, University of Medical Sciences, Poznan, Poland*
[2] *Laboratory of Geriatrics, Department of Palliative Care, University of Medical Sciences, Poznan, Poland*
[3] *Department of Geriatric Medicine and Gerontology, University of Medical Sciences, Poznan, Poland*
[4] *Laboratory of Neuropsychobiology, Department of Psychiatry, University of Medical Sciences, Poznan, Poland*

Correspondence should be addressed to Sławomir Tobis; stobis@ump.edu.pl

Academic Editor: Erna I. Blanche

Background. The question arises how recent developments in robotics can contribute to the care for older people. The study is part of the EU-funded ENRICHME project. *Objectives of Study*. The aim of the study was to investigate opinions of occupational therapy students (OTS), as future professional caregivers, on the use of robots in care for older people. *Methods*. It included 26 OTS from Poznan University of Medical Sciences. To collect data, the Users' Needs, Requirements, and Abilities Questionnaire (UNRAQ) was developed. *Findings*. OTS perceived the robot as "a useful device" and "an assistant" rather than "a companion" ($p < 0.01$). In their opinion, the most important functions of the robot were related to health aspects (emergency alarms, health parameters monitoring, physical activity and memory training, and reminders about medication, drinks, etc.), scored positively by 23–26 OTS. Functions such as mood detection, encouraging to contact with friends, and monitoring of food consumption were accepted by 16-17 OTS. Two statements concerning social functions (accompanying in everyday activities and decreasing the sense of loneliness) were rated positively by less the than half of the participants. *Limitations and Recommendations for Further Research*. A module concerning technology use, including robotics, should constitute an important part of the curricula of both academic and continuous education of OTS.

1. Introduction

World's societies have been ageing rapidly over the last years and older people have already outnumbered the younger cohort. A shortage in both formal and informal caregivers as well as declining resources and capacities is commonly observed [1]. Increasing number of individuals in need of care and limited availability of care professionals call for an implementation of new solutions, allowing for a reduction on the burden of caregivers who are active within the system. Such solutions could be based on the use of robots which would be involved in care and support for older persons living in the community.

If the systems including robots, addressed to the elderly, are to be effective, they have to meet the end users' unique needs and expectations: the health and social ones along with those related to the functioning of the individual in a particular cultural context [2]. For this purpose, the role of the robot must be defined comprehensively, also taking complex ethical and legal issues into consideration.

Similar to health information technology, it is crucial to understand a priori what factors are important in predicting older people's willingness to use robots' assistance [3]. Therefore, caregivers should be aware of those factors as they help promote the use of robots with community-dwelling older adults. Smarr et al. [4] found that older Americans were very imaginative regarding what the robot could do to assist them and were engaged, active, and motivated to discuss the robot's issues. In that study, they even preferred robot's assistance over human assistance, not only in many instrumental activities of daily living (e.g., medication reminder) but also in more complex activities such as new learning and hobbies.

While the majority of available papers are dedicated to the attitude of older people or their potential informal caregivers towards the robot, analysing particularly their expectations and determinants of acceptance [5–7], literature concerning the staff's point of view is sparse. This is surprising, as it is the formal caregivers who are essential to successful implementation and usage of a robot in the older persons' living environments, that is the application of "ageing in place." This term acknowledges that the majority of older people are living independently in their own homes and want to stay there as long as possible, in familiar surroundings, with friends and family [8].

One of the few papers concerning professional caregivers in this aspect was published by Saito et al. who showed that nurses' stress levels at work were lower after the introduction of a seal-shaped "mental commit" robot PARO [9]. In focus groups studies by Zsiga et al. [10], professional caregivers showed a curious and open attitude towards the use of a robot.

In the field of occupational therapy, robotics in the literature is commonly attributed to rehabilitation tasks, mainly within the upper limb function [11, 12]. Many therapeutic techniques consist of showing movements to patients, guiding them through the movement, providing feedback on adequacy of performance, and, then, encouraging the patients to repeat the task until it has been accomplished. Moreover, the occupational therapist takes care of the cognitive status of the subject and provides appropriate exercises for their state [13]. As the key role of occupational therapists in patient-directed application of "ageing in place" is straightforward [14, 15], their interaction with the robot, focused on reaching therapeutic goals in care for older people, is of great importance and should be asked about. This observation was the starting point for our study.

2. Method

The project was approved by the Bioethical Committee of Poznan University of Medical Sciences, Poland (number 785/16).

The study is part of the ENRICHME project (*ENabling Robot and Assisted Living Environment for Independent Care and Health Monitoring of the Elderly*, financed by the European Union within the Horizon 2020 program, 643691) which tackles the progressive decline of cognitive capacity in the ageing population, adopting an integrated platform with a service robot for long-term human monitoring and interaction.

2.1. Participants. The study group consisted of occupational therapy students from Poznan University of Medical Sciences, as potential future formal caregivers for older people. We included only those who were close to finishing their 3-year bachelor curriculum and thus had substantial knowledge of their field. Twenty-six students out of 36 (more than 70%) participated in the study.

2.2. Procedure. To collect the data related to requirements for the robot, the Users' Needs, Requirements, and Abilities Questionnaire (UNRAQ) was developed, based on literature review and the expertise of the ENRICHME project partners. The UNRAQ is a structured questionnaire composed of fixed items used to gather data in the quantitative methodology, which enables categorisation of the answers and their analysis using statistical methods [16]. After a discussion of ENRICHME experts, it was decided to also add an opportunity for participants to comment on each item, as every single contribution of a participant may be of importance and of value while designing the robot. Subsequently, the creativity box was added at the end of UNRAQ for this aim. Therewith, we added elements of qualitative methodology to the questionnaire.

The UNRAQ is composed of three parts. The introductory part provides demographic information of the respondents (e.g., their age, education, and profession). The next section of the questionnaire is constructed of statements to which the participant is asked to express his/her level of agreement-disagreement. These statements pertain to four areas: the interaction with the robot, the role of the robot, social aspects, and assistive role. Answers are structured using 5-point Likert scale (I strongly disagree, I partially disagree, I neither agree nor disagree, I partially agree, and I strongly agree, scored in the range 1–5). This allows for the presentation of results in the form of a mean and a standard deviation (SD). Scores 1-2 are considered negative, score 3 is considered neutral, and scores 4-5 are considered positive. Given the number of participants (26), we used the following categorisation of their agreement, based on the results obtained: excellent agreement (all or all but one agreed, 26 or 25), very good agreement (24 or 23 agreed), and good agreement (17 or 16 agreed).

The final part of UNRAQ is the creativity box. Its purpose is to create an opportunity for the participants to speak out freely. The participant writes down in the creativity box all his/her ideas/suggestions for other functions the robot might have. They are asked to report any observations that come to mind while answering the questionnaire and are not already mentioned as comments to the statements. The free text remarks cited in the following parts of the paper come from both sources (comments to statements and creativity box).

Before completing the questionnaire, pictures of the Kompaï robot [17] were shown to provide the students with a model of the robot concept.

2.3. Statistical Analysis. The statistical analysis was performed with STATISTICA 12.0 software (StatSoft, Poland). Variables were expressed as percentages, frequencies, means ± standard deviation (SD), and medians. Normality in the data distribution was examined with Shapiro-Wilk's test.

Comparison between groups of paired data was made with the Wilcoxon test and differences in the distribution of quality variables between groups, with the χ^2 test with Yates

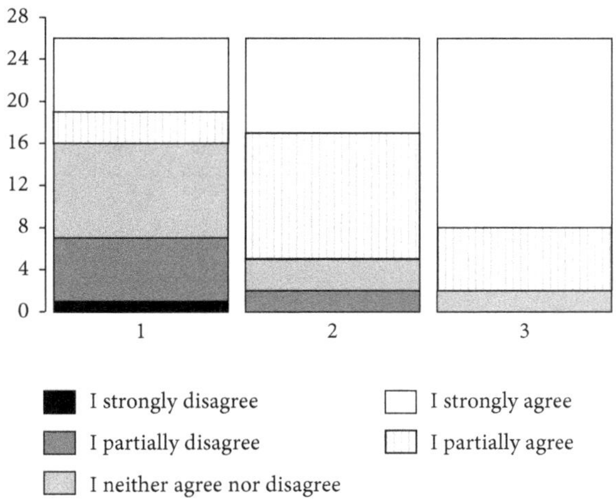

FIGURE 1: Detailed opinions of the participants related to following statements: (1) The robot should be a companion of the elderly person. (2) The robot should be an assistant of the elderly person. (3) The robot should be a useful device of the elderly person (something to be used when needed, with no other interaction).

correction due to small sample size. $p < 0.05$ was considered statistically significant.

3. Results

The mean age of studied group was 21.6 ± 1.2 years (median: 22 years). All students stated that they were familiar with computers and all but one declared being familiar with working with technological systems. Four of them were active as informal caregivers for members of their families.

3.1. Preparedness for the Robot. As for the assessment of the preparedness of older persons for coping with the robot, the majority of students viewed them as unprepared (22 scored the statement *the elderly are prepared to interact with the robot* negatively: 10 strongly disagreed and 12 partially disagreed). The mean score for this statement was only 2.0 ± 1.1 (median 2.0). Nonetheless, the participants were of the opinion that this can be changed, "training on operation of the robot is necessary," and that the introduction of a robot in the life of an older person should be "gradual, allowing for gaining familiarity, increasing the number of available functions." In addition, the students stated that the robot should be "customised and programmed for every individual, since everybody has different needs."

3.2. The Role of the Robot. The statement *the robot should be a companion of the elderly person* was rated positively by 10 students only. On the other hand, the statements *the robot should be a useful device of the elderly person (something to be used when needed, with no other interaction)* and *the robot should be an assistant of the elderly person* were rated positively more often (24 out of 26 and 21 out of 26 individuals strongly agreed with the above statements, $p < 0.0001$ and $p = 0.0042$, resp.). Detailed characteristics are presented in Figure 1.

All analysed functionalities of the robot were viewed favourable with the participants (which was expressed by mean scores above 3.0, Table 1). Seven statements gained positive scores from 25-26 participants (excellent agreement), another seven had 23-24 positive scores (very good agreement), further four were scored positively by 16-17 students (good agreement), and the remaining two were scored positively by 12 students.

Statements with good agreement were related to such functions as mood detection or encouraging to contact with friends and monitoring of food consumption.

In the comments, it was stressed that "the robot would be a potent helper; thank that the caregivers could have more time for the caretakers." On the other hand, it was noted that "the robot should not replace the older person in all activities, as it might lead to higher dependency;" an attitude like "why perform an activity if the robot can do it" could lead to older adults taking a less active role in day to day care and having a potential negative impact on their overall health.

There were as little as two statements which were rated positively by less than half of the students: *the robot should accompany the owner in everyday activities (watching TV, preparing meals)* and *the robot could decrease the sense of loneliness and improve the mood of the elderly person* (Table 1). Notably, as many as nine students had neutral opinion about both these statements. The participants stated "the robot will not replace [human companionship]" but also "it should not be with the older person 24/7 as it would rather be a kind of supervision than company." As far as the reminding function of the robot is concerned, the reminding about fluids intake gained special attention.

The participants broadly accepted the idea of the robot monitoring the health status of its elderly user and collecting their medical history ("the robot should be the source of information – e.g., in case of an emergency team call it could accelerate the help by immediately supplying parameters stored in its memory"). The students also expressed that the robot should react to certain conditions and trigger an alert accordingly ("my grandmother fell, stood up and stated that everything was fine, no need for emergency team, yet afterwards it showed she had a broken leg; the robot should alert that something happened even if seemingly all is OK").

4. Discussion

Occupational therapists facilitate independence and support participation in occupations that are personally meaningful to clients, to enhance the wellbeing and quality of life. One of the core values supporting occupational therapy practice is viewing the patient as a person who acts on the environment [18]. With more and more technology becoming part of a human environment, it is imperative to think of integrating modern technology in the way occupational therapy helps its clients. The progress made in robotics in recent years makes it imaginable to involve robots in various fields of occupational therapy. We thus asked students approaching the end of their occupational therapy curriculum, as the ones who are likely to be soon confronted with this technology in their professional career, about their opinions on the use of

Table 1: Quantitative analysis of the opinions of occupational therapy students related to the statements about the role of the robot in the care for older people, arranged by *number of students who agreed with the statement* and *mean score.*

Statement	Number of students who agreed with the statement (strongly or partially)	The score (mean ± SD; median)
The robot should call the centre in case of emergency	26	4.8 ± 0.4; 5
The robot should increase the safety of the elderly: calling for help when needed, monitoring health parameters (blood pressure, heart rate, etc.)	26	4.8 ± 0.4; 5
The robot should encourage and guide the elderly to perform physical exercises	26	4.6 ± 0.5; 5
The robot should remind the elderly about medication	25	4.8 ± 0.5; 5
The robot should remind the elderly about appointments	25	4.5 ± 0.6; 5
The robot should have entertainment functions (e.g. gaming partner, reading aloud or playing music function)	25	4.4 ± 0.6; 4
The robot should remind about meals times, drinks	25	4.4 ± 0.6; 4
The robot should help the elderly to preserve their memory function for example by playing memory games with them	24	4.6 ± 0.6; 5
The robot should measure physiological parameters (blood pressure, heart rate, body temperature) of the elderly person	24	4.5 ± 0.6; 5
The robot should observe the behaviour of the elderly person to detect falls or changes due to illness	24	4.5 ± 0.6; 5
The robot should monitor the environment (temperature, humidity) and suggest air conditioning adjustment or windows opening	24	4.5 ± 0.6; 5
The robot should increase the safety of the elderly home: for example locking doors, detecting leaking gas and so forth	23	4.5 ± 0.8; 5
The robot should help the owner to find lost objects (e.g. glasses, keys)	23	4.4 ± 0.7; 5
The robot should provide advice about a healthy diet	23	4.3 ± 0.7; 4
The robot should monitor the amount of food and fluid intake of the owner	17	3.8 ± 1.1; 4
The robot could encourage the elderly to enhance their contacts with friends	17	3.9 ± 1.0; 4
The robot should detect the owner's mood (facial expression)	17	4.0 ± 1.1; 4
The robot should initiate contacts with others (calling friends, initiating skype conversations)	16	3.7 ± 1.4; 4
The robot should accompany the owner in everyday activities (watching TV, preparing meals)	12	3.6 ± 1.2; 3
The robot could decrease the sense of loneliness and improve the mood of the elderly person	12	3.4 ± 1.2; 3

robots in elderly care. So far, as suggested by Yerxa [18], the therapists perceived practice as "the profession."

Peek et al. [19], based on literature review, stated that preimplementation acceptance of innovative solutions depends on both the perception of technology (concerns and benefits) and the necessity of technology (need and available alternatives). According to Broadbent et al. [8], healthcare robots can be broadly categorised into those that provide physical assistance, those that provide companionship, and those that monitor health and safety; however, some robotic systems cover more than one of these categories. The students mainly perceived the robot as "a useful device" and "an assistant," significantly more often than "a companion." Additionally, the only statements that were rated positively by less than half of the participants were *the robot could decrease the sense of loneliness and improve the mood of an elderly person* and *the robot should accompany the owner in everyday activities (like watching TV, preparing meals)*. The participants did not seem to express the expectations that the technology at its current level would be sufficient to allow the robot to engage socially in a successful manner. This may, however, also indicate the students' focus on the tasks rather than the social aspects of technology use and may result from their young age/perspective of life. Subsequently, the assistive and monitoring functionalities of the robot were rated higher than the social ones. A comparable pattern of distribution of interests among the young was observed by Zsiga et al. [10].

One may thus speculate that students perceive the robot as a therapy aide, not a substitute for a caregiver, which was additionally reflected in general remarks like "the robot will never replace a human." Similar attitudes were observed by Boissy et al. [20] in focus groups of professional caregivers (among whom there was one occupational therapist) and older persons: "a robotic telepresence service would not replace healthcare professionals or family members, but could supplement them in providing care." In our study, the students noticed that the use of a robot in repeatable activities would allow them to devote more time to their clients. They thus do not have (or at least do not express) the fear of being professionally replaced by the robot. The lack of a feeling of one's job being threatened finds reflection in the study of Frey and Osborne [21], according to which occupational therapy is the profession sixth least endangered by the introduction of computers and robots, out of 702 rated. Dijkers et al. [22] also noted that occupational therapists can quickly adjust to working effectively with this type of equipment.

Wu et al. [23] defined common barriers to robot's acceptance which are uneasiness with technology, feeling of stigmatisation, and ethical issues such as "use or lose it logic" (e.g., if a robot does things for its user, does the user lose some capacities because of not making the effort?). In our study, we found indications of all of them. The students pointed to the necessity of competent pretraining for the older persons for coping with the robot, as they would lack the necessary knowledge and/or experience with technology. They also signalled the risk of losing abilities when certain tasks would be performed by the robot instead of the older subject.

Among the highest scored functions of the robot (25 positive out of 26) were reminders about appointments, medication, and meal times, which fits into the holistic approach to the client, as it encompasses the most significant issues of older individuals. Among them, the danger of dehydration was specifically pointed out as needing special attention. In our opinion, this is worth underlining because dehydration is a common (and often underestimated) risk factor of increasing dependence in age.

Our study has some limitations. The studied population is small, yet we managed to include over 70% of the whole students group, which is a fairly good response rate. In addition, the Poznan University of Medical Sciences is the only university level medical school throughout the country offering a curriculum in occupational therapy. Our students are uniquely prepared to work as members of interprofessional geriatric teams. Secondly, our study was theoretical in the sense that the participants did not have prior interactions with a healthcare robot. It was part of the ENRICHME project, aimed at the definition of necessary and desirable functionalities of the robot to be implemented in the community. Thus, in the next iteration, the participants will have the opportunity to interact with the robot in a real world context which will constitute the base for further investigation of the topic.

Occupational therapists must understand the patient's challenges and/or limitations, have knowledge of different treatment modalities and approaches, and be able to apply them creatively [22]. As robotics makes more therapeutic applications available, both occupational therapy curriculum and continuous education opportunities should take into account the availability of increasingly intelligent robots and how they can help occupational therapy best meet their patients' needs.

Competing Interests

No conflict of interests has been declared by the authors.

Acknowledgments

The study is part of the ENRICHME project, financed by the European Union within the Horizon 2020 program, 643691.

References

[1] World Health Organization, *Global Health and Aging*, National Institutes of Health, 2011, http://www.who.int/ageing/publications/global_health.pdf.

[2] T. Greenhalgh, R. Procter, J. Wherton, P. Sugarhood, S. Hinder, and M. Rouncefield, "What is quality in assisted living technology? the ARCHIE framework for effective telehealth and telecare services," *BMC medicine*, vol. 13, article 91, 2015.

[3] C. K. Or and B. Karsh, "A systematic review of patient acceptance of consumer health information technology," *Journal of the American Medical Informatics Association*, vol. 16, no. 4, pp. 550–560, 2009.

[4] C. A. Smarr, A. Prakash, J. M. Beer, T. L. Mitzner, C. C. Kemp, and W. A. Rogers, "Older adults' preferences for and acceptance of robots assistance for everyday living tasks," *Proceedings of the Human Factors and Ergonomics Society Annual Meeting*, vol. 56, no. 1, pp. 153–157, 2012.

[5] R. Bemelmans, G. J. Gelderblom, P. Jonker, and L. de Witte, "Socially assistive robots in elderly care: a systematic review into effects and effectiveness," *Journal of the American Medical Directors Association*, vol. 13, no. 2, pp. 114–120, 2012.

[6] R. Kachouie, S. Sedighadeli, R. Khosla, and M.-T. Chu, "Socially Assistive Robots in Elderly Care: a mixed-method systematic literature review," *International Journal of Human—Computer Interaction*, vol. 30, no. 5, pp. 369–393, 2014.

[7] H. Robinson, B. MacDonald, and E. Broadbent, "The role of healthcare robots for older people at home: a review," *International Journal of Social Robotics*, vol. 6, no. 4, pp. 575–591, 2014.

[8] E. Broadbent, R. Stafford, and B. MacDonald, "Acceptance of healthcare robots for the older population: review and future directions," *International Journal of Social Robotics*, vol. 1, no. 4, pp. 319–330, 2009.

[9] T. Saito, T. Shibata, K. Wada, and K. Tanie, "Relationship between interaction with the mental commit robot and change of stress reaction of the elderly," in *Proceedings of the IEEE International Symposium on Computational Intelligence in Robotics and Automation (CIRA '03)*, pp. 119–124, Kobe, Japan, July 2003.

[10] K. Zsiga, G. Edelmayer, P. Rumeau, O. Péter, A. Tóth, and G. Fazekas, "Home care robot for socially supporting the elderly: focus group studies in three European countries to screen user attitudes and requirements," *International Journal of Rehabilitation Research*, vol. 36, no. 4, pp. 375–378, 2013.

[11] C. G. Burgar, P. S. Lum, A. M. Erika Scremin et al., "Robot-assisted upper-limb therapy in acute rehabilitation setting following stroke: department of veterans affairs multisite clinical trial," *Journal of Rehabilitation Research and Development*, vol. 48, no. 4, pp. 445–458, 2011.

[12] P. Maciejasz, J. Eschweiler, K. Gerlach-Hahn, A. Jansen-Troy, and S. Leonhardt, "A survey on robotic devices for upper limb rehabilitation," *Journal of Neuroengineering and Rehabilitation*, vol. 11, article no. 3, 2014.

[13] A. Robert, I. Gélinas, and B. Mazer, "Occupational therapists use of cognitive interventions for clients with Alzheimer's disease," *Occupational Therapy International*, vol. 17, no. 1, pp. 10–19, 2010.

[14] W. B. Stav, "Occupational therapy and older drivers: research, education, and practice," *Gerontology and Geriatrics Education*, vol. 29, no. 4, pp. 336–350, 2008.

[15] S. L. Szanton, J. L. Wolff, B. Leff et al., "Preliminary data from Community Aging in Place, Advancing Better Living for Elders, a patient-directed, team-based intervention to improve physical function and decrease nursing home utilization: the first 100 individuals to complete a centers for medicare and medicaid services innovation project," *Journal of the American Geriatrics Society*, vol. 63, no. 2, pp. 371–374, 2015.

[16] G. Kielhofner, *Research in Occupational Therapy: Methods of Inquiry for Enhancing Practice*, F.A. Davies Company, Philadelphia, Pa, USA, 2006.

[17] Robosoft, 2016, http://kompai.com/.

[18] E. J. Yerxa, "In search of good ideas for occupational therapy," *Scandinavian Journal of Occupational Therapy*, vol. 21, no. 1, pp. 11–19, 2014.

[19] S. T. M. Peek, E. J. M. Wouters, J. van Hoof, K. G. Luijkx, H. R. Boeije, and H. J. M. Vrijhoef, "Factors influencing acceptance of technology for aging in place: a systematic review," *International Journal of Medical Informatics*, vol. 83, no. 4, pp. 235–248, 2014.

[20] P. Boissy, H. Corriveau, F. Michaud, D. Labonté, and M.-P. Royer, "A qualitative study of in-home robotic telepresence for home care of community-living elderly subjects," *Journal of Telemedicine and Telecare*, vol. 13, no. 2, pp. 79–84, 2007.

[21] C. B. Frey and M. A. Osborne, "The future of employment: how susceptible are jobs to computerisation?" *Technological Forecasting and Social Change*, vol. 114, pp. 254–280, 2017.

[22] M. P. Dijkers, P. C. deBear, R. F. Erlandson, K. Kristy, D. M. Geer, and A. Nichols, "Patient and staff acceptance of robotic technology in occupational therapy: a pilot study," *Journal of Rehabilitation Research and Development*, vol. 28, no. 2, pp. 33–44, 1991.

[23] Y.-H. Wu, J. Wrobel, M. Cornuet, H. Kerhervé, S. Damnée, and A.-S. Rrigaud, "Acceptance of an assistive robot in older adults: a mixed-method study of human-robot interaction over a 1-month period in the living lab setting," *Clinical Interventions in Aging*, vol. 9, pp. 801–811, 2014.

Integrating Occupational Therapy Specific Assessments in Practice: Exploring Practitioner Experiences

Eric Asaba,[1,2,3] Mio Nakamura,[4] Akie Asaba,[5] and Anders Kottorp[1,6]

[1] *Department of Neurobiology, Care Sciences, and Society (NVS), Division of Occupational Therapy, Karolinska Institutet, Alfred Nobels Allé 23, B4, Huddinge, Sweden*
[2] *Unit for Research, Education, and Development (FoUU), Stockholms Sjukhem Foundation, Stockholm, Sweden*
[3] *Department of Occupational Therapy, Tokyo Metropolitan University, Tokyo, Japan*
[4] *Department of Occupational Therapy, International University of Health and Welfare, Narita, Japan*
[5] *Karolinska University Hospital, Occupational Therapy and Physiotherapy Practice Areas, Huddinge, Sweden*
[6] *Faculty for Health and Society, Malmö University, Malmö, Sweden*

Correspondence should be addressed to Eric Asaba; eric.asaba@ki.se

Academic Editor: Patricia Belchior

Background. Occupational therapists sometimes find it challenging to integrate client-centered and occupational therapy specific assessments in practice. *The aim* of this study was to explore the use of occupational therapy specific assessments such as the Assessment of Motor and Process Skills (AMPS) among occupational therapists in Sweden and Japan. *Methods.* Interviews and qualitative thematic analyses were utilized. *Findings.* Four themes are reported: (1) use it or lose it, (2) simply no space until after hours, (3) biggest barriers can be colleagues, and (4) being more specific: communication. *Conclusion.* In keeping with previous studies, occupational therapists often find it challenging to implement client-centered and occupation-based assessment tools into practice. However, more work is needed to understand how best practices can be incorporated into a changing occupational therapy daily practice.

1. Introduction

Occupational therapists have during many decades used a wide range of formalized assessment tools, including tools borrowed from other disciplines, in order to provide relevant services to clients. During the last 20 years, the profession has seen a steady increase in the development and validation of assessment tools that more distinctly reflect occupational therapy domains of practice such as quality of occupational performance [1, 2], occupational gaps [3], and quality of social interaction [4] to name a few. Occupational therapists use assessment tools with an intended purpose to better guide intervention planning and to provide baseline and outcome measures in order to track progress and/or change among clients. For the purposes of this study, the authors adopt Fisher's [5] differentiation between occupation-centered, occupation-based, and occupation-focused assessments. Occupation-centered assessment refers to the centrality of occupation in informing decisions and action, a perspective; occupation-based assessment refers to situations in which occupation is a fundamental ingredient. Occupation-focused assessment refers to keeping the focus on occupation, with an immediate impact on occupational performance. For instance, an assessment in which occupation is performed as an essential part would by this definition be occupation-based, while an assessment in which goals pertaining to occupational performance are discussed and set, but where the particular occupations are not performed, would be occupation-focused.

2. Background

In a study conducted in northern Sweden, occupational therapists working in an acute hospital facility were interviewed regarding their experiences with integrating client-centeredness and occupation-focus into their practice based on the use of the Occupational Therapy Intervention and Process Model (OTIPM) [6]. Unsurprisingly, occupational therapists experienced a transformation of thought and action as they explicitly worked with a model to critically reflect on their own practices. Their experiences were imbued with both relief from the increased clarity with which they were working and ambiguity from hinders in the healthcare systems and the difficulties in changing organizational culture.

Contrary to the above depiction of deeply engaged therapists spending substantial time in continuing education and reflecting on their practice, it has also been documented that occupational therapists might find it challenging to incorporate specific tools in practice. In one study, 260 occupational therapists were surveyed, finding that occupational therapists most often choose an assessment tool because of availability and ease of administering the assessment (including ease of scoring and time efficiency) or that the tool facilitated client-centeredness [7]. In another study utilizing a survey and follow-up interviews, 50 therapists who had taken an AMPS course in England were asked about incorporating a new assessment in practice. [8]. Barriers to incorporating new assessment skills in clinical practice included the following: lack of support at the workplace, difficulty selecting appropriate clients, time to complete the assessment, and difficulties getting started. It was concluded that the successful implementation of an assessment tool such as AMPS in clinical practice would hinge upon receiving support from managers in the form of time, space for reflection, and invested resources in a continuum of learning [8]. These studies suggest that the utility of occupational therapy assessments might be explained by availability and ease of incorporation in practice rather than the soundness of the psychometric qualities of the assessment [7, 8].

Although client-centeredness and occupation are not new to occupational therapy, occupational therapists still find it difficult to incorporate client-centered and occupation-based or occupation-focused assessments in practice [7–10], even though occupational therapists place value on this type of assessment when asked. It is of importance to study the potential gap between practices in which occupation for different reasons cannot be integrated and a vision in which the value of occupation is central.

It is also relevant from an international perspective. A critique to the importation/exportation of theories (and implicitly assessments grounded in such theories) from one country context to another is well known [11]. It continues to be relevant and important to explore how occupational therapists reflect on their practice [12, 13] in order to situate clinical reasoning in different country/practice settings. Because the utility of assessments from a country/practice perspective is constantly evolving, it is of relevance to periodically and systematically explore experiences of using assessments among occupational therapists in different country/practice contexts.

The aim of this study is to explore the use of occupational therapy specific assessments such as the Assessment of Motor and Process Skills (AMPS) among occupational therapists working in Sweden and Japan.

Table 1: Aggregated demographics.

Demographics	Characteristic	$n = 19$
(i) Sex	Female	14
	Male	5
(ii) Country context	Sweden	7
	Japan	12
(iii) Work experience	General hospital (incl. rehabilitation)	11
	Home visit rehabilitation	1
	Education	3
	Nursing home	2
	Psychiatry facility	2
(iv) Interview style	Individual	8
	Focus group	11

3. Methods

3.1. Design. This study was based on qualitative interviews with occupational therapists from Sweden and Japan who had received training in the Assessment of Motor and Process Skills (AMPS) as well as other occupational therapy specific instruments such as A3 [14]. Data were analyzed in accordance with qualitative thematic analysis [15, 16]. All participants gave informed consent prior to being interviewed. The local ethics committee approved the study.

3.2. Participants. Information about the study was sent to occupational therapists in the A3 course database. The participants (14 women and 5 men) in this study expressed interest by making contact through email or telephone (see Table 1 for overview). Between the years 2004 and 2014, the A3 (formerly AAD) course was held 7 times with a total of 81 course participants (39 men and 42 women) in Japan and 8 times in Sweden with a total of 85 course participants (2 men and 83 women). A3, like the AMPS, requires each occupational therapist to submit 10 cases for calibration upon completion of the course. The validity of the instrument in Japanese and Swedish contexts as well as studies incorporating the assessment has been reported elsewhere [14, 17–23]. Recruitment from the A3 database was seen as relevant because all therapists would have also attended an AMPS course and would have recently taken an initiative to update their knowledge by having attended an A3 course.

All participants were licensed to practice occupational therapy in Japan or Sweden. In addition, all Japanese participants were calibrated AMPS raters. The participants in Japan had between 1 and 7 years of experience using AMPS (mean = 3; SD = 1.95) and participants in Sweden had 4–15 years of experience using AMPS (mean = 9; SD = 3.53). Among the participants, there were both those who used assessments on a regular basis and those who did not. Participant practice areas included the following: physical rehabilitation, home rehabilitation, psychiatry, and education. In order to uphold confidentiality, participant demographics are given in aggregate.

3.3. Data. Data gathering and analysis were iterative. The two country contexts represented geographic areas where there has been a strong interest in AMPS. This was relevant because by identifying challenges and support in integrating assessments such as these in different contexts new knowledge is facilitated in terms of strategies for integrating critical clinical reasoning in practice across different contexts. Moreover, this type of exploration has not previously been conducted over national borders or in Japan and Sweden.

Focus group interviews were initially used to build on the collective experiences of the participants. The method allowed members within the group to build on or refute experiences based on their own practice. However, due to the challenge of finding a common time and place, individual interviews were added to include perspectives that might otherwise be lost. It was possible to probe with questions in both the individual interviews and focus groups in order to integrate and deepen the information gathered.

Semistructured interview questions in conjunction with follow-up questions following general principles of qualitative research were used to gain an understanding of participant experiences [24]. All participants were interviewed on one occasion at a place of their convenience, which included their workplace, a seminar room at a university campus, a conference venue seminar room, or a café. Questions included the following: "can you tell me about how you use client-centered assessments in your practice," "what do you experience as challenges using these assessments," "what has made it possible for you to use these assessments," and "can you describe how these assessments help you in your practice?" The interviewer sometimes used more direct probes such as "can you describe in more detail?" or, in the case of a group interview, "has anyone else shared this experience?" In this way, the interviews were structured to develop richness around particular topics generated by both interviewer and participants. Interviews lasted between 45 and 90 minutes and were digitally recorded and transcribed. All interviews were performed by the first author or a research assistant in the project.

3.4. Data Analysis. The data analysis was based on techniques using thematic analysis [16, 25] and grounded in concepts of analyzing verbal narratives [15]. In keeping with thematic analytic, a back-and-forth process between interviewing and analysis was performed. All audio materials were transcribed near verbatim, retaining pauses, laughter, and nuances of expressions through bracketed qualifiers. These transcripts were carefully read and coded in three steps. All quotations used in this article were translated by the coauthors and the original Japanese text was maintained during the course of the analysis. The software program, Atlas.ti [26], was used during the analysis phase to code and organize data.

The data was analyzed inductively and although this process involved overlapping between steps, the procedure is outlined stepwise here for the purposes of clarity. All Swedish data were independently coded by the first author and all Japanese data were independently coded by the second author. The first author independently coded some of the Japanese data, which served as a way for the first and second authors to discuss and calibrate the coding process. During the analysis, all data were maintained in the original language. The first and second authors had regular meetings to compare and discuss coding during this phase. All data material was finally reviewed by the first author. The translation of quotes was performed by the first, second, and third authors and compared for accuracy. All authors were part of a discussion and interpretations of the findings.

In the first step, open coding entailed identifying and breaking the text into manageable bits that were assigned codes. Codes captured phenomena in one or a few words and were later applied to more segments of the text. Examples of early codes were "no space," "difficult to explain," and "don't have time" to name a few. In the second step, codes were merged and previously coded transcripts were revisited; existing as well as new codes within and across participants were sought by comparison across the data. In this way, both open coding and focused coding were used. Codes such as "don't have time" and "it takes time to prepare" were merged and codes such as "changing the schedule" and "evaluations after hours" contributed to a broader abstraction of the data. In the third step, similar codes were consolidated and organized into coherent groupings, whereby 4 themes were identified. These themes represent possibilities and barriers in using client-centered and occupational therapy specific assessments in practice.

4. Findings

Findings from the thematic analysis are presented in four themes. The title for each theme is taken from participant quotes under each theme. Although the naming of each theme is intended to be representative, each theme encompasses more than the phrase: (1) use it or lose it, (2) simply no space until after hours, (3) biggest barriers can be the work culture, and (4) being more specific communication. The occupational therapists interviewed in this study unanimously communicated an interest in informing their practice with client-centeredness and occupation-focused and/or or occupation-based assessments and interventions. Yet obstacles were also described. Barriers were consistent for occupational therapists in both Swedish and Japanese contexts; however, it is also important to note that some participants in both contexts did not experience these problems. Finally, an interesting finding was that several participants, when pushed to reflect on what they could do to change their situation, reflected that they probably could incorporate more client-centeredness and occupation-based and occupation-focused practice into their work.

5. Use It or Lose It

Something that influenced the choice in what assessments to use was the participant's own familiarity with the assessment as well as the extent to which a particular assessment was situated as routine within their practice. One participant said the following:

> *I simply think, with regard to evaluations, if you don't use it you loose [sic] it and you just don't get it.*

Along the same lines, another participant expressed the following:

> *But often I experience that it is a bit slow in the beginning, but then the more I do the assessments the faster I get...and it takes time to sit with the AMPS bible, one has to look things up, and learn things, if one should put a 4 or a 2 or a 1 for each item...but it takes time, but then when one masters it, then it doesn't take as long.*

All the participants used various assessments in practice but were here referring to occupational therapy specific assessments such as AMPS, A3, and COPM. According to these participants, these occupational therapy specific assessments often required more time and effort to perform than using hospital or facility specific ADL or goal checklists. On the other hand, participants were motivated to use the occupational therapy specific assessments because they felt that using these assessments yielded relevant information and made intervention planning clearer. Another participant says the following:

> *If one does many, it is better to do many AMPS, because the more one does the easier it gets. Because one has all the criteria in ones head. And one, like now when I've been gone for a while, then it's going to take a longer time. But that doesn't mean that I am going to refrain from it...I'll just have to offset some extra time instead, so that I can do it.*

In this way, participants expressed a strong sense of integrity in being able to work according to best practices. However, strategies and priorities in making this work were highly individual for the participants in this study. Moreover, all participants felt that routine was a necessity in making assessments go smoothly.

> *The daily routine is too busy, there are so many things to learn, before I know it I actually cannot use an assessment. If I don't use it I don't know how to do it anymore, especially AMPS I find difficult so I end up not using it as frequently and in the end I might not be using it at all, sort of my situation now.*

Participants expressed a need to create a routine for the use of occupational therapy specific assessments in practice. Moreover, experiences shared here also allude to certain challenges in creating routines, something that is taken up in subsequent themes.

6. Simply No Space until After Hours

Among participants, time was experienced as a significant factor impacting upon choices in day-to-day practices as well as the integration of practices to routines. A scarcity in time to complete all expected tasks within their workloads was one aspect in addition to the amount of time it took to perform an assessment such as AMPS, A3, or COPM to name a few. However, these experiences also need to be nuanced.

> *Well, actually, the staff know about AMPS and A3 and—I'd like to say that I don't have time, but actually if I wanted to make the time I could.*

Participants expressed a subtle reflection about the possibility to actually do more if initiative was to be taken. Yet a common experience and sentiment among the participants was that time was a scare commodity. One participant said the following:

> *So if I do an ADL assessment in preparation for a team planning meeting, so I often do, so I choose Suunnas, because it is quicker. Because if I would do an entire formal AMPS it requires so much more sort of.*

Another participant said the following:

> *And we block, if the patient is in a 4-person room and one chooses to do a shower task and make the bed, well then it takes a long time and then one blocks the bathroom very long.*

Participants illustrated in their shared stories about everyday practices that each day was filled with choices based on weighing the pros and cons of choosing a lengthier versus shorter assessment, perhaps based on requiring observations or longer interviews. In the above situation, the participant reflected no ethical contemplation about the choice but rather expressed this as a matter of practicality. Another therapist summarized the sentiment: "I am simply too busy." However, when therapists felt that they should choose an occupation-based assessment but could not due to time or space, then it introduced a significantly more difficult dilemma. One therapist shared her individual solution to this dilemma:

> *I have to do evaluations outside of working hours. We only have one small rehab room for staff and clients to share, and in the morning we see about 10 clients and in the afternoon about 7 clients. There is simply no space to do an AMPS evaluation until afterhours.*

Strategies such as these can also be seen as reflecting a degree of consideration for peers as well as clients, in avoiding a too great burden. A therapist in another facility responded about how the team solved issues around physical space:

> *But the more we fix our physical spaces to look like home environments, the easier it gets to do assessments. There are ironing boards, a kitchen, a bathroom, a bed to make and so forth. One works actively here so that patients can access familiar occupations, vacuum and so on.*

Similarly, another therapist concurred that environment was an important element in being able to perform assessments such as AMPS.

> *If I tell the kitchen staff 3 days in advance, um, and oh yeah they ask "what do you need," for instance how many slices of bread, and they will prepare it,*

> *and the hospital covers the costs, and so it is sort of that type of environment, it is easy to manage, it is how it is for me but I realize that I should be thankful for the environment.*

All occupational therapists who were interviewed in both Japanese and Swedish contexts concurred that time was scarce in relation to the volume of work that they felt needed to be done. Moreover, the physical environment was also experienced as relevant; however, the environment was to different degrees a barrier or possibility depending on organization.

7. Biggest Barriers Can Be the Work Culture

The impact of the work culture on choice of assessments was expressed as a barrier. When participants worked in teams where they experienced consensus and clear leadership, social conformity was in many ways a positive factor. One participant says the following:

> *One should have consensus, we have two rehabilitation programs and that steers us, because since we work at xx facility, it is a requirement for us to use valid and reliable instruments.*

Another participant says the following:

> *What is there, what we use here is also...it should not just depend on me, what one choses, that one does an assessment.*

Surprisingly, however, some therapists expressed that when this sense of consensus works to create a majority culture that does not include the use of client-centered or occupation-based assessments, the greatest challenge is the team itself. One participant says the following:

> *The biggest barriers are my occupational therapy colleagues. They choose a very biomechanical approach and when their clients see me with my client, they wonder why we are doing things differently and seemingly more fun. Then my colleagues make me feel like I should just do as they do.*

The culture of the work environment is vital for the choices made by therapists. In some cases, this culture serves to strengthen a notion of client-centered practice and in other cases it serves to exclude those that try to introduce these ideas.

8. Being More Specific: Communication

The positive aspect of working in a client-centered and occupation-based manner was the ability to effectively communicate with clients regarding concrete observations in situations where the client had carried out tasks and where there were concrete understandings about where the person might have done well or was in need of assistance. One participant says the following:

> *It used to be difficult for me to communicate about performance concretely, but when using AMPS I can be more specific about what the person did (needed help with) and how it specifically related to real examples from daily life.*

In this way, the use of AMPS provided an added value that could justify the added time or efforts in performing the assessment.

> *To be able to communicate is one thing, not only with the family, but with other staff members, it is sort of easier to explain. Since an actual occupation is used, it is clear what aspects the person is able to do or what the person is not able to do and this is directly connected to everyday life. When someone asks me, before it was difficult to be concrete, but with AMPS data I can be very specific about what I saw and how this is related to the goals and plans. I think this is something important.*

For participants in this study, using an occupation-based assessment such as AMPS required a time investment for both the client and therapist. However, this process also gave the occupational therapist a greater degree of detail on which to base his/her assessment. This in turn led the participants to raise positive experiences about being able to be more concrete about the results of an assessment with an individual client as well as having a richer context around reported outcomes and intervention goals in a team or patient/family setting.

9. Discussion

The main findings from the study highlight what can facilitate and hinder the use of occupational therapy specific assessments in the context of occupational therapy practice in two different country contexts. The findings reflect that incorporating formalized occupational therapy evaluations in practice is challenging on multiple levels. The challenge of integrating new assessments into everyday habits and routines in clinical practice was noteworthy. This is not surprising but it can be concerning that occupational therapists choose assessments based on personal convenience rather than relevance for the case at hand. Given the instruments in focus for recruiting participants to this study, we revisit the Model of Human Occupation.

The Model of Human Occupation (MoHO) [27] can perhaps be useful in informing the lens through which we look when analyzing occupational therapists' experiences. MoHO has been characterized as a body of theory that explains how occupation is motivated, performed, and integrated in daily life. MoHO has primarily been applied to "patient" groups, although by definition applications should be possible to people that for one reason or another experience challenges in performing and/or changing their occupations. Of particular interest, here is the idea of habits and routines. Habitual behavior generally has to do with how people organize occupations in stable and repeatable routines; there is a certain element of automaticity and familiarity which comprises human behavior as habitual within the MoHO. This is of interest because the occupational therapists interviewed in this study raised the dilemma of changing habits in relation to practices in assessment procedures. From the perspective of the human as an occupational being [28, 29], the dilemma raised by the participants in this study can be understood as resistance or as a need to maintain routines in order to be able to work. In the Assessment of Motor and Process Skills (AMPS) manual [2], the need for systematically checking scoring criteria and not relying on habit is desirable for the purposes of validity and reliability of such a standardized evaluation. On the other hand, it is possible as participants in this study purported to establish habits and routines in the use of AMPS, even though the use of AMPS requires the systematic use of a manual. This is a concrete example of the complexity surrounding human occupation when applied to the everyday work of occupational therapists. As illustrated in the findings of this study, on one hand, habit is a necessity for finding a just right challenge and building competencies in performance. On the other hand, habitual action can impact upon the soundness of the results from assessments within occupational therapy practice, thus risking poor outcomes, especially when occupational therapists are implementing changes in their own evaluation practices. Understanding the balance between these two aspects and the need for critical reflection about one's minute practices is of high relevance for evidence-based and person-centered practice.

If occupational therapists choose assessments based more on access than on the immediate needs for the client, there is a risk that the client-centered aspects of practice also are undermined. Shifting power away from the healthcare provider toward the client, prioritizing goals relevant for the client, and focusing on enabling participation in society through occupation are important aspects of client-centeredness here and require the active utilization of relevant assessment tools and intervention models that place the client and his/her needs through occupation into focus. The risk of losing client-centeredness can emerge from small compromises in which a less relevant assessment tool is prioritized because of convenience and in so doing leading to goal setting and intervention planning that neglects empowering the client or focusing on what is most important for him/her [9, 30, 31].

Our findings suggest that the perceptions of the work context largely influenced the choice of a specific assessment. The implementation of new methods is influenced by various social networks. Most of the influencing factors described in our findings are related to individuals or to the organizational environment. Perhaps social networks, when optimal in function, can reduce situations where therapists do not prioritize what they believe is best practice. The participant who said "I'd like to say that I don't have time, but actually if I wanted to make the time I could" reflects something of a dilemma in that the therapist shows a sense of awareness about something lacking in her practice and yet chooses not to prioritize what she considers best practice. Based upon the findings in this study, this phenomenon or trend is something that occupational therapists need to look more carefully at in order to improve possibilities for changing practices and for further work in the integration of research and clinical practice [6, 32]. Although being beyond the scope of this paper, it can also be of interest for occupational therapists to look at implementation science as a way to facilitate the integration of best practices [33].

This study also highlights a discrepancy between how occupational therapists think they should work and how they actually work. The difficulty of incorporating knowledge and changing practice has been reported elsewhere [7, 8, 34, 35]; however, it is interesting to note that incorporating thinking about one's practice seems to be characteristic of therapists who have engaged in continued education [36]. Initially, the authors expected notable differences in experience based on country context; however, the data does not support this assumption. Instead, more generic aspects of practice context and organizational culture appear to have a stronger influence on the implementation process. In order to find innovative strategies to bridge gaps between recommendations and usual practice within clinical settings, it is vital to know what factors impact upon implementation of new methods.

Limitations. There are several limitations to this study. It was not possible to conduct data gathering in two country contexts within the same period, which meant that interview guides could not be revised based on two country contexts. On the other hand, the aim of the study was not to compare country contexts but rather to use Sweden and Japan because both were contexts in which many occupational therapists with AMPS training were active and also were in an active process of learning and implementing additional client-centered and occupation-based or occupation-focused evaluations in practice. The two contexts were thought to contribute with different cultural dimensions. Interestingly, the findings would suggest that Swedish and Japanese contexts have less to do with occupational therapy specific assessments than the practice contexts.

A limitation was that only therapists with initial AMPS and A3 training were recruited. Since there is previous research suggesting that it is difficult to implement time-intensive tools such as AMPS in practice, despite extensive training and in fact also suggested in the findings from this study, then it is of relevance to look at occupational therapists that arguably have optimal conditions. Another limitation is that information about why potential participants did not participate is not available. Information about the study was circulated to course participants in the A3 course database. There can be several reasons for why people did not respond, including the fact that email addresses could have changed, lack of interest in the study, or other competing priorities to name a few. It is possible that those who took initiative to participate were particularly interested in actively pursuing the use of AMPS and A3 in their practices.

Another limitation is that some interview questions were formulated, such as "what do you experience as challenges using these assessments?" or "can you describe how these assessments were helpful in practice?" This can be seen as biasing in that the questions assume that something was challenging or helpful. On the other hand, it is natural in both Swedish and Japanese to talk about challenges and possibilities. If questions had only been about challenges, the bias might have been more limiting; however, in this case, the questions get at two sides of a phenomenon.

Finally, it can be a limitation to have combined individual and focus group interviews because the type of data generated is different. However, the benefits of enriching the data by including individual interviews were seen to outweigh the drawbacks. Some participants had little flexibility in their schedules and therefore found it difficult to participate at the set time and place for a focus group. By incorporating individual interviews, the data also reflects voices among those who would not otherwise have been included.

10. Conclusion

The aim of this study was to explore occupational therapists' experiences in implementing the AMPS in combination with other client-centered and occupation-based or occupation-focused assessments within various clinical practice settings in Sweden and Japan. In keeping with previous studies, occupational therapists in a myriad of clinical and country contexts find it challenging to implement client-centered and occupation-based assessment tools into practice. More work is needed to understand how best practices can be implemented and sustained through the whole continuum of occupational therapy practice.

Conflicts of Interest

The authors declare that there are no conflicts of interest.

Acknowledgments

The authors would like to thank all the participants for sharing their experiences and time. The study was partly funded by a grant from Karolinska Institutet, Center for Caring Sciences (Grant no. 1220/05-226). Special thanks are extended to colleagues at the Division of Occupational Therapy at Karolinska Institutet who have been part of the process and also to those who assisted in the work along the way: Yu Ishibashi, Sanna Edensand, Annikki Jauring, and Peter Bontje. Furthermore, the completion of the manuscript was in part made possible through a mobility grant from Tokyo Metropolitan University where Mio Nakamura was a doctoral student at the time.

References

[1] M. Law, S. Baptiste, M. A. McColl, A. Opzoomer, H. Polatajko, and N. Pollock, "The Canadian occupational performance measure: an outcome measure for occupational therapy," *Canadian Journal of Occupational Therapy*, vol. 57, no. 2, pp. 82–87, 1990.

[2] A. G. Fisher, *Assessment of Motor and Process Skills: Development, Standardization and Administration Manual*, vol. 1, Three Star Press, Fort Collins, Colo, USA, 5th edition, 2003.

[3] G. Eriksson, K. Tham, and J. Borg, "Occupational gaps in everyday life 1–4 years after acquired brain injury," *Journal of Rehabilitation Medicine*, vol. 38, no. 3, pp. 159–165, 2006.

[4] A. G. Fisher and L. A. Griswold, *Evaluation of Social Interaction*, Three Star Press, Fort Collins, Colo, USA, 2009.

[5] A. G. Fisher, "Occupation-centred, occupation-based, occupation-focused: Same, same or different?" *Scandinavian Journal of Occupational Therapy*, vol. 20, no. 3, pp. 162–173, 2013.

[6] M. Sirkka, K. Zingmark, and M. Larsson-Lund, "A process for developing sustainable evidence-based occupational therapy practice," *Scandinavian Journal of Occupational Therapy*, vol. 21, no. 6, pp. 429–437, 2014.

[7] N. M. Alotaibi, K. Reed, and M. S. Nadar, "Assessments used in occupational therapy practice: an exploratory study," *Occupational Therapy in Health Care*, vol. 23, no. 4, pp. 302–318, 2009.

[8] G. Chard, "An investigation into the use of the Assessment of Motor and Process Skills (AMPS) in clinical practice," *The British Journal of Occupational Therapy*, vol 63, no. 10, pp. 481–488, 2000.

[9] J. I. K. Öhman and E. Asaba, "Goal setting in occupational therapy: a narrative study exploring theory and practice in psychiatry," *World Federation of Occupational Therapists Bulletin*, vol. 60, no. 1, pp. 22–28, 2014.

[10] T. Kaneyama and K. Inoue, "A survey of ADL assessment approaches used by occupational therapists in practice," *Okayama Journal of Occupational Therapy*, vol. 19, no. 1, pp. 13–22, 2010 (Japanese).

[11] M. Iwama, "Toward culturally relevant epistemologies in occupational therapy," *American Journal of Occupational Therapy*, vol. 57, no. 5, pp. 582–588, 2003.

[12] C. Mattingly, "In search of the good: Narrative reasoning in clinical practice," *Medical Anthropology Quarterly*, vol. 12, no. 3, pp. 273–297, 1998.

[13] C. Mattingly, *Healing Dramas and Clinical Plots: The Narrative Structure of Experience*, Cambridge University Press, Cambridge, UK, 1998.

[14] E. Asaba, I. Petersson, P. Bontje, and A. Kottorp, "The assessment of awareness of ability (A3) in a Japanese context: A Rasch model application," *Scandinavian Journal of Occupational Therapy*, vol. 19, no. 4, pp. 370–376, 2012.

[15] D. E. Polkinghorne, "Narrative configuration in qualitative analysis," *International Journal of Qualitative Studies in Education*, vol. 8, no. 1, pp. 5–23, 1995.

[16] C. Pope, S. Ziebland, and N. Mays, "Analysing qualitative data," in *Qualitative Research in Healthcare*, C. Pope and N. Mays, Eds., Blackwell Publishing Ltd, Malden, Mass, USA, 3rd edition, 2006.

[17] E. Asaba and A. Asaba, "Towards client-centered and occupation-based evaluation and intervention: A case study," *Okayama Journal of Occupational Therapy*, 2010.

[18] A. G. Fisher, L. A. Griswold, M. Munkholm, and A. Kottorp, "Evaluating domains of everyday functioning in people with developmental disabilities," *Scandinavian Journal of Occupational Therapy*, vol. 24, no. 1, pp. 1–9, 2017.

[19] A. Kottorp, B. Heuchemer, I. P. Lie, and C. H. Gumpert, "Evaluation of activities of daily living ability and awareness among clients in a forensic psychiatry evaluation unit in Sweden," *The*

British Journal of Occupational Therapy, vol. 76, no. 1, pp. 23–30, 2013.

[20] A. Kottorp, L. Ekstam, and I. Petersson Lie, "Differences in awareness between persons with left and right hemispheric stroke," *Scandinavian Journal of Occupational Therapy*, vol. 20, no. 1, pp. 37–44, 2013.

[21] A. Kottorp and I. Petersson, "Psychometric evaluation of an assessment of awareness using two different Rasch models," *Scandinavian Journal of Occupational Therapy*, vol. 18, no. 3, pp. 219–230, 2011.

[22] A. Öhman, L. Nygård, and A. Kottorp, "The relationship between occupational performance and awareness of disability in older adults with cognitive impairment or dementia," *Scandinavian Journal of Occupational Therapy*, vol. 18, pp. 133–142, 2011.

[23] R. L. Anderson, S. E. Doble, B. K. Merritt, and A. Kottorp, "Assessment of awareness of disability measures among persons with acquired brain injury," *Canadian Journal of Occupational Therapy*, vol. 77, no. 1, pp. 22–29, 2010.

[24] I. Seidman, *Interviewing as Qualitative Research: A Guide for Researchers in Education and the Social Sciences*, Teachers College Press, New York, NY, USA, 2nd edition, 1998.

[25] L. Ayres, "Thematic coding and analysis," in *The SAGE Encyclopedia of Qualitative Research Methods*, L. Given, Ed., Sage Publications Inc, Thousand Oaks, Calif, USA, 2008.

[26] T. Muhr, *ATLAS.ti. WIN 4.2 Build 061*, Scientific Software Development, Berlin, Germany, 1997.

[27] G. Kielhofner, *Model of Human Occupation: Theory and Application*, Lippincott Williams & Wilkins, Balitmore, Md, USA, 4th edition, 2008.

[28] A. Wilcock, *An Occupational Perspective of Health*, SLACK Inc, Thorofare, NJ, USA, 1998.

[29] M. P. Cutchin, R. M. Aldrich, A. L. Bailliard, and S. Coppola, "Action theories for occupational science: The contributions of Dewey and Bourdieu," *Journal of Occupational Science*, vol. 15, no. 3, pp. 157–165, 2008.

[30] K. K. Maitra and F. Erway, "Perception of client-centered practice in occupational therapists and their clients," *American Journal of Occupational Therapy*, vol. 60, no. 3, pp. 298–310, 2006.

[31] E. Wressle and K. Samuelsson, "Barriers and bridges to client-centred occupational therapy in Sweden," *Scandinavian Journal of Occupational Therapy*, vol. 11, no. 1, pp. 12–16, 2004.

[32] M. Sirkka, M. Larsson-Lund, and K. Zingmark, "Occupational therapists' experiences of improvement work: A journey towards sustainable evidence-based practice," *Scandinavian Journal of Occupational Therapy*, vol. 21, no. 2, pp. 90–97, 2014.

[33] C. R. May, M. Johnson, and T. Finch, "Implementation, context and complexity," *Implementation Science*, vol. 11, no. 1, article 141, pp. 1–12, 2016.

[34] D. Upton, D. Stephens, B. Williams, and L. Scurlock-Evans, "Occupational therapists' attitudes, knowledge, and implementation of evidence-based practice: A systematic review of published research," *The British Journal of Occupational Therapy*, vol. 77, no. 1, pp. 24–38, 2014.

[35] E. A. Balas and S. A. Boren, "Managing clinical knowledge for health care improvement," in *Yearbook of Medical Informatics 2000: Patient-Centered Systems*, J. Bemmel and A. T. McCray, Eds., pp. 65–70, Schattauer Verlagsgesellschaft, Stuttgart, Germany, 2000.

[36] L. Nygård, A. Kottorp, and L. Rosenberg, "Making use of research: Clinical views on an evaluation of everyday technology use," *Scandinavian Journal of Occupational Therapy*, vol. 22, no. 1, pp. 24–32, 2015.

Permissions

All chapters in this book were first published in OTI, by Hindawi Publishing Corporation, hereby published with permission under the Creative Commons Attribution License or equivalent. Every chapter published in this book has been scrutinized by our experts. Their significance has been extensively debated. The topics covered herein carry significant findings which will fuel the growth of the discipline. They may even be implemented as practical applications or may be referred to as a beginning point for another development.

The contributors of this book come from diverse backgrounds, making this book a truly international effort. This book will bring forth new frontiers with its revolutionizing research information and detailed analysis of the nascent developments around the world.

We would like to thank all the contributing authors for lending their expertise to make the book truly unique. They have played a crucial role in the development of this book. Without their invaluable contributions this book wouldn't have been possible. They have made vital efforts to compile up to date information on the varied aspects of this subject to make this book a valuable addition to the collection of many professionals and students.

This book was conceptualized with the vision of imparting up-to-date information and advanced data in this field. To ensure the same, a matchless editorial board was set up. Every individual on the board went through rigorous rounds of assessment to prove their worth. After which they invested a large part of their time researching and compiling the most relevant data for our readers.

The editorial board has been involved in producing this book since its inception. They have spent rigorous hours researching and exploring the diverse topics which have resulted in the successful publishing of this book. They have passed on their knowledge of decades through this book. To expedite this challenging task, the publisher supported the team at every step. A small team of assistant editors was also appointed to further simplify the editing procedure and attain best results for the readers.

Apart from the editorial board, the designing team has also invested a significant amount of their time in understanding the subject and creating the most relevant covers. They scrutinized every image to scout for the most suitable representation of the subject and create an appropriate cover for the book.

The publishing team has been an ardent support to the editorial, designing and production team. Their endless efforts to recruit the best for this project, has resulted in the accomplishment of this book. They are a veteran in the field of academics and their pool of knowledge is as vast as their experience in printing. Their expertise and guidance has proved useful at every step. Their uncompromising quality standards have made this book an exceptional effort. Their encouragement from time to time has been an inspiration for everyone.

The publisher and the editorial board hope that this book will prove to be a valuable piece of knowledge for researchers, students, practitioners and scholars across the globe.

List of Contributors

Ángel Sánchez-Cabeza
Hospital Universitario Fundación Alcorcón, Madrid, Spain
Department of Physiotherapy, Occupational Therapy, Rehabilitation and Physical Medicine, Universidad Rey Juan Carlos, Madrid, Spain

Elisabet Huertas-Hoyas, Nuria Máximo-Bocanegra, Rosa María Martínez-Piédrola, Marta Pérez-de-Heredia-Torres and Jorge Alegre-Ayala
Department of Physiotherapy, Occupational Therapy, Rehabilitation and Physical Medicine, Universidad Rey Juan Carlos, Madrid, Spain

Rodolfo Morrison, Silvia Gómez, María Jesús Tapia and Laura Rueda
Department of Occupational Therapy and Occupational Science, Faculty of Medicine, University of Chile, Santiago, Chile
Chilean Society of Occupational Science, Santiago, Chile

Enrique Henny
Chilean Society of Occupational Science, Santiago, Chile
Tedes Center, Santiago, Chile

Elelwani Ramugondo and Anande Ferreira
Department of Health and Rehabilitation Sciences, Faculty of Health Sciences, University of Cape Town, Cape Town 7935, South Africa

Donna Chung and Reinie Cordier
School of Occupational Therapy, Social Work and Speech Pathology, Faculty of Health Sciences, Curtin University, Perth 6012, Australia

Si-nae Ahn
Department of Occupational Therapy, Cheongju University, 298 Daesung-ro, Cheongju-si, Republic of Korea

Sujin Hwang
Deparment of Physical Therapy, Division of Health Science, Baekseok University, 76 Munam-ro, Dongnam-gu, Cheonan-si, Chungnam, Republic of Korea

Alexandra Nugent, Nicola Hancock and Anne Honey
The University of Sydney, Cumberland Campus, 74 East St., Lidcombe, NSW2141, Australia

Pragashnie Govender, December M. Mpanza, Tarryn Carey, Kwenzile Jiyane, Bicolé Andrews and Sam Mashele
Discipline of Occupational Therapy, School of Health Sciences, University of KwaZulu Natal,Westville Campus, Westville, South Africa

Larissa Andriske and Debbie Verikios
Barwon Health, Geelong, VIC, Australia

Danielle Hitch
Deakin University, Geelong, VIC, Australia

Lia Lopes Gonçalves, Mariana Callil Voos, Maria Helena Morgani de Almeida and Fátima Aparecida Caromano
Department of Physical Therapy, Speech Therapy and Occupational Therapy Rehabilitation Sciences Post Graduation Program, Medical School, University of S˜ao Paulo, S˜ao Paulo, SP, Brazil

Marieke Lindenschot
Department IQ Healthcare, Research Institute for Health Sciences, Radboud University Medical Center Nijmegen, Postbus 9101, 6500 HB Nijmegen, Netherlands
Department of Occupational Therapy, HAN University of Applied Sciences, Postbus 6960, 6503 GL Nijmegen, Netherlands
Research Group Neurorehabilitation, HAN University of Applied Sciences, Nijmegen, Netherlands
Department of Rehabilitation, Donders Center for Neuroscience, Radboud University Medical Center Nijmegen, Postbus 9101, 6500 HB Nijmegen, Netherlands

Maria W. G. Nijhuis-van der Sanden
Department IQ Healthcare, Research Institute for Health Sciences, Radboud University Medical Center Nijmegen, Postbus 9101, 6500 HB Nijmegen, Netherlands
Department of Rehabilitation, Donders Center for Neuroscience, Radboud University Medical Center Nijmegen, Postbus 9101, 6500 HB Nijmegen, Netherlands

Esther M. J. Steultjens
Department of Occupational Therapy, HAN University of Applied Sciences, Postbus 6960, 6503 GL Nijmegen, Netherlands
Research Group Neurorehabilitation, HAN University of Applied Sciences, Nijmegen, Netherlands

Imelda J. M. de Groot
Department of Rehabilitation, Donders Center for Neuroscience, Radboud University Medical Center Nijmegen, Postbus 9101, 6500 HB Nijmegen, Netherlands

Saskia Koene
Department of Pediatrics, Radboud Center for Mitochondrial Medicine, Radboud University Medical Center Nijmegen, Geert Grooteplein Zuid 10, 6525 GA Nijmegen, Netherlands

Ton Satink
Department of Occupational Therapy, HAN University of Applied Sciences, Postbus 6960, 6503 GL Nijmegen, Netherlands
Research Group Neurorehabilitation, HAN University of Applied Sciences, Nijmegen, Netherlands
European Masters of Science in Occupational Therapy, Amsterdam University of Applied Sciences, Amsterdam, Netherlands

Suchitporn Lersilp and Supawadee Putthinoi
Department of Occupational Therapy, Faculty of Associated Medical Sciences, Chiang Mai University, Thailand

Theeratorn Lersilp
Department of Special Education, Faculty of Education, Chiang Mai Rajabhat University, Thailand

Sean Reilly and Sinéad M. Hynes
Discipline of Occupational Therapy, National University of Ireland Galway, Galway, Ireland

A. Enemark Larsen and B. Rasmussen
Department of Occupational Therapy, Institute of Medwifery and Therapy, University College Copenhagen, Sigurdsgade 26, DK-2200 N Copenhagen, Denmark

J. R. Christensen
Department of Public Health, University of Southern Denmark, JB Winsløwsvej 9A, 5000 Odense, Denmark
Department of Sports Science and Clinical Biomechanics, University of Southern Denmark, Campusvej 55, 5230 Odense, Denmark

Rosa Román-Oyola, Verónica Figueroa-Feliciano, Yoliannie Torres-Martínez, Jorge Torres-Vélez, Keyshla Encarnación-Pizarro, Samariz Fragoso-Pagán and Luis Torres-Colón
University of Puerto Rico, Medical Sciences Campus, School of Health Professions, Occupational Therapy Program, San Juan, PR 00936-5067, USA

Eduardo J. Pedrero-Pérez, Irene León-Frade, Patricia Aldea-Poyo, Marina Alonso-Rodríguez, Jara Pedrero-Aguilar and Sara Morales-Alonso
Institute of Addictions, Madrid Salud, Madrid City Council, Madrid, Spain

Gloria Rojo-Mota
Institute of Addictions, Madrid Salud, Madrid City Council, Madrid, Spain
King Juan Carlos University, Madrid, Spain

José M. Ruiz-Sánchez de León
Complutense University of Madrid, Madrid, Spain

Ann-Charlotte Lindström
Närhälsan Rehabilitation Sörhaga, Alingsås, Sweden

Susanne Bernhardsson
Närhälsan Research and Development Primary Health Care, Region Västra Götaland, Gothenburg, Sweden
Institute of Neuroscience and Physiology, Department of Health and Rehabilitation, Unit of Physiotherapy, University of Gothenburg, The Sahlgrenska Academy, Gothenburg, Sweden

Lucy Jane Miller and Sarah A. Schoen
STAR Institute, 5420 S. Quebec Street, Suite 105, Greenwood Village, CO 80111, USA

Shelley Mulligan
Department of Occupational Therapy, 4 Library Way, University of New Hampshire, Durham, NH03824, USA

Jillian Sullivan
Northeastern University, 312E Robinson Hall, 360 Huntington Ave., Boston, MA 02115, USA

Bryan M. Gee, Jane Strickland and Kelly Thompson
Idaho State University, Pocatello, ID, USA

Lucy Jane Miller
STAR Institute for Sensory Processing Disorder, Greenwood Village, CO, USA
Department of Pediatrics, University of Colorado, Denver, CO, USA

Joo-Hyun Lee, Ji-Hyuk Park, Yeong Jo Kim and Hae Yean Park
Department of Occupational Therapy, Yonsei University, Wonju, Republic of Korea

Sang Heon Lee
Department of Occupational Therapy, Soonchunhyang University, Cheonan, Republic of Korea

Marcel W. M. Post
Brain Center Rudolf Magnus and Center of Excellence in Rehabilitation Medicine, University Medical Center Utrecht and De Hoogstraat Rehabilitation, Utrecht, Netherlands

Lana Bestbier
Priors Court Foundation, Thatcham, UK

Tim I. Williams
Priors Court Foundation, Thatcham, UK
Institute of Education, University of Reading, Reading, UK

Suchitporn Lersilp and Supawadee Putthinoi
Department of Occupational Therapy, Faculty of Associated Medical Sciences, Chiang Mai University, Chiang Mai, Thailand

Sayaka Okahashi
Division of Occupational Therapy, Department of Human Health Sciences, Graduate School of Medicine, Kyoto University, Kyoto, Japan

Ya-Cing Syu
Department of Occupational Therapy, College of Medicine, National Cheng Kung University, Tainan, Taiwan

Ling-Yi Lin
Department of Occupational Therapy, College of Medicine, National Cheng Kung University, Tainan, Taiwan
Institute of Allied Health Sciences, College of Medicine, National Cheng Kung University, Tainan, Taiwan

Daiva Petruseviciene, Daiva Baltaduoniene and Egle Lendraitiene
Department of Rehabilitation, Medical Academy, Lithuanian University of Health Sciences, Kaunas, Lithuania

Deive Surmaitiene
Kulautuva Hospital of Rehabilitation, Hospital of Lithuanian University of Health Sciences Kauno Klinikos, Kaunas, Lithuania

Danit Langer and Adina Maeir
School of Occupational Therapy, Hadassah and Hebrew University, Jerusalem, Israel

Michael Michailevich
Department of Orthopaedics, Sherutay Briut Clalit, Jerusalem, Israel

Shai Luria
Department of Orthopedic Surgery, Hadassah-Hebrew University Medical Center, Jerusalem, Israel

Tore Bonsaksen
Department of Occupational Therapy, Prosthetics and Orthotics, Faculty of Health Sciences, Oslo Met - Oslo Metropolitan University, Oslo, Norway
Faculty of Health Studies, VID Specialized University, Sandnes, Norway
Sławomir Tobis and Mirosława Cylkowska-Nowak
Laboratory of Occupational Therapy, Department of Geriatric Medicine and Gerontology, University of Medical Sciences, Poznan, Poland

Katarzyna Wieczorowska-Tobis
Laboratory of Geriatrics, Department of Palliative Care, University of Medical Sciences, Poznan, Poland

Mariola Pawlaczyk
Department of Geriatric Medicine and Gerontology, University of Medical Sciences, Poznan, Poland

Aleksandra Suwalska
Laboratory of Neuropsychobiology, Department of Psychiatry, University of Medical Sciences, Poznan, Poland

Eric Asaba
Department of Neurobiology, Care Sciences and Society (NVS), Division of Occupational Therapy, Karolinska Institutet, Alfred Nobels Allé 23, B4, Huddinge, Sweden
Unit for Research, Education and Development (FoUU), Stockholms Sjukhem Foundation, Stockholm, Sweden
Department of Occupational Therapy, Tokyo Metropolitan University, Tokyo, Japan

Mio Nakamura
Department of Occupational Therapy, International University of Health and Welfare, Narita, Japan

Akie Asaba
Karolinska University Hospital, Occupational Therapy and Physiotherapy Practice Areas, Huddinge, Sweden

Anders Kottorp
Department of Neurobiology, Care Sciences and Society (NVS), Division of Occupational Therapy, Karolinska Institutet, Alfred Nobels Allé 23, B4, Huddinge, Sweden
Faculty for Health and Society, Malmö University, Malmö, Sweden

Index

www.ingramcontent.com/pod-product-compliance
Lightning Source LLC
LaVergne TN
LVHW060602210926
848485LV00005B/1356